Lu's Basic Toxicology

Fourth Edition

Fundamentals, target organs and risk assessment

Frank C. Lu
Consultant in Toxicology
Miami, Florida
U.S.A.

Sam Kacew
Professor of Pharmacology
University of Ottawa, Ontario
Canada

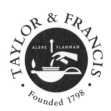

London and New York

First published 2002 by Taylor & Francis
11 New Fetter Lane, London EC4P 4EE

Simultaneously published in the USA and Canada
by Taylor & Francis Inc,
29 West 35th Street, New York, NY 10001

Taylor & Francis is an imprint of the Taylor & Francis Group

© 2002 Frank C. Lu and Sam Kacew

Typeset in Sabon by Wearset Ltd, Boldon, Tyne and Wear
Printed and bound in Great Britain by Biddles Ltd, Guildford and King's
Lynn

Every effort has been made to ensure that the advice and information in
this book is true and accurate at the time of going to press. However,
neither the publisher nor the authors can accept any legal responsibility
or liability for any errors or omissions that may be made. In the case of
drug administration, any medical procedure or the use of technical
equipment mentioned within this book, you are strongly advised to
consult the manufacturer's guidelines.

British Library Cataloguing in Publication Data
A catalogue record for this book is available from the British Library

Library of Congress Cataloging in Publication Data
A catalog record has been requested

ISBN 0-415-24855-8 (HB)
ISBN 0-415-24856-6 (PB)

Contents

About the authors

Frank C. Lu, MD, is a Consulting Toxicologist in Food Additives, Pesticides, and Environmental Chemicals, and the Managing Editor of the journal *Biomedical and Environmental Sciences*. He is also an Honorary Professor at the Chinese Academy of Preventive Medicine. His previous positions include Professor of Pharmacology at the University of Miami, Chief of the Food Additives Unit of the World Health Organization (WHO), and Head of the Pharmacology and Toxicology Section of the Canadian Food and Drug Directorate (FDD). At FDD, he conducted and participated in testing the toxicity of a variety of food additives, contaminants, pesticides, and drugs, and was in charge of assessing their safety. In addition, he was responsible for drafting new sets of Toxicological Requirements for New Drugs and for Food Additives and Pesticides. At WHO, he was the Scientific Secretary to the Joint FAO/WHO Expert Committee on Food Additives and Contaminants, and to the Joint FAO/WHO Meeting on Pesticide Residues. These expert bodies were responsible for assessing the safety of these chemicals on the basis of all available data. He was also the Chief Liaison Officer for WHO to the inter-governmental body, the Codex Alimentarius Commission. A Charter Member of the Society of Toxicology, he is a recipient of the International Achievement Award from the International Society of Pharmacology and Toxicology. In 1994 the Frank C. Lu Foundation for Advancement of Preventive Medicine was established in China to honor him and his work. He received the Magnolia Award in 2000 from the Shanghai Municipal Government for his assistance in the advancement of preventive medicine, especially in the promotion of occupational safety and environmental health. In addition to toxicological testing and assessment, he has given toxicology courses in several countries, notably Canada, China and the U.S.A.

Sam Kacew, PhD, ATS, Professor of Pharmacology at the University of Ottawa. Visiting Professor: Institute of Toxicology, National Taiwan University, Taiper, Taiwan; Joszef Fodor National Center of Public Health,

Budapest, Hungary; Department of Occupational Health, Shanghai Medical University, Shanghai, China; Zhehjiang University, Hangzhou, China and Division of Toxicology, Sung Kyun Kwan University, Colgate-Palmolive Visiting Professor at University of Mexico. Dr Kacew is currently the Editor-in-Chief of the *Journal of Toxicology and Environmental Health, PART A, Current Issues*; Editor-in-Chief of the *Journal of Toxicology and Environmental Health, PART B, Critical Reviews* and Associate Editor of *Toxicology and Applied Pharmacology*. He is a member of the Committee on Toxicology of the National Academy of Sciences of the U.S.A. He has edited several texts on pediatric toxicology and serves on several editorial boards. He has served on subcommittees of NAS/NRC including Flame Retardants and Jet Propulsion-8 Fuels and is a member of Advisory Expert Committee of Canadian Network of Toxicology Centers. He has been a peer reviewer for the EPA on the Integrated Risk Information System (IRIS) documents and National Institutes of Health grant study sections. He has received the Achievement Award of the Society of Toxicology of Canada; Achievement Award, Society of Toxicology; the ICI (Zeneca) Traveling Lectureship Award; the U.S.–China Foundation Award; the Colgate-Palmolive Visiting Professorship Award; National Science Council, Republic of China Visiting Lectureship. He is the author of over 100 papers, reviews and book chapters with emphasis in general toxicology including pediatric, renal, hepatic and pulmonary toxicology.

Preface

Toxicology is an important science. It provides a sound basis for formulating measures to protect the health of workers against toxicants in factories, farms, mines, and other occupational environments. It is also valuable in the protection of public health hazards associated with toxic substances in food, air, and water. Toxicology has played and will continue to play a significant role in the health and welfare of the world. Cognizant of the importance of toxicology, the World Health Organization (WHO) organized a toxicology training course in China in 1982, as part of the ongoing China–WHO collaborative program on medical sciences. One of the authors (FCL) was invited to lectures on basic toxicology. The first edition of this book originated from those lecture notes.

Over the years, a number of important developments have occurred in toxicology. Furthermore, some readers of the book have suggested that discussions on a few groups of important chemicals and toxicants would not only provide some general knowledge of these substances, but also facilitate a deeper appreciation of the various aspects of toxicology. The book has received worldwide acceptance, as evidenced by its repeated editions and reprintings, and by the appearance of six foreign language versions (Chinese, French, Indonesian, Italian, Spanish, and Taiwan Chinese).

This new edition has been further updated and expanded. Thus, there are chapters on lactation, over-the-counter products, occupational toxicology, as well as a section describing the symptomatology of the Gulf War Syndrome and the probable toxicants implicated. A number of other chapters have been updated/expanded, notably those on carcinogenesis, developmental toxicology, immunology, food additives and contaminants, environmental toxicology, and safety/risk assessment. However, details of some toxicity tests have been abbreviated to keep the size of the book within bounds, the retained material is intended to portray more clearly the effects of toxicants.

It is hoped that these additions and updates will enhance the usefulness of the book. In making these changes, the authors have kept in mind the broad aim of the first edition, namely, relatively comprehensive coverage of the subjects and brevity, thereby continuing to serve as an updated introductory text for toxicology students and for those involved in allied sciences who require a background in toxicology. Furthermore, since toxicology is a vast subject and is fast expanding, the book is likely to be useful to those who have become specialized in one or a few areas in toxicology but wish to brush up in other areas. The extensive chemical index and subject index will facilitate the retrieval of specific topics.

Frank C. Lu, MD
Sam Kacew, PhD

Part I

General principles of toxicology

Chapter 1

General considerations

CONTENTS

People are exposed to a great variety of natural and man-made substances. Under certain conditions such exposures cause adverse health effects, ranging in severity from death to subtle biologic changes. Society's ever-increasing desire to identify and prevent these effects has prompted the dramatic evolution of toxicology as a study of poisons to the present-day complex science.

Definition and purpose of toxicology

To state it simply and concisely, toxicology is the study of the nature and mechanism of toxic effects of substances on living organisms and other biologic systems. It also deals with quantitative assessment of the toxic effects in relation to the level, duration and frequency of exposure of the organisms.

The assessment of health hazards of industrial chemicals, environmental pollutants, and other substances represents an important element in the protection of the health of the worker and members of communities.

In-depth studies of the nature and mechanism of the effects of toxicants are invaluable in the invention of specific antidotes and other ameliorative measures. Along with other sciences, toxicology contributes to the development of safer chemicals used as drugs, food additives, pesticides, and many useful industrial chemicals. Even the toxic effects per se are exploited in the pursuit of more effective insecticides, anthelmintics, antimicrobials, and agents used in chemical warfare.

Scope and subdisciplines

Toxicology has a broad scope. It deals with toxicity studies of chemicals used (1) in medicine for diagnostic, preventive, and therapeutic purposes, (2) in the food industry as direct and indirect additives, (3) in agriculture as pesticides, growth regulators, artificial pollinators, and animal feed additives, and (4) in the chemical industry as solvents, components, and intermediates of plastics and many other types of chemicals. It is also concerned with the health effects of metals (as in mines and smelters), petroleum products, paper and pulp, toxic plants, and animal toxins.

Because of its broad scope as well as the need to accomplish different goals, toxicology has a number of subdisciplines. For example, a person may be exposed, accidentally or otherwise, to very large amounts of a toxicant, and become grossly intoxicated. If the identity of the toxicant is not known, *analytical toxicology* will be called upon to identify the toxicant through analysis of body fluids, stomach contents, suspected containers, etc. Those engaged in *clinical toxicology* will administer antidotes, if available, to counter the specific toxicity, and take other measures to ameliorate the symptoms and signs and hasten the elimination of the toxicant from the body. There may also be legal implications, and that will be the task of *forensic toxicology*.

Intoxication may occur as a result of occupational exposure to toxicants. This may result in acute or chronic adverse effects. In either case, the problem is in the domain of *occupational toxicology*. The general public is exposed to a variety of toxicants, via air and water as well as from food as additives, pesticides, and contaminants, often at low levels that may be harmless acutely but may have long-term adverse effects. The sources of these substances, their transport, degradation, and bioconcentration in the environment, and their effects on humans are dealt with in *environmental toxicology*. *Regulatory toxicology* attempts to protect the public by setting laws, regulations, and standards to limit or suspend the use of very toxic chemicals and define use conditions for others. Some of the relevant laws in the U.S.A. are listed in Appendix 1.1.

To set meaningful regulations and standards, extensive profiles of the toxic effects are essential. Such profiles can only be established with a great variety of relevant toxicological studies, which form the foundation of regulatory toxicology. The basic part of such studies is referred to as *conventional toxicology*. In addition, knowledge of the mechanism of action, provided by *mechanistic toxicology*, enhances the toxicological evaluation and provides a basis for other branches of toxicology.

Early developments

The earliest human was well aware of the toxic effects of a number of substances, such as venoms of snakes, the poisonous plants hemlock and aconite, and the toxic mineral substances arsenic, lead, and antimony. Some of these were actually used intentionally for their toxic effects to commit homicide and suicide. For centuries, homicides with toxic substances were not uncommon in Europe. To protect against poisoning, there were continual efforts directed toward the discovery and development of preventive and antidotal measures. However, a more critical evaluation of these measures was only begun by Maimonides (1135–1204) with his famous *Poisons and Their Antidotes*, published in 1198.

More significant contributions to the evolution of toxicology were made in the sixteenth century and later. Paracelsus stated: "No substance is a poison by itself. It is the dose (the amount of the exposure) that makes a substance a poison" and "the right dose differentiates a poison and a remedy." These statements laid the foundation of the concept of the "dose–response relation" and the "therapeutic index" developed later. In addition, he described in his book *Bergsucht* (1533–1534) the clinical manifestations of chronic arsenic and mercury poisoning as well as miner's disease. This might be considered the forefather of occupational toxicology. Orfila wrote an important treatise (1814–1815) describing a systematic correlation between the chemical and biologic information on certain poisons. He also devised methods for detecting poisons and pointed to the necessity for chemical analysis for legal proof of lethal intoxication. The introduction of this approach ushered in a specialty area of modern toxicology, namely forensic toxicology.

Recent developments

In the face of a growing population, modern society demands improvements in health and living conditions, including nutrition, clothing, dwelling, and transportation. To meet this goal, a great variety of chemicals, many of them in large quantities, must be manufactured and used. It has been estimated that tens of thousands of different chemicals are in commercial production in industrialized countries. In one way or another, these chemicals come in contact with various segments of the population: people are engaged in their manufacture, handling, use (e.g., painters, applicators of pesticides), consumption (e.g., drugs, food additives), or misuse (e.g., suicide, accidental poisoning). Furthermore, people may be exposed to the more persistent chemicals via various environmental media and be affected more insidiously. To illustrate the devastating effects of toxicants, some examples of massive acute and long-term poisonings are listed in Appendix 1.2. In some of these episodes, a considerable amount of sophisticated toxicological investigation was done before the etiology was ascertained.

These and other tragic outbreaks of massive chemical poisonings have resulted in intensified testing programs, which have revealed the great diversity of the nature and site of toxic effects. This revelation, in turn, has called for more studies using a greater number of animals, a greater number of indicators of toxicity, etc. There is, therefore, a need to render the task of toxicologically assessing the vast number of chemicals using increasingly more complex testing procedures more manageable. As an attempt to fulfill this need, criteria have been proposed and adopted for the selection of chemicals to be tested according to their priority. In addition, the "tier systems" allow decisions to be made at different stages of toxicologic testing, thus avoiding unnecessary studies. This procedure has been particularly useful in the testing for carcinogenicity, mutagenicity, and immunotoxicity because of the large expenses involved and the great multitude of test systems that are available (Chapters 7, 8, 11, and 25).

Because of the large number of people exposed to these chemicals, society cannot defer appropriate control until serious injuries have appeared. The modern toxicologist, therefore, must attempt to identify, where possible, indicators of exposure, and early, reversible signs of health effects. These will permit the formulation of decisions at the right time to safeguard the health of individuals, either as occupational workers or in exposed communities. The achievements in these areas have assisted responsible personnel in instituting appropriate medical surveillance of occupational workers and other exposed populations. Notable examples are the use of cholinesterase inhibition as an indicator of exposure to organophosphorous pesticides and various biochemical parameters to monitor for lead exposure. Such "biological markers" are intended to measure exposure to toxicants or their effects as well as to detect susceptible population groups (NRC, 1987); they are used for clinical diagnosis, monitoring of occupational workers and facilitating safety/risk assessment (WHO, 1993). Examples of biomarkers are described in the relevant sections.

Advances made in biochemical and toxicokinetic studies, as well as those in genetic toxicology, immunotoxicology, morphologic studies on a subcellular level, and biochemical studies on a molecular level have all contributed to a better understanding of the nature, site, and mechanism of action of toxicants. For example, technological breakthroughs enabled *in vitro* studies to demonstrate that whether the hepatocytes or the non-parenchymal cells are affected by a chemical carcinogen is related to differences in their ability to repair the DNA damage induced by the chemical. Studies using isolated nephrons have provided insight on the site and mode of action of nephrotoxicants (Chapter 14). Various other types of *in vitro* studies have demonstrated the possibility of their use in screening toxicants for specific effects such as mutagenicity and dermal irritancy. Numerous studies have shown that the responses to toxicants are better correlated with the effective dose; that is, the concentration of the toxicant at the site of action, rather than the administered dose. Furthermore, where the effect results mainly or entirely from an active metabolite, the concentration of the metabolite rather than that of the parent chemical is important.

An important function of toxicology is to determine safe levels of exposure to natural and man-made chemicals, thereby preventing the adverse effects of exposures to toxicants. One of the earliest official actions in this field was taken by the U.S. Food and Drug Administration. It stipulated that a 100-fold margin was required for a food additive to be permitted for use. In other words, a chemical additive should not occur in the total human diet in a quantity greater than 1/100 of the amount that is the maximum safe dosage in long-term animal experiments (Lehman and Fitzhugh, 1954). For several reasons this approach was not practicable on an international level (see Chapter 25). While evaluating a number of food additives in 1961, WHO coined the term "acceptable daily intake" (WHO, 1962). Using ADI procedure, WHO has since convened annual meetings of experts on food additives, contaminants, residues of veterinary drugs, and pesticide residues. Assessment of these chemicals has resulted, where appropriate, in the assignment of ADIs (Chapter 25). The term "ADI" and the WHO evaluations have been adopted by regulatory agencies in many nations. The inception, evolution and application of ADI has been outlined by Lu (1988). For toxicants in the occupational settings, quantitative assessment are provided in terms of "threshold limit values" (*Federal Register*, 1971).

These determinations involve comprehensive studies of the toxic properties, demonstration of dosages that produce no observable adverse effects, establishment of dose–effect and dose–response relationships, and toxicokinetic and biotransformation studies.

The greatly increased scope and the multiplicity of subdisciplines as outlined above provide a vivid view of recent progress in toxicology.

Some challenges and successes

The so-called aniline tumors were reported by Rehn (1895), a German surgeon, in the urinary bladders of three men who had worked in an aniline factory. The role of aniline and aniline dyes as the etiologic agents was confirmed only some 40 years later, after much experimental investigation in animals (e.g., Hueper *et al.*, 1938) and extensive epidemiologic studies by Case *et al.* (1954) had been carried out. This discovery led to improved occupational standards and more stringent controls of food colors derived from coal tar.

In the late 1950s, thalidomide was widely used as a sedative. It has a very low acute toxicity and readily met the toxicity testing protocol prevailing at that time. However, a rare form of congenital malformation, phocomelia (the virtual absence of extremities), was observed among some offspring of mothers who had taken this drug during the first trimester (Lenz and Knapp, 1962). This tragedy led to the explosive development of teratology (developmental toxicology), an important specialty area of toxicology. The importance of modifying factors has been dramatized by the tragic effect of cobalt among heavy beer drinkers (see Chapter 5).

The once prevalent lead poisoning in certain areas of industrialized countries has now largely disappeared. This great accomplishment in the field of public health resulted from the implementation of control measures devised on the basis of the knowledge gained from the numerous toxicologic studies of lead.

Many cases of serious illness that culminate in permanent paralysis and death have been reported in Minamata and Niigata in Japan in the 1950s and 1960s, respectively (Study Group on Minamata Disease, 1968; Tsubaki and Irukayama, 1977). The cause of the illness was eventually traced to methylmercury in the fish caught locally. The fish were contaminated with this chemical, which had been discharged as such into the water by a factory, or the contaminant was derived from elemental mercury discharged by the factory and methylated through microorganisms in the mud. Measures to rehabilitate the surviving patients and legal control of the factories have been instituted.

On the other hand, the cause of another mysterious illness in Japan, known as itai-itai disease, remains unsolved, although cadmium apparently played a role. The patients had resided for many years in areas that were in the vicinity of mines and where the cadmium levels in rice and water were excessive.

A more solid foundation in the assessment of risks of chemical carcinogens resulted from recent advances in epidemiologic studies, long-term animal studies, short-term mutagenesis/carcinogenesis tests, and mechanistic studies, as well as the realization that carcinogens differ in their potency, latency, and mode of action (Chapters 7 and 25).

Toxicity vs. other considerations

In general, exposure to toxic substances is to be avoided. However, the severity of the effects vary greatly; some chemicals induce mild, transient, reversible effects, whereas those of others may be irreversible, serious, and even fatal. Exposure to the former type of substances might thus be acceptable, but, as a rule, not the latter. Examples of the exceptions: methyl mercury, which is extremely toxic, is present in many species of fish. Because of the nutritional value of fish, permissible levels of methyl mercury are established to minimize the risk yet not deny this valuable source of nutrients. Aflatoxin B_1 is one of the most potent carcinogens but is present in a variety of foods. Yet the contaminated food is not banned as long as the toxin does not exceed the permissible levels.

The complex nature of assessing the toxicity of a substance in light of its benefits is also exemplified by the toxicology seen in lactation and OTC products. The former involves weighing the benefits of breast feeding vs. the toxicity of certain potential contaminants. OTC products, when improperly used, present toxicologic problems. However, the value of these products in general cannot be ignored. The dilemmas involved in these topics are further described and discussed in other chapters.

Future prospects

The need of new substances will undoubtedly continue. Some of them will treat or prevent a variety of diseases which are currently untreatable or unpreventable. Others will render food more plentiful, tastier, and hopefully more healthy. Still others will improve living conditions in a variety of ways. At the same time, people are more conscious of subtle adverse effects on health, and expect the new substances to be "absolutely safe." Furthermore, the disposal of these substances and their by-products is expected to cause no environmental hazards, adversely affecting humans and the ecosystem.

To satisfy these seemingly irreconcilable societal demands, the toxicologist must carry out a series of studies on each substance: is it readily absorbed, distributed to specific organs, stored, and/or readily excreted? Is it detoxicated or bioactivated? What kind of toxic effects does it induce and what are the host and environmental factors that can alter these effects? How does it produce the effect on a cellular and molecular level? What type of "general toxicity" does it produce? What organs are its targets? What is its predominant mechanism of action? Answers to these and other questions will provide a scientific basis for assessing its safety and risk for the intended use.

It is evident that the multitude of studies involved will place an increasing demand on the limited facilities for toxicologic testing and on the short supply of qualified personnel. It is of utmost importance therefore that toxicity data generated anywhere be accepted internationally. However, to ensure general acceptance, the data must meet certain standards. The "Good Laboratory Practice" promulgated by the U.S. Food and Drug Administration (FDA, 1980) and the Organization of Economic Cooperation and Development (OECD, 1982), should be adopted by all countries involved in toxicological testing.

To streamline the long and costly testing of each chemical separately, there have been schemes that test a representative chemical extensively and verify the results on other members of the group with minimal testing. This practice has been adopted successfully when the substances included in a group are essentially similar. A recent proposal to ban all chlorine compounds, however, appears to have gone too far in ignoring the great diversity of the toxic nature and potency of such a large group of substances (Karol, 1995). It will be a major challenge to determine how diverse a variety of chemicals can be rationally grouped for toxicological testing and assessment purposes.

Other trends designed to simplify and hasten the testing include a reduction in the use of laboratory animals and supplement or supplant them with *in vitro* studies. This is done partly in response to a societal call on humane grounds. Isolated organs, cultured tissues and cells, and lower forms of life will be increasingly used. Furthermore, such test systems will likely be faster and less expensive, and will augment the variety of studies, especially those related to the mechanism of toxicity. An understanding of the mechanism of action of a chemical is often valuable in providing a sounder basis for the assessment of its safety/risk. Other types of improvements of the testing procedure with respect to simplicity and reliability will continue to be made.

As noted earlier, to provide a basis for proper assessment of the safety/risk of a chemical and for a variety of other purposes, toxicology is increasingly becoming a multifaceted science. To facilitate the acquisition of a broad knowledge of toxicology, this book covers four major areas.

Part I describes general topics related to absorption, distribution, and excretion of toxicants, their transformation in the body, the various types of toxic effects they exert, and the host and environmental factors that modify these effects.

Procedures used to determining the general and specific effects are described in Part II.

Part III describes the organ/system-specific toxicants and the procedures commonly used to detect their effects.

Part IV discusses several major groups of toxicants such as food additives and contaminants, pesticides, metals, over-the-counter preparations, various environmental pollutants, and toxicants in the workplace. The last chapter outlines the widely adopted approaches to the assessment of safety/risk of noncarcinogenic and carcinogenic chemicals. In addition, two indices are appended listing chemicals and subjects, respectively, to assist the reader in retrieving relevant parts of the text.

References

Case, R. A. M., Hosker, M. E., McDonald, D. B., and Pearson, J. T. (1954) Tumours of the urinary bladder in workmen engaged in the manufacture and use of certain dyestuff intermediates in the British chemical industry. *Br. J. Ind. Med.* 11:75–104.

Federal Register (1971) *Threshold Limit Values adopted by the American Conference of Governmental Industrial Hygienists, 1968*, vol. 36, no. 105, May 29. Washington, DC: U.S. Government Printing Office.

FDA (1980) *Code of Federal Regulations, Title 21, Food and Drugs.* Part 58. Washington, DC: U.S. Government Printing Office.

Hueper, W. C. *et al.* (1938) Experimental production of bladder tumors in dogs by administration of beta-naphthylamine. *J. Ind. Hyg. Toxicol.* 20:46.

Karol, M. H. (1995) Toxicologic principles do not support the banning of chlorine: A Society of Toxicology position paper. *Fundam. Appl. Toxicol.* 24:1–2.

Lehman, A. J. and Fitzhugh, O. G. (1954) 100-fold margin of safety. *Q. Bull. Assoc. Food Drug Officials U.S.* 18:33–35.

Lenz, W. and Knapp, K. (1962) Thalidomide embryopathy. *Arch. Environ. Health* 5:100–105.

Lu, F. C. (1988) Acceptable daily intakes: Inception, evolution and application. *Regul. Toxicol. Pharmacol.* 8:45–60.

NRC Committee on Biological Markers (1987) Biological markers in environmental health research. *Environ. Health Perspect.* 74:3–9.

OECD (1982) *Good Laboratory Practice in the Testing of Chemicals.* Organization of Economic Cooperation and Development, 75775 Paris Cedex 16, France.

Rehn, L. (1895) Blasengeschwulste bei Fuchsin-Arbeiten. *Arch. Klin. Chir.* 50:588.

Study Group of Minamata Disease (1968) *Minamata Disease.* Minamata, Japan: Minamata University.

Tsubaki, T. and Irukayama, K. (1977) *Minamata Disease: Methyl Mercury Poisoning in Minamata and Niigata, Japan.* New York, NY: Elsevier Scientific.

WHO (1962) *Sixth Report of the Joint FAD/WHO Expert Committee on Food Additives.* Geneva: World Health Organization.

WHO (1993) Biomarkers and Risk Assessment: Concepts and Principles. *Envir. Health Criteria* 155.

Appendix 1.1 U.S. laws that have a basis in toxicology

Responsible agency	Law
Food and Drug Administration (FDA)	Federal Food, Drug, and Cosmetic Act
Environmental Protection Agency (EPA)	Federal Insecticide, Fungicide, and Rodenticide Act
	Clean Air Act
	Safe Drinking Water Act
	Toxic Substances Control Act
Consumer Product Safety Commission (CPSC)	Consumer Product Safety Act
	Federal Hazardous Substances Act
Occupational Safety and Health Administration (OSHA)	Occupational Safety and Health Act

Appendix 1.2 Examples of outbreaks of mass poisoning

Location and year	Toxicant	Adverse effect	Number affected
Detroit, MI., 1930	Tri-o-cresyl phosphate in "ginger jake"	Delayed neurotoxicity	16,000
London, U.K., 1952	Sulfur dioxide and suspended particulate matter in air	Increased deaths from heart and lung diseases	3,000
Toyama, Japan, 1950s	Cadmium in rice	Severe kidney and bone disease	200*
Minamata, Japan, 1950s	Methylmercury in fish	Severe neurological disease ("Minamata disease")	200*†
Southeast Turkey, 1956	Hexachlorobenzene in wheat	Porphyria, neurological diseases	4,000
Morocco, 1959	Tri-o-cresyl phosphate in adulterated oil	Delayed neurotoxicity	10,000
Japan, 1956–1977	Clioquinol	Subacute myelo-opticoneuropathy (SMON)	10,000
Western Europe, late 1950s and early 1960s	Thalidomide	Phocomelia	10,000
Fukuoka, Japan, 1968	Polychlorinated biphenyls (PCB)	Skin disease, general weakness	1,700
Iraq, 1972	Methylmercury in wheat	Deaths from neurological disease	500
		Nonfatal cases	50,000
Madrid, Spain, 1981	Toxic oil in food	Deaths with various symptoms and signs	340
		Nonfatal cases	20,000
Bhopal, India, 1984	Methylisocyanate released into air	Deaths from acute lung disease	6,000
		Nonfatal cases	200,000

Notes
*Many more cases with mild or moderate symptoms and signs of intoxication.
†Hundreds of cases occurred in Niigata, Japan, in 1960s.

Chapter 2

Absorption, distribution, and excretion of toxicants

Introduction

Apart from local effects at the site of contact, a toxicant can cause injury only after it is absorbed by the organism. Absorption can occur through the skin, the gastrointestinal tract, the lungs, and several minor routes. Furthermore, the nature and intensity of the effects of a chemical on an organism depend on its concentration in the target organs. The concentration depends not only on the administered dose but also on other factors, including absorption, distribution, binding, and excretion. For a chemical to be absorbed, distributed, and eventually excreted, a toxicant must pass through a number of cell membranes. A cell membrane generally consists of a biomolecular layer of lipid molecules with proteins scattered throughout the membrane (see Figure 2.1).

There are four mechanisms by which a toxicant may pass through a cell membrane; the most important of them is passive diffusion through the membrane. The others are filtration through the membrane pores, carrier-mediated transport, and engulfing by the cell. The last two mechanisms are different in that the cell takes an active part in the transfer of a toxicant across its membranes.

Passive diffusion

Most toxicants cross cell membranes by simple, passive diffusion. The rate of passage is related directly to the concentration gradient across the membrane, and to the lipid solubility. For example, mannitol is hardly absorbed (<2%); acetylsalicylic acid is fairly well absorbed (21%); and thiopental is even more readily absorbed (67%). It is noteworthy that the chloroform:water partition of the nonionized forms of these chemicals are, respectively, <0.002, 2.0, and 100. For references to this and other examples, see Hogben et al. (1958).

Many toxicants are ionizable. The ionized form is often unable to pene-

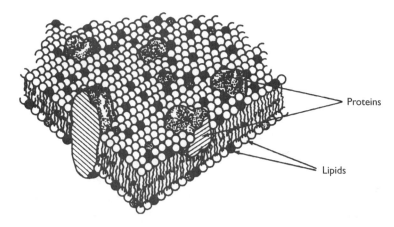

Figure 2.1 Schematic diagram of biologic membrane. Spheres represent head groups (phosphatidylcholine), and zig-zag lines indicate tail ends of lipids. Black, white, and stippled spheres indicate different kinds of lipids. Large bodies represent proteins; some are located on the surface, others within the membrane.

Source: Modified from S. J. Singer and G. L. Nicholson, *Science*, 175:720. By permission of the author and the American Association for the Advancement of Science, © 1972.

trate the cell membrane because of its low lipid solubility. On the other hand, the nonionized form is likely lipid-soluble enough to do so, and its rate of penetration is dependent on the lipid solubility. The extent of ionization of weak organic acids and bases depends on the pH of the medium. Thus, for the former, such as benzoic acid, diffusion is facilitated in acidic environment, where they exist mainly in the nonionized form; for the latter, such as aniline, diffusion is facilitated in basic environment (Figures 2.2 and 2.3).

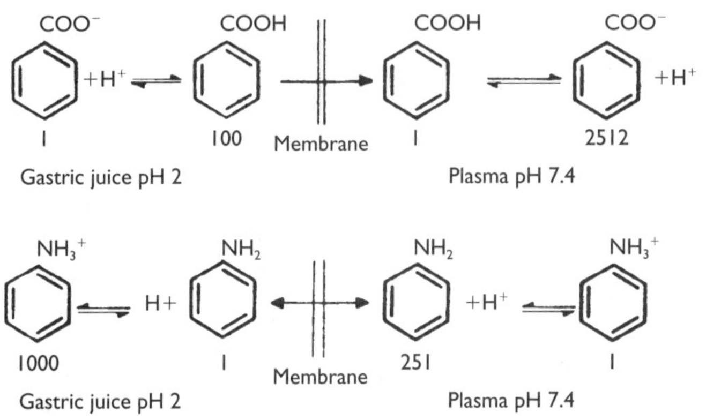

Figure 2.2 Disposition of benzoic acid and aniline in gastric juice and plasma. Figures immediately below the structural formulas represent proportions of ionized and nonionized forms.

Source: Timbrell, 1991, p. 44.

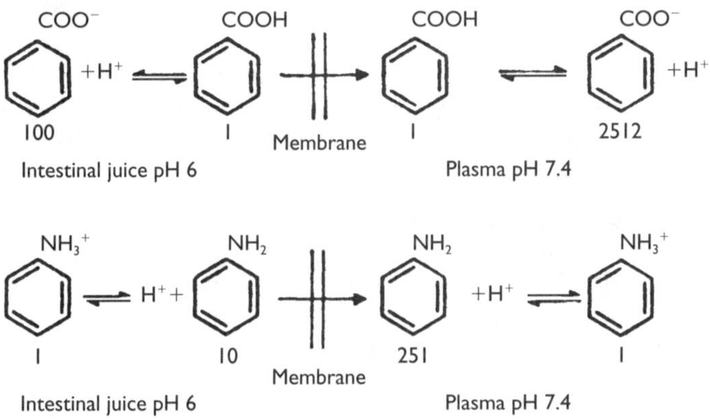

Figure 2.3 Disposition of benzoic acid and aniline in intestinal juice and plasma.

Source: Timbrell, 1991, p. 45.

Filtration

The membranes of the capillaries and the glomeruli have relatively large pores (about 70 nm) and allow molecules smaller than albumin (molecular weight 60,000 dalton) to pass through. Bulk flow of water through these pores results from hydrostatic and/or osmotic pressure and can act as a carrier of toxicants. The pores in most cells, however, are relatively small (about 4 nm) and allow chemicals only up to a molecular weight of 100–200 to pass through. Chemicals of larger molecules, therefore, can filter into and out of the capillaries. They can, therefore, establish equilibrium between the concentrations in the plasma and in the extracellular fluid, but they cannot do so by filtration between the extracellular and intracellular fluids.

Carrier-mediated transport

This involves the formation of a complex between the chemical and a macromolecular carrier on one side of the membrane. The complex then diffuses to the other side of the membrane, where the chemical is released. Thereafter the carrier returns to the original surface to repeat the transport process. The carrier has a limited capacity. When it is saturated, the rate of transport is no longer dependent on the concentration of the chemical and assumes zero order kinetics. Structure, conformation, size, and charge are important in determining the affinity of a chemical for a carrier site, and competitive inhibition can occur among chemicals with similar characteristics.

Active transport involves a carrier that moves molecules across a membrane against a concentration gradient, or, if the molecule is an ion, against an electrochemical gradient. It requires the expenditure of metabolic energy and can be inhibited by poisons that interfere with cell metabolism.

Facilitated diffusion is similar to active transport but does not move molecules against a concentration gradient. Furthermore, it is not energy-dependent, and metabolic poisons will not inhibit this process.

Engulfing by the cell (endocytosis)

Particles may be engulfed by cells. When the particles are solid, the process is called phagocytosis and when they are liquid, it is called pinocytosis. Such special transport systems are important for removal of particulate matter from the alveoli and of certain toxic substances from the blood by the reticuloendothelial system. Absorption of carrageenans (molecular weight about 40,000) from the gut is also by this process.

Absorption

The main routes by which toxicants are absorbed are the gastrointestinal tract, lungs, and skin. However, in toxicologic studies, such special routes as intraperitoneal, intramuscular, and subcutaneous injections are also used.

Gastrointestinal tract

Many toxicants can enter the G.I. tract along with food and water or alone as drugs or other types of chemicals. With the exception of those that are caustic or very irritating to the mucosa, most toxicants do not exert any toxic effect unless they are absorbed. Absorption can take place along the entire G.I. tract. For example, certain drugs are administered as sublingual tablets and suppositories to be absorbed in the mouth and the rectum, respectively. However, the mouth and rectum are, in general, insignificant sites of absorption of environmental chemicals.

The stomach is a significant site of absorption, especially for weak acids, which will exist in the diffusible, nonionized, lipid-soluble form. On the other hand, weak bases will be highly ionized in the acidic gastric juice and therefore not readily absorbable. The difference in absorption is further amplified by the circulating plasma. Weak acids will exist mainly in ionized form in plasma and be carried away, whereas weak bases will exist in nonionized form and can diffuse back to the stomach. The influence of these factors, using benzoic acid and aniline as examples, is shown in Figure 2.2.

In the intestine, weak acids will exist mainly in the ionized form, hence they are less readily absorbable. However, upon entering the blood, they become ionized and thus will not readily diffuse back. On the other hand, weak bases will exist mainly in the nonionized form, hence more readily absorbable, as shown in Figure 2.3. It should be noted that intestinal absorption is further enhanced by the long contact time and the large surface area provided by the villi and microvilli.

In the intestine, there are special carrier-mediated transport systems that are responsible for the absorption of nutrients, such as monosaccharides, amino acids, and such elements as iron, calcium, and sodium. However, a few toxicants, such as 5-fluorouracil, thallium, and lead, are known to be absorbable from the intestine by active transport systems. In addition, particulate matters such as those of the azo dyes and polystyrene latex can enter the intestinal cell by pinocytosis.

Respiratory tract

The main site of absorption in the respiratory tract is the alveoli in the lungs. This is especially true for gases such as carbon monoxide, nitrogen oxides, and sulfur dioxide, and for vapors of volatile liquids such as benzene and carbon tetrachloride. Their ready absorption is related to the large alveolar area, high blood flow, and proximity of the blood to the alveolar air.

The rate of absorption is dependent on the solubility of the gas in the blood: the more soluble it is, the faster the absorption. However, equilibrium between the air and the blood is reached more slowly for more soluble chemicals, such as chloroform, compared to less soluble chemicals such as ethylene. This is because the more soluble a chemical, the more of it can be dissolved in the blood. Since the alveolar air can only carry a limited amount of the chemical, more respirations and hence a longer time will be required to attain equilibrium. It will take even longer if the chemical is also deposited in the fat tissue.

In addition to gases and vapors, liquid aerosols and airborne particles may also be absorbed. In general, large particles (>10 μm) do not enter the respiratory tract; when they do, they are deposited in the nose and disposed of by wiping, blowing, and sneezing. Very small particles (<0.01 μm) are likely to be exhaled. Those in the range of 0.01–10 μm are deposited in various parts of the respiratory tract. The larger ones are likely to be deposited in the nasopharynx and absorbed either through the epithelium of this region or through the gastrointestinal tract epithelium after they are swallowed along with the mucus. Smaller particles are deposited in the trachea, bronchi, and bronchioli and are then either aspirated onto the mucociliary escalator or engulfed by phagocytes. The particles carried up by the escalator will be coughed up or swallowed. The phagocytes with engulfed particles will be absorbed into the lymphatics. Some free particles can also migrate into the lymphatics. Soluble particles may be absorbed through the epithelium into the blood.

A detailed examination of the deposition of particles of various sizes in different parts of the respiratory tract is provided by a Task Group on Lung Dynamics (1966). However, as a rough estimate, 25% of inhaled particles are exhaled, 50% are deposited in the upper respiratory tract, and 25% are deposited in the lower respiratory tract (Morrow et al., 1966).

Skin

In general, the skin is relatively impermeable, and therefore it constitutes a good barrier, separating the organism from its environment. However, some chemicals can be absorbed through the skin in sufficient quantities to produce systemic effects.

A chemical may be absorbed via the hair follicles or through the cells of the sweat glands or those of the sebaceous glands. These are, however, minor routes for absorption since they constitute only a small surface area of the skin. Therefore, the percutaneous absorption of a chemical is essentially through the skin proper, which consists of the epidermis and dermis (see Figure 14.1).

The first phase of percutaneous absorption is diffusion of the toxicant through the epidermis, which, especially its stratum corneum, is the most important barrier. The stratum corneum consists of several layers of thin, cohesive, dead cells that contain chemically resistant material (protein filament). Small amounts of polar substances appear to diffuse through the outer surface of the protein filaments of the hydrated stratum corneum; nonpolar substances dissolve in and diffuse through the lipid matrix between the protein filaments.

In the human stratum corneum, there are significant differences in structure and chemistry from one region of the body to another, which are reflected in the permeability to chemicals. For example, toxicants cross the scrotum readily, cross the abdominal skin less readily, and cross the sole and palm with great difficulty (Zbinden, 1976).

The second phase of percutaneous absorption is diffusion of the toxicant through the dermis, which contains a porous, nonselective, aqueous diffusion medium. Therefore it is much less effective as a barrier than the stratum corneum, and, as a consequence, abrasion or removal of the latter causes a marked increase in the percutaneous absorption. Acids, alkalis, and mustard gases will also increase the absorption by injuring this barrier. Some solvents, notably dimethyl sulfoxide (DMSO), also increase dermal permeability.

Distribution

After a chemical enters the blood, it is distributed rapidly throughout the body. The rate of distribution to each organ is related to the blood flow through the organ, the ease with which the chemical crosses the local capillary wall and the cell membrane, and the affinity of components of the organ for the chemical.

Barriers

The *blood–brain barrier* is located at the capillary wall. The capillary endothelial cells there are tightly joined, leaving few or no pores between these cells (Bradbury, 1984). Thus, the toxicant has to pass through the capillary endothelium itself. A lack of vesicles in these cells further reduces their transport ability. Finally, the protein concentration of the interstitial fluid in the brain is low, in contrast to that in other organs; protein binding therefore does not serve as a mechanism for the transfer of toxicants from the blood to the brain. For these reasons, the penetration of toxicants into the brain is dependent on their lipid solubility. An outstanding example is the toxicant methyl mercury, which enters the brain readily and the main toxicity of which is on the central nervous system. In contrast, inorganic mercury compounds are not lipid-soluble, do not enter the brain readily, and exert their main adverse effects not on the brain but on the kidney.

The *placental barrier* differs anatomically among various animal species. There are six layers of cells between fetal and maternal blood in some species, whereas in others there is only one layer. Furthermore, the number of layers may change as the gestation progresses. Although the relationship of the number of layers of the placenta to its permeability needs quantitative determination, the placental barrier does impede the transfer of toxicants to the fetus, which is therefore protected to some extent. However, the concentration of a toxicant such as methyl mercury may be higher in certain fetal organs, such as the brain, because of the less effective fetal blood–brain barrier. On the other hand, the fetal concentration of the food coloring amaranth is only 0.03–0.06% of that of the mother (Munro and Willes, 1978).

Other barriers are also present in such organs as the eyes and testicles. In addition, the erythrocyte plays an interesting role in the distribution of certain toxicants. For example, its membrane acts as a barrier against the penetration of inorganic mercury compounds but not that of alkyl mercury. Furthermore, there is affinity of the erythrocyte cytoplasm for alkyl mercury compounds. Because of these factors, the concentration of inorganic mercury compounds in the erythrocytes is only about half that in the plasma, whereas that of methyl mercury in the erythrocyte is about ten times that in the plasma (WHO, 1976).

Binding and storage

As noted above, binding of a chemical in a tissue can result in a higher concentration in that tissue. There are two major types of binding. The covalent type of binding is irreversible and is, in general, associated with significant toxic effects. The noncovalent binding usually accounts for a major portion of the dose and is reversible. Therefore, this process plays an important role in the distribution of toxicants in various organs and tissues. There are several types of noncovalent binding as outlined by Guthrie (1980).

Plasma proteins can bind normal physiologic constituents in the body as well as many foreign compounds. Most of the latter are bound to the albumin and are therefore not immediately available for distribution to the extravascular space. However, since the binding is reversible, it permits the bound chemical to dissociate from the protein, thereby replenishing the level of unbound chemical, which may then cross the capillary endothelium. The toxicologic significance of the binding can be illustrated by the possible induction of coma by the administration of sulfonamide drugs to patients who are taking antidiabetic drugs. The antidiabetic drugs are bound to the plasma proteins but can be replaced by the sulfonamide drugs, which have a greater affinity for the plasma protein. The antidiabetic drugs thus released may precipitate a hypoglycemic coma.

The *liver* and *kidney* have a higher capacity for binding chemicals. This characteristic may be related to their metabolic and excretory functions. Certain proteins have been identified in these organs for their specific binding property, such as metallothionein, which is important for the binding of cadmium in the liver and kidney and possibly also for the transfer of the metal from the liver to the kidney. Binding of a substance can increase its concentration in an organ rapidly. For example, 30 minutes after a single administration of lead, its concentration in the liver is 50 times higher than that in the plasma.

The *adipose tissue* is an important storage depot for lipid-soluble substances such as DDT, dieldrin, and polychlorinated biphenyls (PCB). They appear to be stored in the adipose tissue by simple dissolution in the neutral fats. There exists the potential that the plasma concentration of the substances stored in the fat may rise sharply as a result of rapid mobilization of fat following starvation. Conjugation of fatty acid to toxicants such as DDT may also be a mechanism by which these chemicals are retained in the lipid-containing tissues and cells of the body (Leighty *et al.*, 1980).

Bone is a major site for storage for such toxicants as fluoride, lead, and strontium. The storage takes place by an exchange adsorption reaction between the toxicants in the interstitial fluid and the hydroxyapatite crystals of bone mineral. By virtue of similarities in size and charge, F^- may readily replace OH^-, and calcium may be replaced by lead or strontium. These stored substances can be released by ionic exchange and by dissolution of bone crystals through osteoclastic activity.

Excretion

After absorption and distribution in the organism, toxicants are excreted, rapidly or slowly. A generally accepted indicator of the rate of elimination of a toxicant is its "half-life" ($t_{\frac{1}{2}}$), which is the time required for 50% of it to be removed from the bloodstream.

The toxicants are excreted as the parent chemicals, as their metabolites, and/or as conjugates of them. The principal route of excretion is the urine, but the liver and lungs are also important excretory organs for certain types of chemicals. In addition, there are a number of minor routes of excretion.

Urinary excretion

The kidney removes toxicants from the body by the same mechanisms as those used in the removal of end-products of normal metabolism, namely, glomerular filtration, tubular diffusion, and tubular secretion.

The glomerular capillaries have large pores (70 nm); therefore, most toxicants will be filtered at the glomerulus, except those that are very large (greater than 60,000 dalton) or are tightly bound to plasma protein. Once a toxicant enters the glomerular filtrate, it will either be passively reabsorbed across the tubular cells if it has a high lipid/water partition coefficient or remain in the tubular lumen and be excreted if it is a polar compound.

A toxicant can also be excreted through the tubules into the urine by passive diffusion. Since urine is normally acidic, this process plays a role in the excretion of organic bases. On the other hand, organic acids are unlikely to be excreted by passive diffusion through the tubular cells. However, weak acids are often metabolized to stronger acids, thereby increasing the percentage of the ionic forms that are not reabsorbed through the tubular cells and are thus excreted.

Certain toxicants can be secreted by the cells of the proximal tubules into the urine. There are two distinct secretory mechanisms, one for organic acids (e.g., glucuronide and sulfate conjugates) and the other for organic bases. Protein-bound toxicants can also be secreted, provided the binding is reversible. Furthermore, chemicals of similar characteristics compete for the same transport system. For example, probenecid can increase the serum level of penicillin and prolong its activity by blocking its tubular excretion.

Biliary excretion

The liver is also an important organ for the excretion of toxicants, especially for compounds with high polarity (anionic and cationic), conjugates of compounds bound to plasma proteins, and compounds with molecular weights greater than 300. In general, once these compounds are in the bile, they are not reabsorbed into the blood and are excreted via the feces. However, there are exceptions, such as the glucuronide conjugates, which can be hydrolyzed by intestinal flora, enabling the reabsorption of the free toxicants.

The importance of the biliary route of excretion for some chemicals has been well demonstrated in experiments that showed a several-fold increase of the acute toxicity in animals with ligated bile ducts. Such chemicals include digoxin, indocyanine green, ouabain, and, most dramatically, diethylstilbestrol (DES). The toxicity of DES is increased by a factor of 130 in rats with ligated bile ducts (Klaassen, 1973).

Lungs

Substances that exist in the gaseous phase at body temperature are excreted mainly by the lungs. Volatile liquids are also readily excreted via the expired air. Highly soluble liquids such as chloroform and halothane are excreted slowly because of their storage in the adipose tissue and the limited ventilation volume. Excretion of toxicants from the lung is accomplished by simple diffusion through cell membranes.

Other routes

The *gastrointestinal tract* is not a major route of excretion of toxicants. However, because the human stomach and intestine each secretes about 3 liters of fluid per day, some toxicants are excreted along with the fluid. The excretion is mainly by diffusion and thus the rate depends on the pK_a of the toxicant and the pH of the stomach and intestine.

The excretion of toxicants in mother's *milk* is not important as far as the host organism is concerned. However, the presence of toxic substances in milk may be toxicologically significant because they can be passed in the milk from the mother to the nursing child and from cows to humans. The excretion is also via simple diffusion. Since milk is slightly acidic, basic compounds will reach a higher level in milk than in plasma, while the opposite is true with acidic compounds. Lipophilic compounds such as DDT and PCB also reach a higher level in milk because of its higher fat content.

Sweat and *saliva* are also minor routes of excretion of toxicants. The excretion is also by diffusion; thus it is confined to the nonionized, lipid-soluble forms of the toxicants. Substances excreted in the saliva are usually swallowed and then become available for absorption in the G.I. tract.

Levels of toxicants in the body

As noted above, the nature and intensity of the effects of a chemical depend on its concentration at the site of action, namely, the effective dose rather than the administered dose. The level in the target organ is, in general, a function of the blood level. However, binding of a toxicant in a tissue will increase its level, whereas tissue barriers tend to reduce the level. Since the blood level is more readily determined, especially over a time period, it is the parameter often used in toxicokinetic studies.

While the toxicant is being absorbed, its blood level rises. In the meantime, the rates of its excretion, biotransformation (see Chapter 3), and the distribution to other organs and tissues also increase. The curve depicting the blood level against time and the area under that curve (AUC) are useful tools in toxicokinetics. In a series of experimental studies, Smyth and

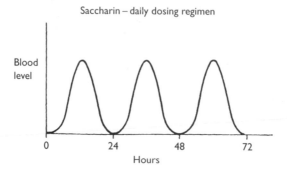

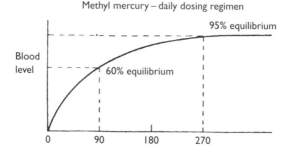

Figure 2.4 Comparative chemobiokinetics of saccharin and methyl mercury chloride.

Source: Adapted from Munro and Willes, 1978, p. 138.

Hottendorf (1980) demonstrated that the AUC for a solution of a chemical is, in general, greater than that for its suspension, and it is greater for acidic than basic chemicals. They also illustrated the effects of the route of administration, dose level, and dosing vehicle on the AUC.

The influence of the rate of excretion on the blood level is vividly shown in Figure 2.4. Saccharin is rapidly excreted; hence its blood level drops rapidly, even after repeated administration. On the other hand, methyl mercury is excreted very slowly; its gradual accumulation culminates in a near plateau only after 270 days (Munro and Willes, 1978).

Methods for determining the rate and extent of absorption, distribution, binding, storage and excretion at various organs and tissues are readily found in the literature. A summary of some of them is given in a WHO publication (WHO, 1986).

References

Bradbury, M. W. B. (1984) The structure and function of the blood–brain barrier. *Fed. Proc.* 43:186–190.

Guthrie, F. E. (1980) Absorption and distribution, in *Introduction to Biochemical Toxicology*, E. Hodgson and F. E. Guthrie (eds), New York, NY: Elsevier.

Hogben, C. A. M., Tocco, D. J., Brodie, B. B., and Schanker, L. S. (1958) On the mechanism of intestinal absorption of drugs. *J. Pharmacol. Exp. Therap.* 125:275–282.

Klaassen, C. D. (1973) Comparison of the toxicity of chemicals in newborn rats to bile duct-ligated and sham-operated rats and mice. *Toxicol. Appl. Pharmacol.* 24:37–44.

Leighty, E. G., Fentiman, A. F., Jr., and Thompson, R. M. (1980) Conjugation of fatty acids to DDT in the rat: Possible mechanism for retention. *Toxicology* 15:77–82.

Morrow, P. E., Hodge, H. C., Newman, W. F., Maynard, E. A., Blanchet, H. J., Jr., Fassett, D. W., Birk, R. E., and Mavrodt, S. (1966) Deposition and retention models for internal dosimetry of the human respiratory tract. *Health Phys.* 12:173–207.

Munro, I. O. and Willes, A. F. (1978) Reproductive toxicity and the problems of *in vitro* exposure, in *Chemical Toxicology of Food*, A. Galli, R. Paoletti and G. Veterazzi (eds), Amsterdam: Elsevier/North Holland.

Singer, S. J. and Nicolson, G. C. (1972) The fluid mosaic model of the structure of cell membranes. *Science* 175:720–731.

Smyth, A. D. and Hottendorf, G. H. (1980) Application of pharmacokinetics and biopharmaceutics in the design of toxicological studies. *Toxicol. Appl. Pharmacol.* 53:179–195.

Task Group on Lung Dynamics (1966) Deposition and retention models for internal dosimetry of the human respiratory tract. *Health Phys.* 12:173–207.

Timbrell, J. A. (1991) *Principles of Biochemical Toxicology*. London: Taylor & Francis.

WHO (1976) *Mercury. Environmental Health Criteria 1*, p. 70. Geneva: World Health Organization.

WHO (1986) *Principles of Toxicokinetic Studies. Environmental Health Criteria 57*. Geneva: World Health Organization.

Zbinden, G. (1976) Percutaneous drug permeation, in *Progress in Toxicology*, vol. 2. New York, NY: Springer-Verlag.

Chapter 3

Biotransformation of toxicants

General considerations

As noted in the previous chapter, a toxicant can be absorbed into an organism via different routes. After absorption it is distributed to various parts of the body, including the excretory organs, and is thus available for excretion. Many chemicals are known to undergo biotransformation (metabolic transformation) while in the organs and tissues. The most important site of such reactions is the liver, the others being the lungs, stomach, intestine, skin, and kidneys.

There are two types of biotransformation:

1   Phase I involving oxidation, reduction, and hydrolysis, may be considered degradation reactions;
2   Phase II involving the production of a compound (a conjugate) that is biosynthesized from the toxicant, or its metabolite, plus an endogenous metabolite may be considered conjugation reactions.

Biotransformation is, therefore, a process that, in general, converts the parent compounds into metabolites and then forms conjugates, but it may involve only one of these reactions. For example, benzene undergoes oxidation, a phase I reaction, to form phenol, which conjugates with sulfate, a phase II reaction. However, when the administered chemical is phenol, it will conjugate with sulfate without a phase I reaction. The metabolites and conjugates are usually more water-soluble and more polar, hence more readily excretable. Biotransformation can therefore be considered a mechanism of detoxication by the host organism.

However, it must be noted that in certain cases the metabolites are more toxic than the parent compounds. Such reactions are known as "bioactivation."

The rate of biotransformation and the type of biotransformation of a toxicant often differ from one species of animal to another and even from one strain to another, a fact that often accounts for the difference of toxicity in these animals (see Chapter 5). The age and sex of the animal and exposures to other chemicals may also alter the biotransformation. Knowledge of such factors is important in the design of toxicologic studies and in the interpretation of health hazards of toxicants to humans.

Phase I (degradation) reactions

The three types of phase I reactions, namely, oxidation, reduction, and hydrolysis, are briefly described.

Oxidation

The biotransformation of a great variety of chemicals involves oxidative processes. The most important enzyme systems catalyzing the processes involve cytochrome P-450 and NADPH cytochrome P-450 reductase. In these reactions, one atom of molecular oxygen is reduced to water and the other is incorporated into the substrate as follows: $SH + O_2 + NADPH + H \rightarrow SOH + H_2O + NAPD$ where S is the substrate.

The cytochrome-linked monooxygenases (oxidases) are located in the endoplasmic reticulum. When a cell is homogenized, the endoplasmic reticulum breaks down to small vesicles known as microsomes. Because of the location of these enzymes and the great variety of chemicals that they may catalyze, they are also known as microsomal, mixed-function oxidases (MFO). The human P-450 MFO system consists of more than 30 isozymes. They catalyze a great variety of chemicals as shown below. In addition, oxidation of a number of toxicants is catalyzed by nonmicrosomal oxidoreductases that are located in the mitochondrial fraction in the 100,000-g supernatant of tissue homogenates.

Oxidation may take place in a variety of reactions, and often more than one metabolite is formed. The following are some examples.

A Microsomal oxidation:
   1 Aliphatic oxidation involves oxidation of the aliphatic side chains of aromatic chemicals: e.g., n-propylbenzene → 3-phenylpropan-1-ol, 3-phenylpropan-2-ol, and 3-phenylpropan-3-ol, as well as aliphatic compounds such as n-hexane.
   2 Aromatic hydroxylation generally proceeds through an epoxide intermediate: e.g., naphthalene → naphthalene-1,2-epoxide → 1-naphthol + 2-naphthol.
   3 Epoxidation: e.g., aldrin → dieldrin.
   4 Oxidative deamination: e.g., amphetamine → phenylacetone.
   5 N-Dealkylation: e.g., N,N-dimethyl-p-nitrophenyl carbamate → N-methyl-p-nitrophenyl carbamate.
   6 O-Dealkylation: e.g., p-nitroanisole → p-nitrophenol.
   7 S-Dealkylation: e.g., 6-methylthiopurine → 6-mercaptothiopurine.
   8 N-Oxidation: e.g., trimethylamine → trimethylamine oxide.
   9 N-Hydroxylation: e.g., aniline → phenylhydroxylamine.
  10 P-Oxidation: e.g., diphenylmethylphosphine → diphenylmethylphosphine oxide.
  11 Sulfoxidation: e.g., methiocarb → methiocarb sulfone.
  12 Desulfuration involves the replacement of S by O: e.g., parathion → paraoxon.

B Nonmicrosomal oxidations catalyzed by enzymes in mitochondria, cytosol and nuclei:
   1 Amine oxidation: Monoamine oxidase is located in mitochondria and diamine oxidase is a cytosolic enzyme. Both are involved in the oxidation of the primary, secondary, and tertiary amines, such as 5-hydroxytryptamine and putrescine, into corresponding aldehydes.
   2 Alcohol and aldehyde dehydrogenations are catalyzed, respectively, by alcohol dehydrogenase and aldehyde dehydrogenase: e.g., ethanol → acetaldehyde → acetic acid.

Reduction

Toxicants may undergo reductions through the function of reductases. These reactions are less active in mammalian tissues but more so in intestinal bacteria. A notable example is the reduction of prontosil to sulfanilamide converting an inactive chemical to an effective antibacterial drug.

A Microsomal reduction:
    1 Nitro reduction: e.g., nitrobenzene → nitrosobenzene → phenylhydroxylamine → aniline.
    2 Azo reduction: e.g., azobenzene → aniline.

B Nonmicrosomal reductions occur via the reverse reaction of alcohol dehydrogenases (see "Oxidation," B2 above).

Hydrolysis

Many toxicants contain ester-type bonds and are subjects to hydrolysis. These are essentially esters, amides, and compounds of phosphate. Mammalian tissues, including the plasma, contain a large number of nonspecific esterases and amidases, which are involved in hydrolysis. The esterases, usually located in the soluble fraction of the cell, may be broadly categorized into four classes:

1 Arylesterases, which hydrolyze aromatic esters
2 Carboxylesterases, which hydrolyze aliphatic esters
3 Cholinesterases, which hydrolyze esters in which the alcohol moiety is choline
4 Acetylesterases, which hydrolyze esters in which the acid moiety is acetic acid.

In contrast to esterases, amidases cannot be classified according to substrate specificity. Furthermore, enzymatic hydrolysis of amides proceeds much more slowly than that of esters, probably a result of the lack of substrate specificity.

Phase II (conjugation) reactions

Phase II reactions involve several types of endogenous metabolites that, as noted above, may form conjugates with the toxicants per se or their metabolites. These conjugates are generally more water-soluble and more readily excretable. This is because the physiological transport mechanisms for the endogenous metabolites also recognize the conjugates and hence facilitate their excretion.

Glucuronide formation

This is the most common and most important type of conjugation. The enzyme catalyzing this reaction is UDP-glucuronyl transferase (uridine diphosphate glucuronyl transferase) and the coenzyme is UDPGA (uridine-5'-diphospho-α-D-glucuronic acid). This enzyme is also located in the endoplasmic reticulum. There are four classes of chemical compounds that are capable of forming conjugates with glucuronic acid: (1) aliphatic or aromatic alcohols, (2) carboxylic acids, (3) sulfhydryl compounds, and (4) amines.

Sulfate conjugation

This reaction is catalyzed by sulfotransferases. These enzymes are found in the cytosolic fraction of liver, kidney, and intestine. The coenzyme is PAPS (3'-phosphoadenosine-5'-phosphosulfate). The functional groups of the foreign compounds for sulfate transfer are phenols and aliphatic alcohols as well as aromatic amines.

Methylation

This reaction is catalyzed by methyl transferases. The coenzyme is SAM (S-adenosylmethionine). Methylation is not a major route of biotransformation of toxicants because of the broader availability of UDPGA, which leads to the formation of glucuronides. Furthermore, it does not always increase the water solubility of the methylated products.

Acetylation

Acetylation involves transfer of acetyl groups to primary aromatic amines, hydrazines, hydrazides, sulfonamides, and certain primary aliphatic amines. The enzyme and coenzyme involved are, respectively, N-acetyl transferases and acetyl coenzyme A. In certain cases, such as isoniazid, acetylation results in a decrease in water solubility of an amine and an increase in toxicity.

Amino acid conjugation

This conjugation is catalyzed by amino acid conjugates and coenzyme A. Aromatic carboxylic acids, arylacetic acids, and aryl-substituted acrylic acids can form conjugates with α-amino acids, mainly glycine, but also glutamine in humans and certain monkeys and ornithine in birds.

Glutathione conjugation

This important reaction is effected by glutathione S-transferases and the cofactor glutathione. Glutathione conjugates subsequently undergo enzymatic cleavage and acetylation, forming N-acetylcysteine (mercapturic acid) derivatives of the toxicants, which are readily excreted. Examples of chemicals such as epoxides and aromatic halogens that conjugate with glutathione are shown in Figure 3.1. In addition, glutathione can conjugate unsaturated aliphatic compounds and displace nitro groups in chemicals.

In the process of biotransformation of toxicants, a number of highly reactive electrophilic metabolites are formed. Some of these metabolites can react with cellular constituents and cause cell death, induce tumor formation, or affect immune function. The role of glutathione is to react with the electrophilic metabolites and thus prevent their harmful effects on the cells. However, exposure to very large amounts of such reactive substances can deplete the glutathione, thereby resulting in marked toxic effects. An example of the depletion of glutathione by acetaminophen and the concomitant increase in covalent binding to macromolecules is shown in Figure 3.2. Similarly, 3-methylindole is bioactivated mainly in lungs and, after depleting the glutathione, will induce lung damages (Adams *et al.*, 1988). Furthermore, certain glutathione conjugates may become toxic (Anders *et al.*, 1988).

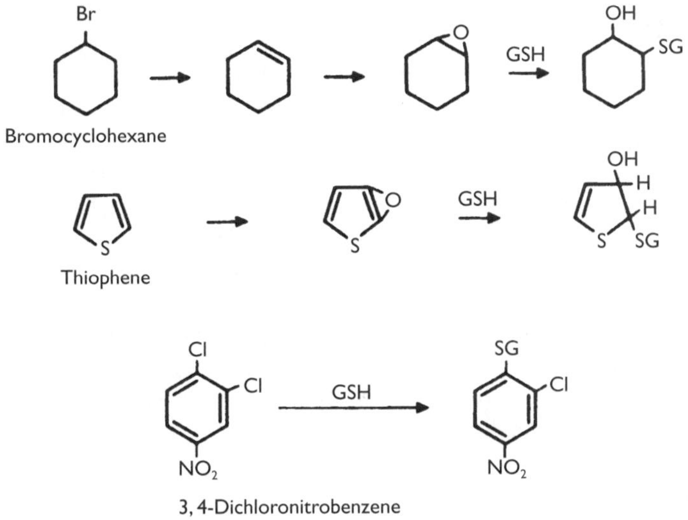

Figure 3.1 Conjugation of epoxide and dehalogenation catalyzed by glutathione (GSH) transferase.

Source: Timbrell, 1991.

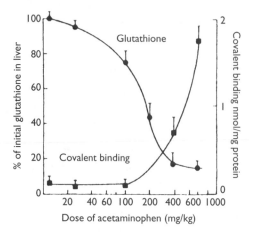

Figure 3.2 Protective effect of glutathione against covalent binding of acetaminophen to liver proteins.

Source: Wills, 1981.

For additional information on the biological functions of glutathione in
the conjugation of electrophiles and as antioxidant, see DeLeve and
Kaplowitz (1991) and Commandeur *et al.* (1995).

Bioactivation

Certain chemically stable compounds can be converted to chemically reactive metabolites. The reactions are generally catalyzed by cytochrome
P-450-dependent monooxygenase systems, but other enzymes, including
those of the intestinal flora, are involved in certain cases. Furthermore,
additional phase I or phase II reactions may be required. The reactive
metabolites, such as epoxides, can become covalently bound to cellular
macromolecules and cause necrosis and/or cancer. Others, such as free
radicals, can cause lipid peroxidation resulting in tissue damage. Descriptions of the bioactivation of various classes of chemicals are available in
the literature, such as the book edited by Anders (1985). The following are
some notable examples. Appendix 3.1 lists a number of chemicals that are
known to be bioactivated.

Epoxide formation

Many aromatic compounds are converted to epoxides by microsomal
mixed-function oxygenase systems. The biotransformation of bromobenzene to its epoxide and subsequent reactions serve as an interesting

example of bioactivation and its consequences. These are depicted in Figure 3.3.

Although bromobenzene epoxide may become covalently bound to tissue macromolecules and cause injury, the alternative routes of metabolism may prevent or reduce the injury. The most important of these routes is the conjugation with glutathione. This reaction is important in that it serves as a protective mechanism. Only after the hepatic levels of reduced glutathione have been greatly depleted will the bromobenzene epoxide significantly bind to macromolecules and result in hepatic necrosis. Depletion of glutathione occurs when a huge dose of bromobenzene is present or when there has been an induction of microsomal enzymes; both conditions increase the amount of bromobenzene epoxide. Other reactions include a nonenzymatic arrangement to form p-bromophenol and the formation of 3,4-dihydro-3,4-dihydroxy-bromobenzene catalyzed by hydrase.

Other chemicals that undergo epoxidation include aflatoxin B_1, benzene, benzo{a}pyrene, furosemide, olefins, polychlorinated and polybrominated biphenyls, trichloroethylene, and vinyl chloride. The bioactivation takes place mainly in the liver, and the resulting reactive metabolites induce toxicity through covalent binding with macromolecules in the tissue, resulting in necrosis or cancer formation.

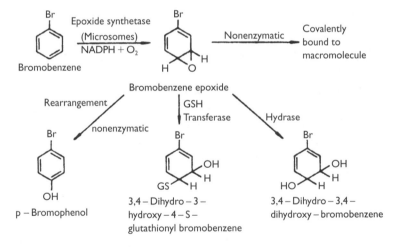

Figure 3.3 The bromobenzene epoxide formed from the parent chemical may covalently bind to macromolecules, but such binding may be minimal when the other metabolic routes are predominant.

Source: Gillette and Mitchell, 1975.

N-hydroxylation

Microsomal enzymes from many tissues can N-hydroxylate a variety of chemicals. Some of the N-hydroxy metabolites, such as those of acetaminophen, 2-AAF, urethane, and certain aminoazo dyes, can cause cancer or tissue necrosis through covalent binding, whereas others, such as certain aromatic amines, can induce hemolysis or methemoglobinemia.

N-hydroxy metabolites are also subject to conjugation reactions. Their conjugates with glucuronic acid are readily excreted; those formed with sulfuric or acetic acid, however, may be unstable and thus can be mutagenic, carcinogenic, and highly toxic (Weisburger and Weisburger, 1973).

Free radical and superoxide formation

Certain halogen-containing compounds undergo metabolism to form free radicals. For example, carbon tetrachloride forms trichloromethyl radical, which causes peroxidation of polyunsaturated lipid as well as covalently binds to protein and unsaturated lipid. These initial reactions are followed by disturbances of various cellular components, as described in Chapter 12. Halothane and bromotrichloromethane are other examples of chemicals that may form free radicals. The herbicide paraquat is known to produce superoxide radicals (Halliwell *et al.*, 1992).

Other pathways

Ethanol can be oxidized by a dehydrogenase to acetaldehyde, which has been implicated in some of the manifestations of alcohol toxicity. Pyrrolizidine alkaloids are dehydrogenated to reactive pyrrole derivatives, which are carcinogenic. There is evidence confirming that the acute toxicity of aliphatic nitriles is attributable to the cyanide released through hepatic microsomal enzyme activities (Willhite and Smith, 1981).

Activation in the G.I. tract

Nitrites and certain amines can react in the acidic environment of the stomach to form nitrosamines, many of which have been shown to be potent carcinogens, and nitrates, which, under certain conditions, can be converted to nitrites that may induce methemoglobinemia. The artificial sweetener cyclamate is converted by intestinal bacteria to cyclohexylamine, which can induce testicular atrophy. Cycasin is converted to its aglycone, methylazoxymethanol, which is hepatotoxic and can induce tumors.

Complex nature of biotransformation

Toxicants generally undergo several types of biotransformation, resulting in a variety of metabolites and conjugates. Some of the various metabolites and conjugates of bromobenzene are shown in Figure 3.3. Organophosphorous insecticides, such as fenithrothion, chlorofenvinphos, and omethoate, can be metabolized through dealkylation, oxidation, desulfuration, or hydrolysis, yielding ten or more different metabolites.

Parathion, an organophosphorous pesticide, is bioactivated in the liver to paraoxon, which is a much more potent cholinesterase inhibitor. Infusion of parathion by way of the vena cava, bypassing the liver, therefore produced little cholinesterase inhibition, but a moderate effect was induced following infusion by way of the portal vein. On the other hand, infusion of paraoxon via the vena cava nearly completely blocked the cholinesterase activity, whereas it had negligible effect after an infusion via the portal vein, since it is detoxicated in the liver (Westermann, 1961).

A reactive metabolite formed in a phase I reaction can be further metabolized, such as carbon tetrachloride and halothane. Such a metabolite may also be followed by a phase II reaction to produce another reactive metabolite. 2-Acetylaminofluorene, for example, after N-hydroxylation can undergo acetylation or form sulfate or glutathione conjugates, all of which are highly reactive.

The relative importance of various types of biotransformation of a toxicant depends on many host, environmental, and chemical factors as well as the dose of the toxicant. Since the metabolites resulting from different biotransformations are often markedly different in their effects, the toxicity of a chemical can be greatly altered by these factors, as will be discussed in Chapter 5.

Some of the metabolic reactions take place in sequence; hence interference with the normal metabolic pathway may have considerable influence on the toxic effects. For example, ethanol is normally metabolized through the intermediary product acetaldehyde. In normal humans the acetaldehyde formed is rapidly further metabolized to acetate, which in turn is converted to carbon dioxide and water. However, if the aldehyde dehydrogenase is inhibited, such as after the administration of disulfiram, the level of acetaldehyde rises and results in distress symptoms such as nausea, vomiting, headache, and palpitations.

A toxicant may be transformed in one organ to a stable proximate metabolite, which is transported to another organ and metabolizes to the ultimate toxic metabolite (Cohen, 1986).

Reeves (1981) provides a number of examples of biotransformations of "typical" chemicals, as well as a limited generalization of the typical routes of foreign compound metabolism in humans (Figure 3.4).

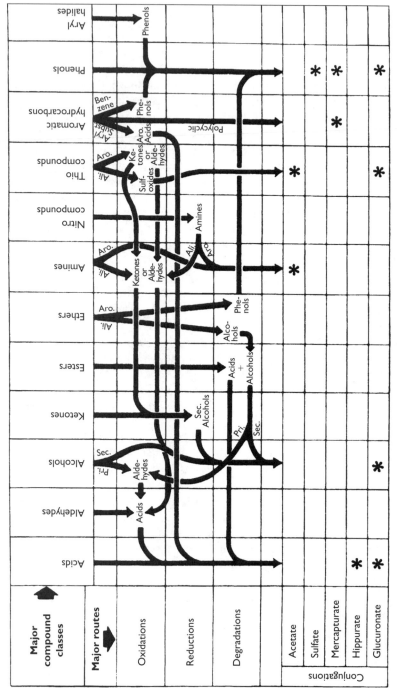

Figure 3.4 Typical routes of foreign compound metabolism in humans.

Source: Reeves, 1981.

References

Adams, J. D., Jr., Laegreid, W. W., Huijzer, J. C., Hayman, C., and Yost, G. S. (1988) Pathology and glutathione status in 3-methylindole-treated rodents. *Res. Commun. Chem. Pathol. Pharmacol.* 60:323–336.

Anders, M. W. (ed.) (1985) *Bioactivation of Foreign Compounds.* New York, NY: Academic Press.

Anders, M. W., Lash, L., Dekant, W., Elfarra, A. E., and Dohn, D. R. (1988) Biosynthesis and biotransformation of glutathione *S*-conjugates to toxic metabolites. *CRC Crit. Rev. Toxicol.* 18:311.

Cohen, G. M. (1986) Basic principles of target organ toxicity, in *Target Organ Toxicity*, G. M. Cohen (ed.), Boca Raton, FL: CRC Press.

Commandeur, J. N. M., Stijntjes, G. J., and Vermeulen, N. P. E. (1995) Enzymes and transport systems involved in the formation and disposition of glutathione *S*-conjugates. *Pharmacol. Revs.* 47:271–330.

DeLeve, L. D. and Kaplowitz, N. (1991) Glutathione metabolism and its role in hepatotoxicity. *Pharmacol. Ther.* 52:287–305.

Gillette, J. R. and Mitchell, J. R. (1975) Drug actions and interactions: Theoretical considerations, in *Handbook of Experimental Pharmacology. New Series*, vol. 28, O. Eichler, A. Farah, H. Herken and A. D. Welch (eds), New York, NY: Springer-Verlag pp. 359–382.

Halliwell, B., Gutteridge, J. M. C., and Cross, C. E. (1992) Free radicals, antioxidants and human diseases – where are we now? *J. Lab. Clin. Med.* 119:598–620.

Reeves, A. L. (1981) The metabolism of foreign compounds, in *Toxicology: Principles and Practices, Vol. 1*, A. L. Reeves (ed.), New York, NY: John Wiley.

Timbrell, J. A. (1991) *Principles of Biochemical Toxicology.* London: Taylor & Francis.

Weisburger, J. H. and Weisburger, E. K. (1973) Biochemical formation and pharmacological, toxicological and pathological properties of hydroxylamines and hydroxyamic acids. *Pharmacol. Rev.* 25:166.

Westermann, E. O. (1961) Bioactivation of parathion. *Proc. Internat. Pharmacol. Meeting* 6:205. Summarized in *Introduction to General Toxicology*, E. J. Ariens, A. M. Simmonis, and J. Offermeier (eds), New York, NY: Academic Press, p. 147.

Willhite, C. C. and Smith, R. P. (1981) The role of cyanide liberation in the acute toxicity of aliphatic nitriles. *Toxicol. Appl. Pharmacol.* 59:589–602.

Wills, E. D. (1981) The role of glutathione in drug metabolism and the protection of the liver against toxic metabolites, in *Testing for Toxicity*, J. W. Gorrod (ed.), London: Taylor & Francis.

Appendix 3.1 Examples of bioactivation*

Parent compound	Toxic metabolite	Mechanism of toxicity	Toxic effect
Acetaminophen	N-hydroxy derivative	Covalent binding	Hepatic necrosis
2-Acetylaminofluorene (AAF)	N-hydroxy-AAF, Sulfate ester	Covalent binding	Cancers
Aflatoxin B₁	Aflatoxin-8,9-epoxide	Covalent binding	Hepatic cancer
Allyl formate	Acrolein	Covalent binding	Hepatic necrosis
Amygdalin	Mandelonitrile, gut flora	Cyanide formation	Cytotoxic hypoxia
Benzene	Benzene epoxide	Covalent binding	Bone marrow depression
Benzo-a-pyrene (BaP)	BaP-7,8-epoxide → BaP-7,8-diol-9, 10-epoxide	Covalent binding Covalent binding	Cancers
Bromobenzene	Bromobenzene epoxide	Covalent binding	Hepatic, renal, bronchiolar necrosis
Carbon tetrachloride	Trichloromethane free radical	Covalent binding	Hepatic necrosis, hepatic cancer
Carcinogenic alkylnitrosamines	α-Hydroxylation	Alkylation	Hepatic cancer
Carcinogenic aminoazo dyes	N-hydroxy derivatives	Covalent binding	Hepatic cancer
Carcinogenic polycyclic hydrocarbons	Epoxides, many organs	Covalent binding	Cancers, cytotoxicity
Chloroform	Phosgene	Covalent binding	Hepatic, renal necrosis
Cycasin	Methylazoxymethanol, gut flora	Alyklation	Cancers, hepatic necrosis
Cyclophosphamide	Many proposed	Alkylation	Cytotoxic
Fluoroacetate	Fluorocitrate	Enzyme inhibition	General toxicity
Furosemide	Epoxide?	Covalent binding	Hepatic, renal necrosis
Halothane	Free radical	Covalent binding	Hepatic necrosis
Isoniazid	Acetylhydrazine (metabolite of)	Covalent binding	Hepatic necrosis
Methemoglobin-producing aromatic amines and nitro compounds	N-hydroxy metabolites	Cyclic oxidoreduction	Methemoglobinemia
Methoxyflurane	Inorganic fluoride	Enzyme inhibition	Renal failure
Naphthylamine	N-hydroxy naphthylamine	Covalent binding	Bladder cancer
Nitrates	Nitrites, gut flora	Hemoglobin oxidation	Methemoglobin
Nitrites plus secondary or tertiary amines	Nitrosamines	Alkylation	Hepatic, pulmonary cancers
Parathion	Paraoxon	Covalent binding to cholinesterase	Neuromuscular paralysis
Purine and pyrimidine base analogues	Mononucleotides, nucleotide triphosphates	Lethal synthesis, lethal incorporation	Cytotoxicity
Safrole	1'-Hydroxysafrole (metabolite of)	Covalent binding	Cancers
Urethane	N-hydroxyurethane	Alkylation	Cancers, cytotoxicity
Vinyl chloride	Epoxide	Covalent binding	Liver cancer

Note
*Site of bioactivation is the liver except as otherwise noted.

Chapter 4

Toxic effects

CONTENTS

General considerations

Toxic effects are greatly variable in nature, potency, target organ, and mechanism of action. A better understanding of their characteristics can improve assessment of the associated health hazards. It can also facilitate the development of rational preventive and therapeutic measures.

All toxic effects result from biochemical interactions between the toxicants (and/or their metabolites) and certain structures of the organism. The structure may be nonspecific, such as any tissue in direct contact with corrosive chemicals. More often it is specific, involving a particular subcellular structure. A variety of structures may be affected.

The nature of effects may vary from organ to organ. The organ-specific effects will be discussed in some detail in the chapters in Part III. In some cases, the reason why a particular organ is affected is known. This knowledge is useful in many ways. A few examples are described in this chapter.

Spectrum of toxic effects

The great variety of toxic effects can be grouped according to the target organ, mechanism of action, or other characteristics such as those discussed below.

Local and systemic effects

Certain chemicals can cause injuries at the site of first contact with an organism. These local effects can be induced by caustic substances on the gastrointestinal tract, by corrosive materials on the skin, and by irritant gases and vapors on the respiratory tract.

Systemic effects result only after the toxicant has been absorbed and distributed to other parts of the body. Most toxicants exert their main effects on one or a few organs. These organs are referred to as the "target organs" of these toxicants. A target organ does not necessarily have the highest concentration of the toxicants in the organism. For example, the target organ of DDT is the central nervous system, but it is concentrated in adipose tissues.

Reversible and irreversible effects

Reversible effects of toxicants are those that will disappear following cessation of exposure to them. Irreversible effects, in contrast, will persist or even progress after exposure is discontinued. Certain effects are obviously irreversible. These include carcinomas, mutations, damage to neurons, and liver cirrhosis.

Certain effects are considered irreversible even though they disappear some time after cessation of exposure. For example, the "irreversible" cholinesterase-inhibiting insecticides inhibit the activity of this enzyme for a period of time that approximates that required for the synthesis and replacement of the enzyme.

The effect produced by a toxicant may be reversible if the organism is exposed at a low concentration and/or for a short duration, whereas irreversible effects may be produced at higher concentrations and/or for longer durations of exposure.

Immediate and delayed effects

Many toxicants produce immediate toxic effects, which develop shortly after a single exposure, a notable example being cyanide poisoning. Delayed effects occur after a lapse of some time. Carcinogenic effects generally become manifest 10–20 years after the initial exposure in humans; even in rodents, a lapse of many months is required. To determine these and other delayed effects of toxicants, long-term studies are essential.

Morphologic, functional, and biochemical effects

Morphologic effects refer to gross and microscopic changes in the morphology of the tissues. Many of these effects, such as necrosis and neoplasia, are irreversible and serious. Functional effects usually represent reversible changes in the functions of target organs. Functions of the liver and kidney (e.g., rate of excretion of dyes) are commonly tested in toxicologic studies.

Functional effects are in general reversible, whereas morphologic effects are not, and functional changes are generally detected earlier or in animals exposed to lower doses than those with morphologic changes. In addition, functional tests are valuable in following the progress of effects on target organs in long-term studies in animals and humans. However, the results are often more variable.

Although all toxic effects are associated with biochemical alterations, in routine toxicity testing, "biochemical effects" usually refer to those without apparent morphologic changes. An example of such effects is the cholinesterase inhibition following exposure to organophosphate and carbamate insecticides. ALAD inhibition in lead poisoning is another example (see Chapters 19 and 21).

Allergic and idiosyncratic reactions

Allergic reaction (also known as hypersensitivity and sensitization reaction) to a toxicant results from previous sensitization to that toxicant or a chemically similar one. The chemical acts as a hapten and combines with an endogenous protein to form an antigen, which in turn elicits the formation of antibodies. A subsequent exposure to the chemical will result in an antigen-antibody interaction, which provokes the typical manifestations of allergy. Thus this reaction is different from the usual toxic effects, first because a previous exposure is required, and second because a typical sigmoid dose–response curve is usually not demonstrable with allergic reactions. Nevertheless, threshold doses were demonstrable for the induction as well as the challenge in dermal sensitization (Koschier *et al.*, 1983).

Generally an idiosyncratic reaction is a genetically determined abnormal reactivity to a chemical. Some patients exhibit prolonged muscular reaction and apnea following a standard dose of succinylcholine. These patients have a deficiency of serum cholinesterase, which normally degrades the muscle relaxant rapidly. Similarly, people with a deficiency in NADH methemoglobinemia reductase are abnormally sensitive to nitrites and other chemicals that produce methemoglobinemia.

Graded and quantal responses

Effects on body weight, food consumption, and enzyme inhibition are examples of graded responses. On the other hand, mortality and tumor formation are examples of quantal (all-or-none) responses. Both types of responses can be statistically analyzed as illustrated in Chapter 6.

The relationship between dose and response usually follows an S-shaped curve. Figure 4.1 is a schematic representation of most chemicals (B) and that of certain essential nutrients (A). The latter is exemplified by thiamine

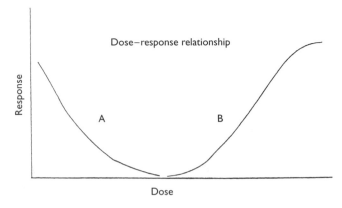

Figure 4.1 Schematic representation of dose–response relationship. Curve A: certain essential nutrients, with which the response (deficiency syndrome) increases along with decreased intake. Curve B: Most chemicals with which the response (toxic effects) increases along with increased intake. Certain substances, e.g., selenium, exhibit both types of responses.

and ascorbic acid. Insufficient intake of these vitamins will induce deficiency syndromes, but higher intakes will be readily eliminated in the urine. Selenium is an essential element but excessive intake will be toxic (see Chapter 21); therefore its dose–response relationship is represented by curves A and B.

Another type of dose–response relationship consists of an effect observable at doses lower than the NOAEL (see Chapter 25) and is opposite to the main toxic effect (e.g., stimulation vs. inhibition). It is known as "hormesis" and has been reported for a number of chemicals (Calabrese and Baldwin, 2001).

As the dose of a toxicant increases, so does the response, either in terms of the proportion of the population responding or in terms of the severity of graded responses. Furthermore, additional toxic effects may also appear along with increased doses. For example, methyl mercury induces paresthesia at low doses, but it also induces ataxia, dysarthria, deafness and death at higher doses, as shown in Figure 21.2, which depicts both *dose–response* and *dose–effect* relationships.

Target organs

Toxicants do not affect all organs to the same extent. An understanding of the mechanisms that determine organ specificity will assist in the advancement of various aspects of toxicology. While the reason is not always clear, the probable mechanisms by which many toxicants act specifically on certain organs are known. In general, the underlying mechanism is either a greater susceptibility of the target organ or a higher concentration of the chemical and/or its metabolite at the site of action. The higher concentration may arise under a variety of conditions.

Sensitivity of the organ

Neurons and myocardium depend primarily on adenosine triphosphate (ATP) generated by mitochondrial oxidation with little capacity for anaerobic metabolism, and there are rapid ionic shifts through the cell membrane. They are, therefore, especially sensitive to lack of oxygen resulting from disorders of the vascular system or of hemoglobin (e.g., carbon monoxide poisoning).

Rapidly dividing cells, such as those in the bone marrow and the intestinal mucosa, are more susceptible to mitotic poisons (e.g., methotrexate).

Distribution

The respiratory tract and the skin are target organs of industrial and environmental toxicants because these are the sites of absorption. An example is provided by bischloromethyl ether. It produces skin tumors in humans when applied topically, but will induce tumors in the respiratory tract after exposure by inhalation.

On a unit weight basis, the liver and kidney have a higher volume of blood flow, and thus they are in general exposed to toxicants to a greater extent. In addition, these organs have greater metabolic and excretory functions, which also render them more susceptible to toxicants. Being lipophilic, methylmercury can cross the blood–brain barrier and exert its toxic effects on the nervous system. Inorganic mercury compounds, in contrast, are not able to cross the blood–brain barrier and are not neurotoxic.

Radiation may damage DNA and induce tumors. Ultraviolet light has little penetrating power and therefore will only produce skin tumors, whereas ionizing radiation may penetrate tissues and cause leukemia and other types of cancer.

Selective uptake

Certain cells have a high affinity for selected chemicals. For example, in the respiratory tract, the type I and type II alveolar epithelial cells, which have an active uptake system for endogenous polyamines, will take up paraquat, a structurally similar chemical. This process can result in local tissue damage even when paraquat is administered orally.

Melanin is present in the eye, inner ear, etc. Drugs such as chloroquine and kanamycin that have an affinity for melanin may accumulate, after prolonged administration, in these organs and cause damage. Strontium-90 is selectively deposited in the bone and can induce tumors of the bone.

Biotransformation

As a result of *bioactivation*, reactive metabolites are formed. Liver, being a major site of biotransformation, is susceptible to the action of many toxicants. However, there are exceptions. For example, certain metabolites are sufficiently stable; they may affect other organs after being transported there. Thus bromobenzene, though bioactivated in the liver, can affect the kidney.

With some toxicants, the bioactivation at certain sites predominates their effects. For example, the organophosphorothioate insecticides, such as parathion, are bioactivated mainly in the liver, but the abundance of detoxifying enzymes and of reactive but noncritical binding sites there prevents any overt signs of toxicity. On the other hand, nervous tissue has much less bioactivating enzymes, but because the bioactivation takes place near the critical target sites, that is, the synapses, the main toxic manifestations of this group of toxicants arise from the nervous system.

The bioactivating enzymes are not necessarily evenly distributed in an organ or tissue. For example, the Clara cells (nonciliated bronchiolar epithelial cells) constitute only 1% of the cells in the lung, yet they contain a major portion of the pulmonary cytochrome P-450. They are therefore more susceptible to damage by such toxicants as 4-ipomeanol and CCl_4. A similar situation exists in the kidney. The proximal tubules, especially the S_3 cells, which are located in the pars recta portion of these tubules, have the highest concentrations of this enzyme system, hence the most susceptible parts of the kidney are the proximal tubules, especially its pars recta portion.

Repair mechanism

A toxicant may affect a specific organ because of a lack of the required repair mechanism. For example, N-methyl-N-nitrosourea (MNU) produces tumors in the rat mainly in the brain, occasionally in the kidney, but not in the liver. Kleihues and Cooper (1976) demonstrated that the liver is capable of enzymatically excising the O_6-alkyl-guanine induced by MNU from the DNA, whereas the brain is deficient in this respect. The capacity of the kidney falls between those of the liver and brain.

Mechanisms of action

While the mechanisms of action of all toxicants are not fully understood, a number of biochemical reactions are likely involved. The underlying processes/subcellular sites are listed, along with some exemplary toxicants, in Table 4.1. The table clearly shows the diverse nature of the mechanisms as well as the multiple processes/sites that are involved in the action of a number of toxicants. For many of the toxicants listed in Table 4.1, the mechanisms will be described, along with their toxic manifestations, in the relevant chapters.

Of the various mechanisms of action, disturbance of calcium homeostasis merits special mention because of its importance and complexity. The extracellular level of Ca^{2+} is more than 10 times higher than that in the cytosol.

The ionic differential is maintained by a variety of mechanisms including the Ca^{2+} transporting ATPase at the plasma membrane, the store in the endoplasmic reticulum, mitochondria and nucleus as well as the binding with intracellular calmodulin. Increases of cytosolic Ca^{2+} may be caused via different mechanisms. For example, CCl_4 and bromobenzene act through inhibition of Ca^{2+} ATPase, acetaminophen and CCl_4 through damage of plasma membrane, and cadmium by release of Ca^{2+} from mitochondria. The rise in cytosolic Ca^{2+} may affect cytoskeleton thereby damage cellular integrity either directly or through Ca^{2+}-activated

Table 4.1 Some mechanisms of toxic action*

Mechanism of action	Process/subcellular site	Examples of toxicants
Interference with normal receptor–ligand interaction	Neurotransmitters	Botulinum toxin, organophosphate pesticides
	Hormone receptors	Amitrole, DES, retinoic acid, TCDD
	Enzymes	Fluoroacetate, cyanide, organophosphate pesticides
	Transport proteins	CO, nitrites
Interference with membrane function	Excitable membrane-ion influx	DDT, saxitoxin, tetrodotoxin
	Membrane-fluidity	Organic solvents (e.g., CCl_4, chloroform), ethanol
	Lysosomal membranes	CCl_4, phosphorus, phalloidin
	Mitochondrial membranes	CCl_4, organotins, phosphorus
Interference with cellular energy production	Hemoglobin	CO, nitrites
	Oxidative phosphorylation-uncoupling	Dinitrophenol, organotins
	Electron transport-inhibition	Cyanide, rotenone
	Carbohydrate metabolism-inhibition	Fluoroacetate
Covalent binding to biomolecules	Lipids-peroxidation	CCl_4, ozone, paraquat, phenytoin
	Glutathione-depletion	Acetaminophen
	Protein thiols-oxidation	Acetaminophen, phenytoin
	Nucleic acids	Carcinogens, mutagens, teratogens
Perturbation of calcium homeostasis	Cytoskeleton, etc.	Arsenic, cobalt, doxorubicin, microcystin, paraquat, phalloidin
	Apoptosis	TCDD

Note
*The toxic effects of a number of the toxicants are described in other sections. For the relevant page, refer to the Chemical Index.

proteases. Oxidant stress produces injury in lung through an increase in Ca^{2+} in alveolar macrophages by a Ca-mediated signaling. In addition, TCDD may promote "apoptosis" (programmed cell death) by combining with Ah receptor, increasing intracellular Ca^{2+} activating endonuclease and causing DNA breakdown (Timbrell, 1992; Halliwell and Cross, 1994).

Most of the reactions take place at various subcellular sites. Table 13.1 lists a number of hepatotoxicants along with the organelles that they affect.

Molecular targets: chemical nature

Proteins

Receptors

Receptors are located across plasma membrane, or in cytosol or nucleus, and serve to transmit physical or chemical signals to the cell. There are many types of receptors serving a variety of functions. Some of them are known to be affected by toxicants (see next Section, p. 50).

Enzymes

Enzymes are common targets of toxicants. The enzyme effects may be specific, such as the inhibition of acetylcholinesterase. They may be reversible, such as the case with a number of carbamate insecticides on cholinesterase. Irreversible enzyme inhibition is exemplified by DFP (diisopropyl fluorophosphate), which covalently bind with the enzymes.

The effects may be nonspecific. For example, lead and mercury are inhibitors of a great variety of enzymes. However, some enzymes are more susceptible: for example, δ-aminolevulinic acid dehydrase is especially sensitive to lead, and its activity in erythrocytes is used as an early indicator of lead poisoning.

The last step of the oxidation of many chemicals is catalyzed by the cytochrome oxidase chain. Hydrocyanic acid (HCN) can bind with the iron in these enzymes and block their redox function. The aerobic respiration of cells is then arrested and biochemical asphyxia ensues.

An enzyme can also be inhibited by a chemical derived by synthesis from the toxicant such as fluoroacetic acid and its derivatives. The process is known as *lethal synthesis*. Fluoroacetic acid is metabolized as acetic acid in the citric acid cycle, and fluorocitric acid is synthesized, instead of citric acid. Since fluorocitric acid is an inhibitor of aconitase, further metabolism, and consequently the energy production, is blocked.

In a somewhat similar manner, amino acid antagonists (e.g., azaserine and fluorophenylalanine) can interfere with the utilization of specific amino acids in the synthesis of proteins.

The energy that is liberated by biochemical oxidation is normally stored in the form of high-energy phosphates. *Uncoupling agents* such as dinitrophenol interfere with the synthesis of energy-rich phosphates, and thus the energy is liberated as heat instead of being stored.

Carriers

Carriers such as hemoglobin can be affected by a toxicant through preferential binding. For example, carbon monoxide can bind hemoglobin at the site where oxygen is normally bound. Because of its greater affinity for hemoglobin, it can inactivate hemoglobin and cause manifestations of oxygen deficiency in tissues.

Oxygen transport can also be impaired by an accumulation of methemoglobin, which is an oxidation product of hemoglobin with no oxygen-binding ability. In normal individuals the trace amount of methemoglobin is readily reduced to hemoglobin. Certain toxicants, such as nitrites and aromatic amines, can enhance the formation of methemoglobin and overwhelm the normal process of its reduction to hemoglobin. People with glucose-6-phosphatase dehydrogenase deficiency have a lower capacity to regenerate hemoglobin from methemoglobin and are thus prone to have methemoglobinemia.

Structural proteins

Extracellular structural proteins such as collagen are unlikely to be affected by toxicants. However, toxicants such as ozone and asbestos may cause an increase in fibroblasts and deposition of collagen in the lung (Chapter 11). Intracellular structural proteins, such as cytoskeleton, may be damaged by toxicants, e.g., arsenic and paraquat (Li *et al.*, 1987; Li and Chou, 1992).

Coenzymes

Coenzymes are essential for the normal function of enzymes. Their levels in the body can be diminished by toxicants that inhibit their synthesis. For example, pyrithiamine can inhibit thiamine kinase, which is responsible for the formation of the coenzyme thiamine pyrophosphate. NADPH can be destroyed in the presence of free radicals, which can be produced by such toxicants as carbon tetrachloride.

Metal-dependent enzymes can be inhibited by chelating agents (e.g., cyanides and dithiocarbamates) through removal of metal coenzymes such as copper and zinc.

Lipids

Peroxidation of polyenoic fatty acids has been suggested as a mechanism of the necrotizing action of a number of toxicants, such as carbon tetrachloride.

Cell membrane derangement may result after exposure to various types of toxicants. The general anesthetics ether and halothane as well as many other lipophilic substances can accumulate in the cell membranes and thereby interfere with transport of oxygen and glucose into the cell. The cells of the central nervous system are especially susceptible to a lowering of oxygen tension and glucose level and are therefore among the first to be deleteriously affected by these substances. Membrane dissolution can follow contact with organic solvents and amphoteric detergents. The ions of mercury and cadmium can complex with phospholipid bases and expand the surface area of the membrane, thereby altering its function. Lead ion can increase the fragility of erythrocytes and result in hemolysis. The oxygen-carrying function of hemoglobin is lost after it escapes from the hemolyzed erythrocytes.

Nucleic acids

Covalent binding between a toxicant (such as alkylating agents) and replicating DNA and RNA can cause cancer, mutation, and teratogenesis. Such toxicants may also exert immunosuppressive effects.

Antimetabolites such as aminopterin and methotrexate may be incorporated into DNA and RNA and then interfere with their replication.

Others

Hypersensitivity reactions result from repeated exposure to a particular substance or to its chemically related substances. The latter phenomenon is referred to as cross sensitization. The substance, if it is a large polypeptide, acts as an antigen and stimulates the body to form antibodies. Otherwise, the substance acts as a hapten and combines with proteins in the body to form antigens. The reaction between an antigen from a later exposure and the corresponding antibodies results in the release of histamine, bradykinin, and others. The reaction has a typical pattern irrespective of the nature of the antigen. Photosensitization reaction is somewhat similar except sunlight is also required for its induction (see Chapters 11, 12, and 15).

Corrosive agents such as strong acids and bases can destroy local tissues by precipitating cellular proteins. Irritation of the underlying tissues occurs as a consequence.

Blockade of renal and biliary tubules may follow the precipitation of relatively insoluble toxicants or their metabolites. For example, acetyl-sulfapyridine, a metabolite of sulfapyridine, may block renal tubules, and harmol glucuronide from harmol may cause cholestasis.

Receptors

Historical notes

It has long been observed that a number of poisons and toxins exert certain specific biologic effects. John N. Langley proposed in 1905 the concept of a "receptive substance." That the receptors are protein in nature was first suggested by Welsh and Taub (1951).

To demonstrate the protein nature of acetylcholine receptors, Lu (1952) showed that the stimulant effect of acetylcholine on isolated rabbit ileum was lost after the ileum was treated with the proteolytic enzyme trypsin (10 mg/100 ml, for 30 minutes). That the effect was on the receptor rather than the muscle was demonstrated by the fact that the treated ileum still responded to barium chloride, a direct-acting muscle stimulant. In 1971, Cuatrecasas observed that trypsin, at the same concentration as that used by Lu, eliminated the activity of insulin receptor.

In the 1970s cholinergic receptors (ChR) were solubilized, isolated, and characterized by several groups of investigators. The amino acid composition of ChR was reported by Heilbronn et al. (1975). They also found that ChR contained about 6% carbohydrates. While it has been generally agreed that the ligand-receptor complex would initiate responses in the cells, it was Rodbell et al. (1971) who proposed a "transducer" was required to act between the receptor and the effector. This "transducer" was later confirmed as the G-proteins (see Gilman, 1987).

Functional categories

There are many types of receptors, located either in the cell membrane, the cytosol or the nucleus. They serve a variety of functions such as metabolism, secretion, muscular contraction, neural activity and proliferation. In general they are placed in the categories listed below.

Neurotransmitter receptors include the cholinergic (nicotinic, located in ganglia and skeletal muscles, and muscarinic in smooth muscles and brain), α- and β-adrenergic, dopamine, opiates (e.g., endorphin), and histamine (H_1 and H_2) receptors.

Hormone receptors are for insulin, cortisone, ACTH, thyrotropin, estrogen, progesterone, angiotensin, glucagon, prostaglandin, and others.

Certain chemicals such as antidepressants and antitumor agents bind with specific macromolecules that may be considered as "drug receptors." These receptors may well have endogenous messengers (such as endorphins and enkephalins for opiates) but these are as yet undiscovered. Another example of such agents is benzodiazepine, for which receptors, and possible endogenous effectors, have been discovered. Furthermore, antagonists have been synthesized (Lal *et al.*, 1988).

Other receptors are located on *enzymes* and *carrier proteins*. They may also be affected by toxicants as listed in Table 4.1.

Structure and signal transduction

The various functional categories of receptors described above exert their biological effects upon binding with an appropriate ligand, which may be an endogenous or exogenous substance. These effects are preceded by a series of biochemical activities, the signaling, which vary according to the structural characteristics of the receptor. Structurally they may be placed in four classes of receptors. These are (1) G-protein coupled receptors, (2) ligand-gated ion channels, (3) voltage-gated channels, and (4) intracellular receptors.

With the G-protein coupled receptors (Figure 4.2: 1), binding with a

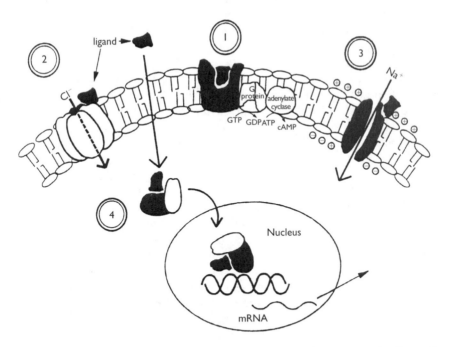

Figure 4.2 Schematic representation of the four classes of receptors. 1. G-protein coupled receptor, 2. Ligand-gated ion channel, 3. Voltage-gated ion channel, and 4. Intracellular receptor.

Source: Adapted from Mailman and Lawler, 1944.

ligand results in the activation of the G-protein, converting GTP (guanosine triphosphate) to GDP (guanosine diphosphate), which activates or inhibits a specific enzyme (adenylate cyclase or phospholipase C), followed by the formation of a "second messenger," e.g., cAMP (from ATP), diacylglycerol or phosphoinositol. The second messenger then initiates the cellular response: the biologic effect. Typical ligands for this class of receptors are adrenergic, muscarinic, cholinergic, and dopaminergic neurotransmitters and their analogs (e.g., ephedrine), as well as others such as diphtheria toxin.

The second class of receptors are transmembrane proteins with an ion channel (Figure 4.2: 2). Upon binding with a ligand, the receptor undergoes conformational changes resulting in the opening of the channel. This process allows changes of Na^+, K^+, Cl^- or Ca^{2+} concentrations across the plasma membrane. Nicotinic cholinergic and $GABA_A$ receptors belong to this class. In addition, glutamate and chemicals such as kainate, diazepam, barbiturates and picrotoxin also act on this type of ion-channel receptors.

The voltage-gated conductance channels (Figure 4.2: 3) are located across plasma membranes of excitable cells such as neurons and their axons. At present, no endogenous ligands are known. However, the neurotoxins tetrodotoxin and saxitoxin (see Chapter 17) bind to a site near the extracellular opening of the $Na+$ channel and block the entry of Na^+ through the channel, thereby interfering with the conduction of nerve impulse.

Intracellular receptors are located in the cytosol or nucleus (Figure 4.2: 4). The main endogenous ligands are estrogens, androgens, progestins, glucocorticoids and mineralocorticoids. A representative toxicant that binds with this type of receptor is TCDD. It binds with the Ah receptor in the cytosol, but moves to the nucleus after the binding (see p. 53). For additional details see Mitchell (1992), Mailman and Lawler (1994).

The ligand that binds with the receptor may be an "agonist" or an "antagonist." An agonist induces the "physiologic" function of the receptor, whereas an antagonist blocks its functions. For example, methacholine is an agonist interacting with certain cholinergic receptors, mimicking the effects of acetylcholine, whereas atropine, an antagonist, blocks these effects. Both types of effects may be adverse to health. In addition, an agonist may cause a toxic effect by failing to dissociate from the receptor readily enough, thereby preventing further action of the endogenous messenger, and an antagonist can compete with the messenger for the site on the receptor and block the action of the latter. In addition, a toxicant may induce tolerance to its toxicity by reducing the number of receptors, as shown by Costa *et al.* (1981) with the chronic treatment with an organophosphate acetylcholinesterase inhibitor.

Receptors in toxicology

The receptor concept has been valuable in advancing our understanding of certain biochemical, physiologic, and pharmacologic effects, as well as facilitating the development of drugs. Its role in toxicology is evidenced by an increasing number of receptors being recognized as mediators of effects of toxicants.

Poland and Knutson (1982) reviewed the extensive literature on TCDD (2,3,7,8-tetrachlorodibenzo-p-dioxin) and related halogenated aromatic hydrocarbons with respect to their toxicity, their ability to induce AHH (aryl hydrocarbon hydroxylase), and their affinity for a cytosol receptor. It was suggested that TCDD binds with the Ah (aromatic hydrocarbon) receptor. The TCDD-receptor complex translocates to the nucleus and there interacts with specific genomic recognition sites. This initiates the transcription and translation of the specific genes that code for AHH. A preponderance of evidence suggests that most of the TCDD toxicities are receptor-mediated. It was also noted that the concentration of this cytosol receptor is much higher in the liver of C57BL/6 mice than that of DBA/2 mice and that the former strain of mice was much more susceptible than the latter with respect to TCDD-induced thymus involution, teratogenesis, and hepatic porphyria. Furthermore, the genetic evidence indicated that the *Ah* locus in mice was the structural gene for the cytosol receptor (see also Whitlock, 1990; Okey *et al.*, 1994).

Many neurotoxicants act through receptors on CNS, PNS and autonomic nervous systems. For example, certain organophosphorus compounds act not only through acetylcholine but also on muscarinic receptors (Huff *et al.*, 1994).The receptors for TPA (12,0-tetradecanoyl phorbol 13-acetate) and retinoic acid are worth noting. TPA, a tumor promoter, binds with a receptor that initiates a chain of events leading to selected replication of initiated cells (Blumberg *et al.*, 1983). Retinoic acid, as TCDD, acts on an estrogen receptor to exert teratogenic and other effects (see Lu *et al.*, 1994). A few examples of toxicants that act through receptors are mentioned in the previous section. Peroxisome proliferators such as the hypolipidemic drug clofibrate and the plasticizers phthalate esters are active on the receptors that are involved in the metabolism of polyunsaturated fatty acids. Furthermore, many immunotoxicants act through specific receptors on T cell, B cell, cytokine, polymorphonuclear cells and monocytes (Lad *et al.*, 1995). Aberrant expression and regulation of insulin-like growth factor binding protein 3 regulates normal and malignant cell growth (Zou *et al.*, 1998).

References

Blumberg, P. M., Delcos, B. K., Dunn, J. A., Jaken, S., Leach, K. L., and Yeh, E. (1983) Phorbol ester receptors and the *in vitro* effects of tumor promoters. *Ann. NY Acad. Sci.* 407:303–315.

Calabrese, E. J. and Baldwin, L. A. (2001) The frequency of U-shaped dose responses in the toxicological literature. *Toxicol. Sci.* 62:330–338.

Costa, L. G., Schwab, B. W., Hand, H., and Murphy, S. D. (1981) Reduced [H³] quinuclidinyl benzilate binding to muscarinic receptors in disulfoton-tolerant mice. *Toxicol. Appl. Pharmacol.* 60:441–450.

Cuatrecasas, P. (1971) Perturbation of the insulin receptor of isolated fat cells with proteolytic enzymes. *J. Biol. Chem.* 246:6522–6531.

Gilman, A. G. (1987) G-proteins: Transducers of receptor-generated signals. *Ann. Rev. Biochem.* 56:615–649.

Halliwell, B. and Cross, C. E. (1994) Oxygen-derived species: Their relation to human disease and environmental stress. *Environ. Health Persp*, 102 (Suppl. 10):5–12.

Heilbronn, E., Mattsson, C., and Elfman, L. (1975) Biochemical and physical properties of the nicotinic ACh receptor from *Torpedo marmorata*, in *Properties of Purified Cholinergic and Adrenergic Receptors*, vol. 37, M. Wollemann (ed.), New York, NY: Elsevier.

Huff, R. A., Corcoran, J. J., Anderson, J. K., and Abou-Donia, M. B. (1994) Chloropyrifos oxon binds directly to muscarinic receptors and inhibits cAMP accumulation in rat striatum. *J. Pharmacol. Exper. Therap.* 269:329–335.

Kleihues, P. and Cooper, H. K. (1976) Repair excision of alkylated bases from DNA *in vivo*. *Oncology* 33:86–88.

Koschier, F. J., Burden, E. J., Brunkhorst, C. S., and Friedman, M. A. (1983) Concentration-dependent elicitation of dermal sensitization in guinea pigs treated with 2,4-toluene diisocyanate. *Toxicol. Appl. Pharmacol.* 67:401–407.

Lad, P. M., Kapstein, J. S., and Lin, C. E. (eds) (1995) *Signal Transduction in Leukocytes. G-Protein-Related and Other Pathways*. Boca Raton, FL: CRC Press.

Lal, H., Kumer, B., and Forster, M. J. (1988) Enhancement of learning and memory in mice by a benzodiazepine antagonist. *FASEB J.* 2:2707–2711.

Li, W. and Chou, I. N. (1992) Effects of sodium arsenite on the cytoskeleton and cellular glutathione levels in cultured cells. *Toxicol. Appl. Pharmacol.* 114:132–139.

Li, W., Zhao, Y., and Chou, I. N. (1987) Paraquat-induced cytoskeletal injury in cultured cells. *Toxicol. Appl. Pharmacol.* 91:96–106.

Lu, F. C. (1952) The effects of proteolytic enzymes on the isolated rabbit intestine. *Br. J. Pharmacol.* 7:624–640.

Lu, Y., Wang, X., and Safe, S. (1994) Interaction of 2,3,7,8-tetrachlorodibenzo-*p*-dioxin and retinoic acid in MCF-7 human breast cancer cells. *Toxicol. Appl. Pharmacol.* 127:1–8.

Mailman, R. B. and Lawler, C. P. (1994) Toxicant–receptor interactions: Fundamental principles, in *Introduction to Biochemical Toxicology*, E. Hodgson and P. E. Levi (eds), Norwalk, CT: Appleton & Lange.

Mitchell, R. H. (1992) Inositol lipids in cellular signalling mechanisms. *Trends in Biochem. Sci.* 17:274–276.

Okey, A. B., Riddick, D. S., and Harper, P. A. (1994) The Ah receptor: mediator of the toxicity of 2,3,7,8-tetrachlorodibenzo-*p*-dioxin (TCDD) and related compounds. *Toxicol. Lett.* 70:1–22.

Poland, A. and Knutson, J. C. (1982) 2,3,7,8-Tetrachlorodibenzo-*p*-dioxin and related halogenated aromatic hydrocarbons: Examination of the mechanism of toxicity. *Annu. Rev. Pharmacol. Toxicol.* 22:517–554.

Rodbell, M., Birnbaumer, L., Pohl, S. L., and Kraus, H. M. J. (1971) The glycagon sensitive adenyl cyclase system in plasma membranes of rat liver. V. An obligatory role of guanyl nucleotides in glucagon action. *J. Biol. Chem.* 246:1877–1887.

Timbrell, J. A. (1991) *Principles of Biochemical Toxicology*. London: Taylor & Francis.

Welsh, J. H. and Taub, R. (1951) The significance of the carbonyl group and ether oxygen in the reaction of acetylcholine with receptor substance. *J. Pharmacol. Exp. Ther.* 103:62–73.

Whitlock, J. P., Jr. (1990) Genetic and molecular aspects of 2,3,7,8-tetrachlorodibenzo-*p*-dioxin action. *Ann. Rev. Pharmacol. Toxicol* 30:251–277.

Zou, T., Fleisher, A. S., Kong, D. *et al.* (1998) Sequence alterations of insulin-like growth factor binding protein 3 in neoplastic and normal gastrointestinal tissues. *Cancer Res.* 58:4802–4804.

Chapter 5

Modifying factors of toxic effects

General considerations

While toxicity is an inherent property of a substance, the nature and extent of the toxic manifestations in an organism that is exposed to the substance depend on a variety of factors. The obvious ones are the dose and duration of exposure.

They also include such less obvious host factors as the species and strain of the animal, its sex and age, and its nutritional and hormonal status.

Various environmental (physical and social) factors also play a part. In addition, the toxic effect of a chemical may be influenced by simultaneous and consecutive exposure to other chemicals.

The toxic effects may be modified in a number of ways: alterations of the absorption, distribution, and excretion of a chemical; an increase or decrease of its biotransformation; and changes of the sensitivity of the receptor at the target organ.

A clear understanding of the existence of these factors and of their mode of action is important in designing the protocols of toxicologic investigation. It is equally important in evaluating the significance of the toxicologic data and in assessing the safety/risk to humans under specified conditions of exposure.

The most common mechanism underlying various modifying factors is differences in the rate of detoxication. However, differences in bioactivation, and toxicokinetic, toxicodynamic physiologic, and anatomic characteristics are responsible for a number of modifying factors. Examples are listed in Appendix 5.1.

Host factors

Species, strain, and individual

In general, different species of animals respond similarly to most toxicants. However, differences of toxic effect from one species to another have long been recognized. Knowledge in this field has been used to develop, for example, pesticides, which are more toxic to pests than to humans and other mammals. Among various species of mammals, most effects of toxicants are somewhat more similar. This fact forms the basis of predicting the toxicity to humans from results obtained in toxicologic studies conducted in other mammals, such as the rat, mouse, dog, rabbit, and monkey. There are, however, notable differences in toxicity even among mammals (Williams, 1974).

Some of these differences can be attributed to variations in detoxication mechanisms. For example, the sleeping time induced in several species of laboratory animals by hexobarbital shows marked differences, which are obviously attributable to the activity of the detoxication enzyme as shown in Table 5.1.

Differences in response to hexobarbital, although less marked, also exist among various strains of mice (Jay, 1955). Other examples include ethylene glycol and aniline. Ethylene glycol is metabolized to oxalic acid, which is responsible for the toxicity, or to carbon dioxide. The magnitude of the toxicity of ethylene glycol in animals is in the following order: cat > rat > rabbit, and this is the same for the extent of oxalic acid production. Aniline is metabolized in the cat and dog mainly to o-aminophenol,

Table 5.1 Species differences in duration of action and metabolism of hexobarbital. Dose of barbiturate 50 mg/kg in dogs, 100 mg/kg in the other animals

Species	Duration of action (min)	Plasma half-life (min)	Relative enzyme activity [(μg/g/h)]	Plasma level on awakening (μg/ml)
Mouse	12	19	598	89
Rabbit	49	60	196	57
Rat	90	140	135	64
Dog	315	260	36	19

Source: Reprinted with permission from Quinn et al. Species, strain and sex differences in metabolism of hexobarbitone, amidopyrine, antipyrine and aniline. Biochemical Pharmacology, Vol. 1. © 1958, Pergamon Press plc.

which is more toxic, but it is metabolized mainly to p-aminophenol in the rat and hamster, which are less susceptible to aniline (Timbrell, 1992).

Differences in bioactivation also account for many dissimilarities of toxicity. A notable example is 2-naphthylamine, which produced bladder tumors in the dog and human but not in the rat, rabbit, or guinea pig. Dogs and humans, but not the others, excrete the carcinogenic metabolite 2-naphthyl hydroxylamine (Miller et al., 1964). Acetylaminofluorene (AAF) is carcinogenic to many species of animals but not to the guinea pig. However, the N-hydroxy metabolite of AAF is carcinogenic to all animals including the guinea pig, demonstrating that the difference between the guinea pig and the other animals is not in their response to the toxicant but in the bioactivation (Weisburger and Weisburger, 1973).

Although differences in biotransformation, including bioactivation, account for species variation in susceptibility to a great majority of chemicals, other factors such as absorption, distribution, and excretion also play a part. In addition, variations in physiologic functions are important in toxic manifestations in response to such toxicants as squill. This toxic chemical is a good rodenticide because rats cannot vomit, whereas humans and many other mammals can eliminate this poison by vomiting (Doull, 1980). Anatomic differences may also be responsible, such as with BHA (see Chapter 19).

With the diversity in the number of rat strains available, it should not be surprising that there are differences in chemical-induced sensitivities. In general, each chemical will induce a change in all rat strains, but the degree of the effect will vary amongst strains (as in all science, there are no exceptions). However, there may be no response in humans. Clearly there are hormonal differences between males and females, but the precise role of these hormones in strain-associated chemical-induced outcomes still remains to be established. It should be noted that the reproductive cycle in female F344 rats is dramatically different from that of Sprague-Dawley rats. Consequently, the incidence of spontaneous and chemical-induced mammary tumorigenesis is markedly higher in Sprague-Dawley rats as this stock possesses greater estrogen levels. The human does not resemble the Sprague-Dawley strain and thus findings cannot be applied to humans. In comparing both males and females of the same strain, in general, chemicals including nitrosamines, decalin, hydroquinone, chloroform, etc., induce markedly greater responses in the male. It is of interest that in studies where males and females of different strains are compared, the males of certain strains are far more susceptible to adverse effects.

Apart from the differences in susceptibility that exist from one species to another and from one strain to another, there are also variables among individuals of the same species and same strain. While the magnitude of such individual variations is usually relatively small, there are exceptions. This phenomenon has been widely studied among humans. For example, there are "slow inactivators," who are deficient in acetyltransferase. Such individuals acetylate isoniazid only slowly and are thus likely to suffer from peripheral neuropathy resulting from an accumulation of isoniazid. On the other hand, people with more efficient acetyltransferase require larger doses of isoniazid to obtain its therapeutic effect and are thus more likely to suffer from hepatic damage.

Differences in response to succinylcholine provide another example. Individuals with an atypical or a low level of plasma cholinesterase may exhibit prolonged muscular relaxation and apnea following an injection of a standard dose of this muscle relaxant. Glucose-6-phosphate dehydrogenase deficiency and altered stability of reduced glutathione are responsible for hemolytic anemia in subjects exposed to primaquine, antipyrine, and similar agents. A more extensive list of potentially hemolytic chemicals and drugs has been compiled by Calabrese et al. (1979).

Less dramatic but more consistently greater susceptibility to many drugs have been reported to exist among Indonesians, and perhaps also other Asians (Darmansjah and Muchtar, 1992).

Sex, hormonal status, and pregnancy

Male and female animals of the same strain and species usually react to toxicants similarly. There are, however, notable quantitative differences in their susceptibility, especially in the rat. For example, many barbiturates induce more prolonged sleep in female rats than in males. The shorter duration of action of hexobarbital in male rats is related to the higher activity of the liver microsomal enzymes to hydroxylate this chemical. This higher activity can be reduced by castration or pretreatment with estrogen. Similarly, male rats demethylate aminopyrine and acetylate sulfanilamide faster than females, and the males are thus less susceptible.

Female rats are also more susceptible than the males to such organophosphorus insecticides as azinphosmethyl and parathion. Castration and hormone treatment reverse this difference. Furthermore, weaning rats of both sexes are equally susceptible to these toxicants. However, unlike hexobarbital, parathion is metabolized more rapidly in the female rat than in the male. This faster metabolism of parathion results in a higher concentration of its metabolite, paraoxon, which is more toxic than the parent compound. This higher toxicity resulting from greater bioactivation in female rats, compared to males, is also true with aldrin and heptachlor, which undergo epoxidation. The female rat is also more susceptible to warfarin and strychnine. On the other hand, male rats are more susceptible than females to ergot and lead.

Differences in susceptibility between the sexes are also seen with other chemicals. For example, chloroform is acutely nephrotoxic in the male mouse but not in the females. Castration or the administration of estrogens reduces this effect in the males, and treatment with androgens enhances susceptibility to chloroform in the females. The greater susceptibility of male mice was explained on the basis of a much higher concentration of cytochrome P-450 (Smith et al., 1983). Strain and sex also play an important role in hyalin droplet nephropathy. Administration of decalin to male F-344, SD, Buffalo, or BN rats increased $\alpha2_u$-globulin content associated with hyalin droplet formation. In contrast, female F-344, SD, Buffalo, and BN rats showed no evidence of hyalin droplet formation or accumulation of $\alpha2_u$-globulin. It is of interest that both male and female NCI-Black-Reiter (NBR) rats resembled female responsiveness, as there was no hyalin droplet nephropathy. Clearly, the decalin-induced hyalin droplet nephropathy is strain-related, but the role of male hormones is difficult to decipher due to the lack of response noted in NBR male rats. However, there are marked differences in endogenous circulating testosterone levels among strains and this may account for the differences between NBR and other strains. It is also conceivable that NBR male rats, unlike SD or F-344, lack the gene necessary to synthesize $\alpha2_u$-globulin. Nicotine is also more toxic to the male mouse, and digoxin is more toxic to the male dog. However, the female cat is more susceptible to dinitrophenol and the female rabbit is more so to benzene.

Imbalances of non-sex hormones can also alter the susceptibility of animals to toxicants. Hyperthyroidism, hyperinsulinism, adrenalectomy, and stimulation of the pituitary–adrenal axis have all been shown to be capable of modifying the effects of certain toxicants (Doull, 1980; Hodgson, 1987).

Age

It has long been recognized that neonates and very young animals in general are more susceptible to toxicants such as morphine. For a great majority of toxicants, the young are 1.5–10 times more susceptible than adults (Goldenthal, 1971).

The available information indicates that the greater susceptibility of the young animals to many toxicants can be attributed to deficiencies of various detoxication enzyme systems. Both phase I and phase II reactions may be responsible. For example, hexobarbital at a dose of 10 mg/kg induced a sleeping time of longer than 360 min in 1-day-old mice compared to 27 min in the 21-day-old. The proportion of hexobarbital metabolized by oxidation in 3 hours in these animals was 0% and 21–33%, respectively (Jondorf et al., 1959). On the other hand, chloramphenicol is excreted mainly as a glucuronide conjugate. When a dose of 50 mg/kg was given to 1- or 2-day-old infants, the blood levels were 15 µg/ml or higher over a period of 48 hours. In contrast, children aged 1–11 years maintained such blood levels for only 12 hours (Weiss et al., 1960).

However, not all chemicals are more toxic to the young. Certain substances, notably CNS stimulants, are much less toxic to neonates. Lu et al. (1965) reported that the LD_{50} of DDT was more than 20 times greater in newborn rats than in adults, in sharp contrast to the effect of age on malathion (Table 5.2). This insensitivity to the toxicity of DDT may be reassuring in assessing the potential risk of this pesticide, because of the very much larger intake in young babies via breast feeding and cow's milk, especially on the unit body weight basis.

The effect of age on the susceptibility to other CNS stimulants, including other organochlorine insecticides (e.g., dieldrin) appears less marked (generally in the range of 2–10 times). Most organophosphorous pesticides such as malathion are more toxic to the young; Schradan (octamethyl pyrophosphoramide) and phenylthiourea are notable exceptions (Brodeur and DuBois, 1963).

Apart from differences in biotransformation, other factors also play a

Table 5.2 Effect of age on acute toxicity of malathion, DDT, and dieldrin in rats

Pesticide	Age	LD_{50} (mg/kg) with 95% confidence limits	
Malathion	Newborn	134.4	(94.0–190.8)
	Pre-weaning	925.5	(679.01–261.0)
	Adult	3,697.0	(3,179.0–4,251.0)
DDT	Newborn	>4,000.0	
	Pre-weaning	437.8	(346.3–553.9)
	Adult	194.5	(158.7–238.3)
Dieldrin	Newborn	167.8	(140.8–200.0)
	Pre-weaning	24.9	(19.7–31.5)
	Adult	37.0	(27.4–50.1)

Source: Reprinted with permission from Lu et al. Toxicity of pesticides in young versus adult rats. Food and Cosmetics Toxicology, vol. 3. © 1965, Pergamon Press plc.

role. For example, a lower susceptibility at the receptor has been found to be the reason for the relative insensitivity of young rats to DDT (Henderson and Woolley, 1969).

Certain toxicants are absorbed to a greater extent by the young than by the adult. For example, young children absorb four to five times more lead than adults (McCabe, 1979) and 20 times more cadmium (Sasser and Jarbor, 1977). The greater susceptibility of the young to morphine is attributable to a less efficient blood–brain barrier, as is vividly illustrated in Figure 5.1 (Kupferberg and Way, 1963). Penicillin and tetracycline are excreted more slowly and hence are more toxic in the young (Lu, 1970). Ouabain is about 40 times more toxic in the newborn than in the adult rat because the adult rat's liver is much more efficient in removing this cardiac glycoside from the plasma. The higher incidence of methemoglobinemia in young infants has been explained on the basis that their lower gastric acidity allows upward migration of intestinal microbial flora and the reduction of nitrates to a greater extent. Furthermore, they have a higher proportion of fetal hemoglobin, which is more readily oxidized to methemoglobin (WHO, 1977).

There is evidence that the newborn is more susceptible to such carcinogens as aflatoxin B_1. Furthermore, the fetuses, but not the embryos, of

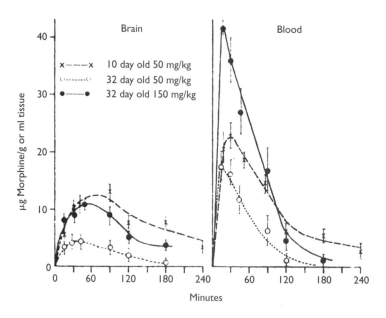

Figure 5.1 Brain and blood levels of free morphine at specific time intervals after intraperitoneal injections of morphine. Bracketed vertical lines show the standard error, using four animals per point.

Source: Kupferberg and Way, 1963.

rodents are much more susceptible. For example, there was a 50-fold increase in the potency of ethylnitrosourea. This is also true with non-human primates, except the maximal effects occur during the first third of gestation. If this is true with human fetuses, then they may be exposed to carcinogens before the mothers are aware of their pregnancies (Rice, 1979).

Old animals and humans are also more susceptible to certain chemicals. This problem has not been studied as extensively as in the young. However, the available evidence indicates that the aged patients are generally more sensitive to many drugs. The possible mechanisms include reduced detoxication and an impaired renal excretion (Goldstein, 1990). In addition, the distribution of chemicals in the body may also be altered because of increased body fat and decreased body water (Jarvik *et al.*, 1981). A number of drugs have been found to be likely to induce more severe signs of toxicity. These include most CNS depressants, certain antibiotics, cardiac glycosides, and hypotensive agents (WHO, 1981; Rochon *et al.*, 1999).

Nutritional status

The principal biotransformation of toxicants, as noted in Chapter 3, is catalyzed by the microsomal mixed-function oxidases (MFO). A deficiency of essential fatty acids generally depresses MFO activities. This is also true with protein deficiency. The decreased MFO has different effects on the toxicity of chemicals. For example, hexobarbital and aminopyrine are detoxicated by these enzymes and are thus more toxic to rats and mice with these nutrient deficiencies. On the other hand, the toxicities of aflatoxin, carbon tetrachloride, and heptachlor are lower in such animals because of their depressed bioactivation of these toxicants. Rats fed low-protein diets were 2–26 times more sensitive to a variety of pesticides (Boyd, 1972). MFO activities are decreased in animals fed high levels of carbohydrates.

A number of carcinogenesis studies have demonstrated that restriction of food intake decreases tumor yield. Deficiency of protein generally lowers tumorigenicity of carcinogens, such as aflatoxin B_1 and dimethyl-nitrosamine. The importance of diet on carcinogenesis is further demonstrated by the fact that rats and mice fed diets rich in fats have higher tumor incidences compared to those that are given a restricted diet.

Vitamin A deficiency depresses the MFO. In general, this is also true with deficiencies of vitamins C and E. But thiamine deficiency has the opposite effect. Vitamin A deficiency, in addition, increases the susceptibility of the respiratory tract to carcinogens (Nettesheim *et al.*, 1979).

Some foods contain appreciable amounts of chemicals that are strong inducers of MFO, such as safrole, flavones, xanthines, and indoles. In addition, potent inducers such as DDT and polychlorinated biphenyls (PCB) are present as contaminants in many foods.

Diseases

The liver is the main organ wherein biotransformation of chemicals takes place. Such diseases as acute and chronic hepatitis, cirrhosis of the liver, and hepatic necrosis often decrease the biotransformation. The microsomal and nonmicrosomal enzyme systems as well as the phase II reactions may be affected.

Renal diseases may also affect the toxic manifestations of chemicals. This effect stems from disturbances of the excretory and metabolic functions of the kidney. Heart diseases, when severe, can increase the toxicity of chemicals by impairing the hepatic and renal circulation, thus affecting the metabolic and excretory functions of these organs. Respiratory tract disorders such as asthma render the subjects much more susceptible to air pollutants such as SO_2.

Environmental factors

Physical factors

Changes in temperature may alter the toxicity. For example, colchicine and digitalis are more toxic to the rat than to the frog. But their toxicity to the frog can be increased by raising the environmental temperature. The duration of the response, however, is shorter when the temperature is higher. The effect of environmental temperature on the magnitude and duration of the response is apparently related to the temperature-dependent biochemical reactions responsible for the effect and for the biotransformation of the chemical.

Interest in the effect of barometric pressure on the toxicity of chemicals stems from human exposure to them in space and in saturation diving vehicles. At high altitudes, the toxicity of digitalis and strychnine is decreased, whereas that of amphetamine is increased. The influence of changes in barometric pressure on the toxicity of chemicals seems attributable mainly, if not entirely, to the altered oxygen tension rather than to a direct pressure effect.

Whole-body irradiation increases the toxicity of CNS stimulants but decreases that of CNS depressants. However, it has no effect on analgesics such as morphine. More details and literature citations have been provided by Doull (1980).

The effects of toxicants often show a diurnal pattern that is mainly related to the light cycle. In the rat and the mouse, the activities of cytochrome P-450 are greatest at the beginning of the dark phase.

Social factors

It is well known that animal husbandry and a variety of social factors can modify the toxicities of chemicals: the handling of the animals, the housing (singly or in groups), the types of cage, the supplier, and bedding materials are all important factors. Some examples of the influence of environmental factors on toxicity are given in Chapter 6.

Chemical interaction

Types of interaction

The toxicity of a chemical in an organism may be increased or decreased by a simultaneous or consecutive exposure to another chemical (Table 6.1). If the combined effect is equal to the sum of the effect of each substance given alone, the interaction is considered to be *additive*; for example, combinations of most organophosphorous pesticides on cholinesterase activity. If the combined effect is greater than the sum, the interaction is considered to be *synergistic*; for example, carbon tetrachloride and ethanol on the liver and asbestos exposure and cigarette smoking on the lung. In the latter example, Selikoff *et al.* (1968) reported that there was a five-fold increase in lung cancer incidence among asbestos workers, an 11-fold increase among cigarette smokers, and a 55-fold increase among asbestos workers who were cigarette smokers. The term *potentiation* is used to describe the situation in which the toxicity of a substance on an organ is markedly increased by another substance that alone has no toxic effect on that organ. For example, isopropanol has no effect on the liver, but it can increase considerably the hepatotoxicity of carbon tetrachloride.

Similarly, trichloroethylene, which has little effect on the liver, increases the hepatotoxicity of carbon tetrachloride, as measured by the release of liver enzymes ALT, SDH and AST (Borzelleca *et al.*, 1990).

The exposure of an organism to a chemical may reduce the toxicity of another. *Chemical antagonism* denotes the situation wherein a reaction between the two chemicals produces a less toxic product, for example, chelation of heavy metals by dimercaprol. *Functional antagonism* exists when two chemicals produce opposite effects on the same physiologic parameters, such as the counteraction between CNS stimulants and depressants. *Competitive antagonism* exists when the agonist and antagonist act on the same receptor, such as the blockade of the effects of nicotine on ganglia by ganglionic blocking agents. *Noncompetitive antagonism* exists when the toxic effect of a chemical is blocked by another not acting on the same receptor. For example, atropine reduces the toxicity of acetylcholinesterase (AChE) inhibitors not by blocking the receptors on the AChE, but by blocking the receptors for the ACh accumulated.

Mechanisms of action

Chemical interactions are achieved through a variety of mechanisms. For instance, nitrites and certain amines can react in the stomach to form nitrosamines, the majority of which are potent carcinogens, and thus greatly increase the toxicity. On the other hand, the action of many antidotes is based on their interaction with the toxicants; for example, thiosulfate is used in cases of cyanide poisoning. Furthermore, a chemical may displace another from its binding site on plasma protein and thereby increase its effective concentration. A chemical may modify the renal excretion of weak acids and weak bases by altering the pH of urine. Competition for the same renal transport system by one chemical can hinder the excretion of another. A notable example is the administration of probenecid along with penicillin to reduce the renal excretion of the antibiotic, thereby prolonging its duration of action.

One important type of interaction involves the binding of chemicals with their specific receptors. An antagonist blocks the action of an agonist, such as a neurotransmitter or a hormone, by preventing the binding of the agonist to the receptor.

Another important type of interaction results from alterations of the biotransformation of a chemical by another. Some chemicals are *inducers* of xenobiotic-metabolizing enzymes. They augment the activities of these enzymes, perhaps mainly by de novo synthesis. The common inducers include phenobarbital, 3-methylcholanthrene (3-MC), PCB, DDT, and BaP. The inducers may lower the toxicity of other chemicals by accelerating their detoxication. For example, pretreatment which phenobarbital shortens the sleeping time induced by hexobarbital and the paralysis induced by zoxazolamine. Such pretreatment also reduces the plasma level of aflatoxins (Wong *et al.*, 1981). In addition, 3-MC pretreatment greatly reduces the liver necrosis produced by bromobenzene, probably by increasing the activity of the epoxide hydrase (see Figure 3.3). On the other hand, pretreatment with phenobarbital augments the toxicity of acetaminophen and bromobenzene, apparently by increasing the toxic metabolites formed. Repeated administration of a chemical may induce its metabolizing enzymes, as has been shown with vinyl chloride.

Piperonyl butoxide, isoniazid, and SKF 525A and related chemicals are *inhibitors* of various xenobiotic-metabolizing enzymes. For instance, piperonyl butoxide increases the toxicity of pyrethrum in insects by inhibiting their MFO that detoxifies this insecticide. Isoniazid, when taken along with diphenylhydantoin, lengthens the plasma half-life of the antiepileptic drug and increases its toxicity. Iproniazid inhibits monoamine oxidase and increases the cardiovascular effects of tyramine, which is found in cheese and which is normally readily metabolized by the oxidase.

Characteristics of enzyme induction

Because of the importance of the effect of enzyme induction, much work has been done on certain inducers, notably phenobarbital and polycyclic aromatic hydrocarbons (PAHs). These two types of inducers differ in several respects. For example, phenobarbital markedly increases the liver weight and the smooth endoplasmic reticulum, but PAHs such as 3-MC and BaP have little effect on these parameters. Phenobarbital augments mainly the amounts of cytochrome P-450 and NADPH-cytochrome c reductase. PAHs have little effect on these enzymes, but they increase the amount of cytochrome P-448, which is also known as P_1-450, and aryl hydrocarbon hydroxylase (AHH), as discussed on p. 53. These isozymes have different substrate specificity and hence alter the effects of toxicants differently (see Sipes and Gandolfi, 1993).

Interaction as toxicologic tools

Studies on chemical interaction are conducted not only to determine the effects of combinations of chemicals, but the data thereof are useful in assessing health hazards associated with exposures to such combinations. These studies are also done to elucidate the nature and the mode of action of the toxicity of a chemical by the administration of another, as well as to bring out weak or latent effects of chemicals.

References

Borzelleca, J. F., O'Hara, T. M., Gennings, C., Granger, R. H., Sheppard, M. A., and Condie, L. W. (1990) Interactions of water contaminants. *Fundam. Appl. Toxicol.* 14:477–490.

Boyd, E. M. (1972) *Protein Deficiency and Pesticide Toxicity.* Springfield, IL: Charles C. Thomas.

Brodeur, J. and DuBois, K. P. (1963) Comparison of acute toxicity of anti-cholinesterase insecticides to weanling and adult male rats. *Proc. Soc. Exp. Biol. Med.* 114:509–511.

Calabrese, E. J., Moore, G., and Brown, R. (1979) Effects of environmental oxidant stressors on individuals with a G-6-PD deficiency with particular refer-ence to an animal model. *Environ. Health Perspect.* 29:49–55.

Darmansjah, I. and Muchtar, A. (1992) Dose–response variation among different populations. *Clin. Pharmacol. Therap.* 52:449–452.

Doull, J. (1980) Factors influencing toxicology, in *Casarett and Doull's Toxicology*, J. Doull, C. D. Klaassen and M. O. Amdur (eds), New York, NY: Macmillan.

Goldenthal, E. I. (1971) A compilation of LD_{50} values in newborn and adult animals. *Toxicol. Appl. Pharmacol.* 18:185–207.

Goldstein, R. S. (1990) Drug-induced nephrotoxicity in middle-aged and senescent rats, in *Proceedings of the V International Congress of Toxicology.* London: Taylor & Francis.

Henderson, G. L. and Woolley, D. A. (1969) Studies on the relative insensitivity of the immature rat to the neurotoxic effects of DDT. *J. Pharmacol. Exp. Ther.* 170:173–180.

Hodgson, E. (1987) Modification of metabolism, in *Modern Toxicology*, E. Hodgson and P. E. Levi (eds), New York, NY: Elsevier.

Jarvik, L. F., Greenblatt, D. J., and Harman, D. (1981) *Clinical Pharmacology and the Aged Patient*. New York, NY: Raven Press.

Jay, G. E., Jr. (1955) Variation in response of various mouse strains to hexobarbital (Evipal). *Proc. Soc. Exp. Biol. Med.* 90:378–380.

Jondorf, W. R., Maickel, R. P., and Brodie, B. B. (1959) Inability of newborn mice and guinea pigs to metabolize drugs. *Biochem. Pharmacol.* 1:352–354.

Kupferberg, H. J. and Way, E. L. (1963) Pharmacologic basis for the increased sensitivity of the newborn rat to morphine. *J. Pharmacol. Exp. Ther.* 141:105–112.

Lu, F. C. (1970) Significance of age of test animals in food additive evaluation, in *Metabolic Aspects of Food Safety*, F. J. C. Roe (ed.), Oxford: Blackwell Scientific.

Lu, F. C., Jessup, D. C., and Lavellee, A. (1965) Toxicity of pesticides in young versus adult rats. *Food Cosmet. Toxicol.* 3:591–596.

McCabe, E. B. (1979) Age and sensitivity to lead toxicity: A review. *Environ. Health Perspect.* 29:29–33.

Miller, E. C., Miller, J. H., and Enomotor, M. (1964) The comparative carcinogenetics of 2-acetylaminofluorene and its N-hydroxy metabolite in mice, hamsters and guinea pigs. *Cancer Res.* 24:2018–2032.

Nettesheim, P., Snyder, C., and Kim, J. C. S. (1979) Vitamin A and the susceptibility of respiratory tract tissues to carcinogenic insult. *Environ. Health Perspect.* 29:89–93.

Quinn, G. P., Axelrod, J., and Brodie, B. B. (1958) Species, strain and sex differences in metabolism of hexobarbitone, amidopyrine, antipyrine and aniline. *Biochem. Pharmacol.* 1:152–159.

Rice, J. M. (1979) Perinatal period and pregnancy: Intervals of high risk for chemical carcinogens. *Environ. Health Perspect.* 29:23–27.

Rochon, P. A., Anderson, G. M., Tu, J. V. *et al.* (1999) Age and gender-related use of low dose drug therapy. *J. Am. Geriatr. Soc.* 47:954–959.

Sasser, L. B. and Jarbor, G. E. (1977) Intestinal absorption and retention of cadmium in neonatal rat. *Toxicol. Appl. Pharmacol.* 41:423–431.

Selikoff, I. J., Hammond, E. C., and Churg, J. (1968) Asbestos exposure, smoking, and neoplasia. *J. Am. Med. Assoc.* 204:106–112.

Sipes, I. G. and Gandolfi, A. J. (1993) Biotransformation of toxicants, in *Casarett and Doull's Toxicology*, M. O. Amdur, J. Doull and C. D. Klaassen (eds), New York, NY: McGraw-Hill.

Smith, J. H., Maita, K., Adler, V., Schacht, T., Sleight, S. D., and Hook, J. B. (1983) Effect of sex hormone status on chloroform nephrotoxicity and renal drug metabolizing enzymes. *Toxicol. Lett.* 28(Suppl. 1):23.

Timbrell, J. A. (1991) *Principles of Biochemical Toxicology*. London: Taylor & Francis.

Weisburger, J. H. and Weisburger, E. K. (1973) Biochemical formation and pharmacological, toxicological and pathological properties of hydroxylamines and hydroxamic acids. *Pharmacol. Rev.* 25:166.

Weiss, C. G., Glazko, A. J., and Weston, A. (1960) Chloramphenicol in the newborn infant. A physicologic explanation of its toxicity when given in excessive doses. *N. Engl. J. Med.* 262:787–794.

WHO (1977) Nitrates, nitrites and N-nitroso compounds. *Environmental Health Criteria 5.* Geneva: World Health Organization.

WHO (1981) Health care in the elderly: Report of the technical group on use of medicaments by the elderly. *Drugs* 22:279–294.

Williams, R. T. (1974) Inter-species variations in the metabolism of xenobiotics. *Biochem. Soc. Trans.* 2:359–377.

Wong, Z. A., Wei, Ching-I, Rice, D. W., and Hsieh, D. P. H. (1981) Effects of phenobarbital pretreatment on the metabolism and toxicokinetics of aflatoxin B_1 in the rhesus monkey. *Toxicol. Appl. Pharmacol.* 60:387–397.

Appendix 5.1 Mechanisms* underlying certain modifying factors

Toxicant	Responsible mechanism	Toxic response
1. *Bioactivation differences*		
2-Naphthylamine	2-Naphthyl hydroxylamine	Bladder tumor in dog, human, but not rat, mouse
Acetylaminofluorene	N-hydroxy metabolite	Carcinogenic in rat, mouse and hamster, but not in guinea pigs
2. *Toxicokinetic characteristics*		
Lead, cadmium	Greater *absorption* in the young	Greater toxic effects
Penicillin, tetracycline	Slower *excretion* in the young	Longer half-life
Morphine	Blood–brain barrier inefficient in the young	Greater CNS effect
3. *Toxicodynamic characteristics*		
DDT	Susceptibility of receptor	Less susceptible in the young
4. *Anatomic characteristics*		
BHA, BHT	Presence of forestomach in rat	Hyperplasia of forestomach
5. *Physiologic characteristics*		
Squill	Vomiting reflex	Absence in rat leading to toxic effect

Note
*Other than detoxication.

Appendix 5.2 Strain-related differences in drug-induced responses

| Parameter | Tissue | Strain/stock | |
		Resistant	Susceptible
Ciprofibrate-induced peroxisomal proliferation	Liver	Sprague-Dawley	Long-Evans
Acetaminophen-induced necrosis	Kidney	Sprague-Dawley	F344
Streptozotocin-induced autoimmune reactivity	Popliteal lymph node	F344	Sprague-Dawley or Wistar
Amiodarone-induced phospholipidosis	Lung	Sprague-Dawley	F344
Diethylstilbesterol-induced carcinoma	Mammary tissue	COP	F344
Saccharin-induced histopathologic changes	Urinary bladder	Sprague-Dawley	Wistar
Mepirizole-induced ulceration	Duodenum	DONYRU	Sprague-Dawley or F344
Azaserine-induced carcinoma	Pancreas	F344	Wistar
B-Adrenoceptor suppression of lipolysis	Adipocyte	Wistar	Sprague-Dawley
Diethylstilbesterol-induced prolactin secretion	Pituitary	Sprague-Dawley	F344

Note
Adapted from S. Kacew and M. F. W. Festing (1995). Role of rat strain in the differential sensitivity to pharmaceutical agents and naturally occurring substances. *Journal of Toxicology and Environmental Health* 47:1–30. Resistant does not imply a lack of effect but a significantly lower responsiveness than susceptible.

Part II

Testing procedures for conventional and nontarget organ toxicities

Chapter 6

Conventional toxicity studies

CONTENTS

Introduction

Usefulness

As noted in prior chapters, toxicants vary greatly in their potency, target organ, and mode of action. To provide proper orientation for additional in-depth targeted studies, conventional toxicity studies are generally carried out first. These studies are designed to provide indications of the appropriate dosage range, the probable adverse effect, and the target organ (e.g., liver), system (e.g., respiratory), or special toxicity (e.g., carcinogenicity).

In addition to providing preliminary information for proper orientation of additional investigations, however, the conventional toxicity studies per se yield data that can be used to assess the nature of the adverse effects and the "no-observed-adverse-effect level" (NOAEL) of the toxicant, which are required in the safety assessment described in Chapter 25. For example, approximately half of the pesticides evaluated by the WHO Expert Committee on Pesticide Residues in the past 30 years have been based on conventional toxicity studies, in spite of the extensive database that is also available (Lu, 1995).

Categories

In order to examine the different effects associated with various lengths of exposure, the conventional studies are generally divided into three categories: (1) *Acute toxicity studies* involve either a single administration of the chemical under test or several administrations within a 24-hour period. (2) *Short-term* (also known as subacute and subchronic) toxicity studies involve repeated administrations, usually on a daily or five times per week basis, over a period of about 10% of the life-span, namely three months in rats and one or two years in dogs. However, shorter durations such as 14- and 28-day treatments have also been used by some investigators. (3) *Long-term* (also known as chronic) toxicity studies involve repeated administrations over the entire life-span of the test animals or at least a major fraction of it, for example, 18 months in mice, 24 months in rats, and seven to ten years in dogs and monkeys.

Importance of selection of rat strains

In the search for compounds to enhance our living standards, there is a necessity for understanding normal human functions and mechanisms which underlie dysfunction in these processes. Utilization of a suitable animal model which simulates humans is necessary in order to develop new pharmaceutical agents to alleviate diseases or chemicals to enhance lifestyle. It is incumbent upon investigators to choose a species in which pharmacokinetic principles are established and resemble those of humans. The choice of rodent has specific advantages in that there are similar pharmacodynamic parameters resembling those in humans. Other advantages include availability, low cost, ease of breeding, and an extensive literature database to enable comparisons to present findings. Factors which need to be recognized as playing an important role in chemical-induced outcomes include strain, supplier, sex, and dietary intake. This is especially critical in the risk assessment process.

In an effort to establish animal models to extrapolate to human responses, one must be apprised in that choosing the rat, strain can affect the responses observed under normal or chemically-altered conditions. Even by limiting genetic variability by simply using the same strain, factors such as supplier and dietary intake can bring about differences in responsiveness of one strain as well as between strains. Further, the rodent may be susceptible while the human is nonresponsive.

Acute toxicity studies

These studies are designed either to determine the median lethal dose (LD_{50}) of the toxicant or a rough estimate of it. The LD_{50} has been defined as "a statistically derived expression of a single dose of a material that can be expected to kill 50% of the animals." In addition, such studies may also indicate the probable target organ of the chemical and its specific toxic effect and provide guidance on the doses to be used in the more prolonged studies.

In certain cases, especially those with low acute toxicities, it may not be necessary to determine precise LD_{50}s. Simple lethality data can serve useful purposes. For example, synergistic and antagonistic effects can be demonstrated using a few animals as shown by the data presented in Table 6.1. Furthermore, even the information that a sufficiently large dose causes

Table 6.1 Using lethality in demonstrating chemical interaction

Lethality (number of deaths/number on test)			
$KBrO_3$ (mg/kg)	Control (saline)	Cysteine* (400 mg/kg)	Diethyl maleate[†] (0.7 ml/kg)
169	5/5	0/5	
130	5/5	0/5	
49	0/5		4/5
29	0/5		4/5

Source: Adapted from Kurakawa et al. (1987).

Notes
With five animals per dose group, the interactions between $KBrO_3$ and the "antagonist" (cysteine) and a "synergist" (diethyl maleate) are evident.
*Antagonistic.
[†]Synergistic.

few or no deaths may suffice. This *limit test* has been applied. For example, a number of food colors were given to rats at a dose of 2 g/kg. Since none of the rats died, it was considered sufficient to rule out any serious acute toxicity and no LD_{50} was determined (Lu and Lavallée, 1965). This view was accepted by the Joint FAO/WHO Expert Committee on Food Additives (WHO, 1966). EPA (1994) recommends the use of 5 g/kg.

When the route of exposure is inhalation, the end point is then either the median lethal concentration (LC_{50}) with a given duration of exposure or the median lethal time (LT_{50}) with a given concentration of the chemical in the air.

Experimental design

Selection of species of animal

In general, the rat, and sometimes the mouse, are selected for use in determining the LD_{50}. Their preference stems from the fact that they are economical, readily available, and easy to handle. Further, there are more toxicologic data on these species of animals, a fact that facilitates comparisons of toxicities to other chemicals.

Sometimes a nonrodent species is desirable. This is true especially when the LD_{50} values in rats and mice are markedly different or when the pattern or rate of biotransformation in humans is known to be significantly different from rats and mice.

The LD_{50} determination is preferably done in animals of both sexes, and also in adult and young animals, because of their differences in susceptibility.

Route of administration

Generally, the toxicant is administered by the route by which humans would be exposed. The oral route is most commonly used. The dermal and inhalation routes are used increasingly, not only for chemicals that are intended for human use by such routes but also for chemicals whose health hazards to personnel handling these chemicals are to be assessed (see Chapters 12 and 15). Parenteral routes are mainly used in assessing the acute toxicity of parenteral drugs. In addition, immediate or very prompt and complete or nearly complete absorption generally follow intravenous and intraperitoneal injection.

Dosage and number of animals

To properly ascertain an LD$_{50}$, it is necessary to try to select a dose that would kill about half of the animals, another that would kill more than half (preferably less than 90%), and a third dose that would kill less than half (preferably more than 10%) of the animals. OECD (1992), among others, recommends a "Sighting" study to aid in the selection of the doses, which can be accomplished with no more than five animals. Dosing of the animals is done sequentially, with at least a 24-hour interval to allow adjustment of the dose that the next animal is to receive.

To determine a relatively precise LD$_{50}$, 40–50 animals are used, with a ratio of 1.2 between successive doses (Lu and Lavallée, 1965). For most chemicals, however, approximate LD$_{50}$s are adequate. These doses can be estimated using six to nine animals (Bruce, 1985).

Observations and examinations

After administering the toxicant to the animals, they should be examined for the number and time of death in order to estimate the LD$_{50}$. More importantly, their signs of toxicity should be recorded. Table 6.2 provides a list of body organs and systems that might be affected, along with the specific signs of toxicity. The observation period should be sufficiently long so that delayed effects, including death, would not be missed. The period is usually 7–14 days but may be much longer.

Gross autopsies should be performed on all animals that have died as well as at least some of the survivors, especially those that are morbid at the termination of the experiment. Autopsy can provide useful information on the target organ, especially when death does not occur shortly after the dosing. Histopathologic examination of selected organs and tissues may also be indicated.

Multiple endpoint evaluation

To derive additional information concerning the chemical on test, the toxic signs, such as those listed in Table 6.2, should be critically observed and recorded for evaluating non-lethal endpoints. These endpoints may assist in characterizing the nature of the toxicant.

Evaluation of the data

Dose–response relationship

When the mortality, or the frequency of other effects expressed in percentages, is plotted against the dose on a logarithmic scale, an S-shaped curve is obtained (Figure 4.1, curve B). The central portion of the curve (between

Table 6.2 Relationship between toxic signs and body organs or systems

System	Toxic signs
Autonomic	Relaxed nictitating membrane, exophthalmos, nasal discharge, salivation, diarrhea, urination, piloerection.
Behavioral	Sedation, restlessness, sitting position – head up, staring straight ahead, drooping head, severe depression, excessive preening, gnawing paws, panting, irritability, aggressive and defensive hostility, fear, confusion, bizarre activity.
Sensory	Sensitivity to pain; righting, corneal, labyrinth, placing, and hind limb reflex; sensitivity to sound and touch; nystagmus, phonation.
Neuromuscular	Decreased and increased activity, fasciculation, tremors, convulsions, ataxia, prostration, straub tail, hind limb weakness, pain and hind limb reflexes (absent or diminished), opisthotonos, muscle tone, death.
Cardiovascular	Increased and decreased heart rate, cyanosis, vasoconstriction, vasodilation, hemorrhage.
Respiratory	Hypopnea, dyspnea, gasping, apnea.
Ocular	Mydriasis, miosis, lacrimation, ptosis, nystagmus, cycloplegia, pupillary light reflex.
Gastrointestinal, gastrourinary	Salivation, retching, diarrhea, bloody stool and urine, constipation, rhinorrhea, emesis, involuntary urination and defecation.
Cutaneous	Piloerection, wet dog shakes, erythema, edema, necrosis, swelling.

Source: McNamara (1976).

16% and 84% response) is sufficiently straight for estimating the LD_{50} or ED_{50}. However, a much wider range of the curve can be straightened by converting the percentages to probit units. This procedure is especially useful in estimating, for example, the LD_{01} or LD_{99}, when the extreme ends of this curve have to be used.

The probit units correspond to normal equivalent deviations around the mean, for example, $+1$, $+2$, $+3$ ... and -1, -2, -3 ... deviations, whereas the mean value itself has a zero deviation. However, to avoid negative numbers, the probit units are obtained by adding five to these deviations. The corresponding figures in these systems are as follows:

Deviations	Probit	% Response
−3	2	0.1
−2	3	2.3
−1	4	15.9
0	5	50.0
1	6	84.1
2	7	97.7
3	8	99.9

Table 6.3 Acute LD_{50} values for a variety of chemical agents

Agent	Species	LD_{50} (mg/kg body weight)
Ethanol	Mouse	10,000
Sodium chloride	Mouse	4,000
Ferrous sulfate	Rat	1,500
Morphine sulfate	Rat	900
Phenobarbital, sodium	Rat	150
DDT	Rat	100
Picrotoxin	Rat	5
Strychnine sulfate	Rat	2
Nicotine	Rat	1
d-Tubocurarine	Rat	0.5
Hemicholinium-3	Rat	0.2
Tetrodotoxin	Rat	0.1
Dioxin (TCDD)	Guinea pig	0.001
Botulinum toxin	Rat	0.00001

Source: Loomis (1978).

Detailed methods for estimating the LD_{50} and its standard errors are given in many papers and books on statistics, including those of Bliss (1957), Finney (1971), and Weil (1952).

Relative potency

The potency of toxicants varies significantly. Table 6.3 illustrates the range of LD_{50} values.

To render the LD_{50} values more meaningful, it is advisable to also determine their standard errors (or the confidence limits) and the slopes of the dose–response curves. The importance of the slope can be readily appreciated when comparing two substances with similar LD_{50}s. The one with a flatter slope will likely cause more deaths than the other at doses smaller than the LD_{50}s (Figure 6.1, chemicals C and D). The examples in Table 6.4 illustrate the marked differences in slopes.

Table 6.4 Dose–response relationships*

Aflatoxin B₁[†]		Botulinum toxin[‡]			
Dose (ppb)	Response (tumor)	Dose (pg)	Response (death)	Dose (pg)	Response (death)
0	0/18	1	0/10	34	11/30
1	2/22	5	0/10	37	10/30
5	1/22	10	0/30	40	16/30
15	4/21	15	0/30	45	26/30
50	20/25	20	0/30	50	26/30
100	28/28	24	0/30	55	17/30
		27	0/30	60	22/30
		30	4/30	65	20/30

Notes
*Note relatively shallow dose–response relationship with aflatoxin B₁ wherein a 100-fold increase existed between the minimal and maximal effective doses, in contrast to the steep slope of botulin toxin, wherein there was a mere 50% increase.
[†]Data quoted from Food Safety Council (1980).
[‡]Data supplied by E. J. Schantz (Food Research Institute, University of Wisconsin, Madison, WI 53706). Part of the data also appears in the Report of Food Safety Council (1980).

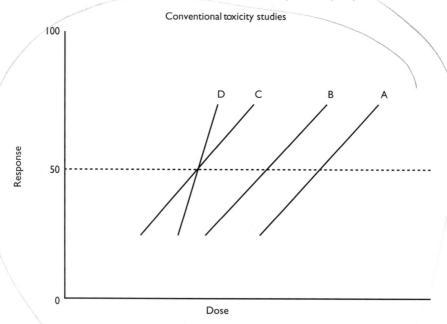

Figure 6.1 Median lethal doses and slopes of the dose–response (death) relationships of four chemicals. Chemical A is less toxic than the others. Chemical C is as toxic as D at the median lethal dose level but is more toxic at lower dose levels. Chemical B is less toxic than D at the median lethal dose level, but it may be more or less so at lower doses.

Uses of LD_{50} values and signs of toxicity

These values are useful in a number of ways.

1 Classification of chemicals according to relative toxicity. A common classification is as follows:

Category	LD_{50}
Supertoxic	5 mg/kg or less
Extremely toxic	5–50 mg/kg
Highly toxic	50–500 mg/kg
Moderately toxic	0.5–5 g/kg
Slightly toxic	5–15 g/kg
Practically nontoxic	>15 g/kg

2 Other uses include evaluation of the hazard from accidental overdosage; planning subacute and chronic toxicity studies in animals; providing information about (a) variations in response among different animal species and strains, (b) the susceptibility of a particular animal population, and (c) quality control of chemical products, to detect toxic impurities, etc.

For toxicants with important health implications (e.g., TCDD), LD_{50}s are determined in several species of animals. The extent of variation of these values indicates the range of differences in the toxicokinetics and/or toxicodynamics among these species.

Guidelines for acute oral, dermal, and inhalation toxicity studies have been published by various national and international agencies (e.g., EPA, 1994). However, the prevailing advice is to estimate approximate LD_{50}s unless otherwise indicated.

Short-term and long-term toxicity studies

Humans are more often exposed to chemicals at levels much lower than those that are acutely fatal, but they are exposed over longer periods of time. To assess the nature of the toxic effects under these more realistic situations, short-term and long-term toxicity studies are conducted. These studies are also known as subacute (or subchronic) and chronic toxicity studies. The procedures involved in these two types are very similar except their duration.

Experimental design

Species and number

Generally, two or more species of animals are used. Ideally, the animals chosen should biotransform the chemical in a manner essentially identical to humans. Since this is often unattainable, the rat and the dog are usually selected. This preference is based on their appropriate size, ready availability, and the great preponderance of toxicologic information on chemicals in these animals. As noted in Chapter 5, different strains of rats may respond markedly differently to toxicants.

Equal numbers of male and female animals should be used. Generally, 10–50 rats are used in each dose group as well as in the control group. As a rule, this procedure will provide data that are statistically analyzable. Smaller numbers of dogs (48 per group) are used because of the greater number of examinations that can be made on each animal and because of their size and the expense involved.

Route of administration

The chemical should be administered by the route of the intended use or exposure in humans. For most chemicals, the common route is oral. The preferred procedure is to incorporate the chemical in the diet, although the drinking water is sometimes used as the vehicle. The latter method is advisable when the chemical may react with a component in the diet. The chemical, especially if it is reactive, volatile, or unpalatable, is often administered by gavage or in gelatin capsules, a procedure more often used in dogs. The daily dose of the chemical may also be incorporated in a bolus of canned dog food.

Dermal application, exposure by inhalation, and parenteral routes are used for special purposes, such as industrial and agricultural products and drugs.

Dosage and duration

Since the aims of these studies are to determine the nature and site of the toxic effects as well as the "no-observed-adverse-effect level," it is advisable to select three doses: a dose that is high enough to elicit definite signs of toxicity but not high enough to kill many of the animals, a low dose that is expected to induce no toxic effect, and an intermediate dose. Sometimes, one or more additional doses are included to ensure that the above objectives are achieved. As noted earlier, a control group should be included. These animals will not receive the chemical under test but must be given any vehicle used.

The doses are generally selected on the basis of the information obtained in the acute toxicity studies, using both the LD_{50} and the slope of the dose–response curve. Any information on related chemicals and on their metabolism, especially the presence or absence of bioaccumulation, is also taken into account. A range-finding study is sometimes done. It consists of dosing five rats of each sex at each of three or four dose levels for seven days. The criteria for toxic effects were mortality, body weight gain, relative liver and kidney weights, and feed consumption. The results from seven-day tests are generally better than the LD_{50} values in predicting the dose levels for the longer-term toxicity study.

In studies in rats, the dose levels may be constant concentrations and expressed in mg/kg diet (ppm) or constant dosage and expressed in mg/kg body weight of the animals. As the animal grows, there are changes in the body weight as well as in the food consumption. For the constant dose regimen, the concentration of the chemical must therefore be adjusted periodically to maintain a relatively constant dose in mg/kg body weight. This is usually done at weekly intervals during the period of rapid growth and biweekly thereafter.

In the short-term studies, the duration in rats is generally 90 days. In the dog, the duration is often extended to six months or even one year. The duration of long-term studies in rats is generally 24 months, and seven or more years in dogs.

Observations and examinations

Body weight and food consumption

These should be determined weekly. Decreased body weight gain is a simple yet sensitive index of toxic effects. Food consumption is also a useful indicator. In addition, a marked decrease in food consumption can induce effects that mimic or aggravate the toxic manifestations of the chemical. In such cases, *paired feeding* or parenteral feeding may have to be instituted. Where the animals receiving the toxicant are affected more than those maintained on a reduced feed alone, the toxicant, apart from the undernutrition, is responsible for the effect.

General observations

These should include appearance, behavior, and any abnormality. Dead and moribund animals should be removed from the cages for gross and possibly microscopic examination. Frequent observation is necessary to minimize cannibalism.

Laboratory tests

Hematologic examinations usually include hematocrit, hemoglobin, erythrocyte count, total leukocyte count, and differential leukocyte count. All dogs should be sampled before the initiation of treatment and at one week, one month, and at the end. Tests at other intervals may be warranted. Because of the small blood volume of rats, only half of them are sampled at various intervals, while the others are sampled only at the end. Special tests such as reticulocyte count, platelet count, methemoglobin, and glucose-6-phosphate dehydrogenase (G-6-PD) may be indicated.

Clinical laboratory tests usually include fasting blood glucose, serum aspartate aminotransferase (AST or SGOT), alanine aminotransferase (ALT or SGPT), alkaline phosphatase (AP), total protein, albumin, globulin, blood urea nitrogen (BUN), and such elements as sodium, potassium, calcium, and chloride. Other tests may be done where indicated. For example, cholinesterase activity is assessed when testing organophosphorus and carbamate pesticides.

Urinalysis usually includes color, specific gravity, pH, protein, glucose, ketones, formed elements (red blood cells, etc.) and crystalline and amorphous materials.

Postmortem examination

Whenever possible, all animals that are found dead or dying should be subjected to a gross pathologic examination. If the state of the tissue permits, histologic examinations should also be done. In addition, the weights of a number of organs, either in absolute values or in terms of the body weights, should be determined as they serve as useful indicators of toxicity.

The organs that are usually weighed are liver, kidneys, adrenals, heart, brain, thyroid, and testes or ovaries. Those that are histologically examined are the following: all gross lesions, brain (three levels), spinal cord, eye and optic nerve, a major salivary gland, thymus, thyroid, heart, aorta, lung with a bronchus, stomach, small intestine (three levels), large intestine (two levels), adrenal gland, pancreas, liver, gallbladder (if present), spleen, kidney, urinary bladder, skeletal muscle, and bone and its marrow.

A list indicating the correlation between general observations, clinical laboratory tests, and postmortem examinations is produced as Appendix 6.1.

Guidelines for short-term and long-term studies have been published by WHO (1978, 1990), and the U.S. Environmental Protection Agency (EPA, 1994), among others.

Evaluation

Comprehensive short-term and long-term toxicity studies, using the various parameters of observations and examinations described above, usually yield information on the toxicity of the chemical under test, with respect to the target organs, the effects on these organs, and the dose–effect and dose–response relationships. Such information often provides indication on the additional specific types of studies that should be conducted. The quantitative data from the short-term and other studies have been suggested for use in the determination of the "no-observed-adverse-effect level" (NOAEL). This suggestion, however, has not been widely accepted because it is considered more prudent to use the data from long-term studies. This is especially true for chemicals (e.g., food additives, pesticides, environmental pollutants) to which humans may be subjected to life-time exposure. On the other hand, short-term studies may suffice in testing such chemicals: as most pharmaceuticals are used for short durations.

The NOAEL from the long-term studies, along with data on their acute toxicity and metabolism as well as information from genetic, reproductive, and any other studies, is used in determining their "acceptable intakes" (ADI) for humans. For further discussion on the procedure used for this purpose, see Chapter 25.

Good laboratory practice

In 1975 and 1976, the U.S. Food and Drug Administration (FDA) raised questions about the integrity of toxicologic data received from certain laboratories. On inspecting these facilities, FDA discovered a number of unacceptable laboratory practices, such as selective reporting, underreporting, lack of adherence to a specified protocol, poor animal care procedures, poor recordkeeping, and inadequate supervision of personnel. In an attempt to improve the validity of the data, FDA proposed a set of regulations for good laboratory practice in 1978. These were later included in the Regulation for the Enforcement of the Federal Food, Drug, and Cosmetic Act.

These regulations (FDA, 1987) contain detailed guidance on provisions for the following:

1 Personnel, stipulating the responsibilities of the study director, testing facility management, and quality assurance unit.
2 Facilities for animal care, animal supply, and handling test and control chemicals.
3 Equipment, regarding its design, maintenance, and calibration.
4 Testing facilities operation, including standard operating procedures, reagents and solutions, and animal care.

5   Test and control chemicals, such as their characterization and handling.
6   The protocol and conduct of a laboratory study.
7   Records, their storage, retrieval, and retention, as well as the preparation and contents of reports.
8   Disqualifications of testing facilities.

The U.S. Environmental Protection Agency also proposed a set of good laboratory practice standards. They contain provisions similar to those of the FDA regulation regarding health effects testing. However, the EPA standards also contain provisions for environmental effects testing (EPA, 1989). At an international level, OECD (1982) has also produced a set of similar guidelines.

References

Bliss, C. L. (1957) Some principles of bioassay. *Am. Sci.* 45:449–466.

Bruce, R. D. (1985) An up-and-down procedure for acute toxicity testing. *Fundam. Appl. Toxicol.* 5:151–157.

EPA (1994) *Health Effects Test Guidelines. Hazard Evaluation.* Code of Federal Regulations, Title 40, Parts 792 and 798.

FDA (1987) Good laboratory practice regulations; Final rule. *Fed. Reg.* 52:33768–33782.

Finney, D. J. (1971) *Probit Analysis.* Cambridge: Cambridge University Press.

Food Safety Council (1980) Proposed system for food safety assessment. *Food Cosmet. Toxicol.* 16, Suppl. 2.

Kurakawa, Y., Takamura, N. *et al.* (1987) Comparative studies on lipid peroxidation in the kidney of rats, mice and hamsters and the effect of cysteine, glutathione and diethyl maleate treatment on mortality and nephrotoxicity after administration of potassium bromate. *J. Am. Coll. Toxicol.* 6:487–501.

Loomis, T. (1978) *Essentials of Toxicology,* 3rd edn. Philadelphia: Lea & Febiger.

Lu, F. C. (1995) A review of the acceptable daily intakes of pesticides assessed by WHO. *Regul. Toxicol. Pharmacol.* 21:352–364.

Lu, F. C. and Lavallée, A. (1965) The acute toxicity of some synthetic colors used in drugs and foods. *Can. Pharm. J.* 97:30.

McNamara, B. P. (1976) Concepts in health evaluation of commercial and industrial chemicals, in *New Concepts in Safety Evaluation,* M. A. Mehlman, R. E. Shapiro and H. Blumenthal (eds), Washington, DC: Hemisphere.

OECD (1982) *Good Laboratory Practice in the Testing of Chemicals.* Organization of Economic Cooperation and Development. 75775 Paris Cedex 16, France.

OECD (1992) *OECD Guidelines for Testing Chemicals. Acute oral toxicity.* Organization of Economic Cooperation and Development. 75775 Paris Cedex 16, France.

Weil, C. S. (1952) Tables for convenient calculation of median effective dose (LD_{50} or ED_{50}) and instructions for their use. *Biometrics* 8:249–263.

WHO (1966) *Specifications for Identity and Purity and Toxicological Evaluation of Food Colors*, WHO/Food Add./66.25. Geneva: World Health Organization.

WHO (1978) *Principles and Methods for Evaluating the Toxicity of Chemicals. Part I*, Environmental Health Criteria 6. Geneva: World Health Organization.

WHO (1990) Principles for toxicological assessment of pesticide residues in food. *Envir. Health Criteria.* 104: Geneva, World Health Organization.

Workshop on Subchronic Toxicity Testing (1980) *Proceedings of the Workshop EPA-560/11-80-028*, N. Page, D. Sawbney and M. G. Ryon (eds), Springfield, VA: National Technical Information Service.

Additional reading

Ecobichon, D. J. (1992) *The Basis of Toxicity Testing.* Boca Raton, FL: CRC Press.

Appendix 6.1 General observations, clinical laboratory tests, and pathology examinations that may be used in short- and long-term toxicity studies

Organ or organ system	General observations	Clinical laboratory tests on blood	Pathology examination*
Liver	Discoloration of mucus membranes, edema, ascites	ALT (SGPT), AP, AST (SGOT), cholesterol, total protein, albumin, globulin	Liver†
Urinary system	Urine volume, consistency, color	BUN, total protein, albumin, globulin	Kidney and urinary bladder†
Gastrointestinal (G.I.) system	Diarrhea, vomit, stool, appetite	Total protein, albumin, globulin, sodium, potassium	Stomach, G.I. tract, gallbladder (if present), salivary gland, pancreas
Nervous system	Posture, movements, responses, behavior		Brain, spinal cord, and sciatic nerve
Eye	Appearance, discharge, ophthalmologic examination		Eye and optic nerves
Respiratory system	Rate, coughing, nasal discharge	Total protein, albumin, globulin	One lung with a major bronchus
Hematopoietic system	Discoloration of mucus membranes, lethargy, weakness	Packed red cell volume, hemoglobin, erythrocyte count, total and differential leukocyte count, platelet count, prothrombin time, activated partial thromboplastin time	Spleen, thymus, mesenteric lymph nodes, bone marrow smear and section
Reproductive system	Appearance and palpation of external reproductive organs	FSH, LH, estrogen, testosterone	Testes and epididymis or ovaries. Uterus or prostate and seminal vesicles†
Endocrine system	Skin, hair coat, body weight, urine, and stool characteristics	Glucose, Na, K, AP (dog), cholesterol	Thyroid, adrenal, pancreas
Skeletal system	Growth, deformation, lameness	Calcium, phosphorus, AP	Bone and breakage strength
Cardiovascular system	Rate and characteristic of pulse, rhythm, edema, ascites	AST	Heart, aorta, small arteries in other tissues
Skin	Color, appearance, odor, hair coat	Total protein, albumin, globulin	Only in dermal studies
Muscle	Size, weakness, wasting, decreased activity	AST creatine phosphokinase	Only if indicated by observations, clinical chemistry, or gross lesions

Source: Adapted from: Workshop on Subchronic Toxicity Testing, 1980.

Notes
*All animals should undergo thorough gross examination; organs or tissues listed should be examined microscopically.
†These organs should also be weighed.

Chapter 7

Carcinogenesis

CONTENTS

Introduction

Historical background

The relation between cancer and exposure to chemicals have long been noted. Thus, in 1761 Hill found users of tobacco snuff had a high rate of nasal cancer, and Pott observed in 1775 that exposure to soot by chimney sweeps induced cancer of the scrotum. Twenty years later, Sommering noted that cancer of the lip was often associated with pipe smoking. Rehn discovered in 1895 that bladder tumors occurred among workers in aniline dye factories. In the twentieth century, cancers induced by a variety of chemicals under different exposure conditions have been observed.

In view of the seriousness of carcinogenesis, and the rapid development of new chemicals, many governmental agencies as well as academic and industrial laboratories have undertaken extensive research and testing in laboratory animals. These endeavors have provided leads for further epidemiological studies.

Definition and identification

The term *chemical carcinogenesis* is generally defined to indicate the induction or enhancement of neoplasia by chemicals. Although in the strict etymologic sense this term means the induction of carcinomas, it is widely used to indicate tumorigenesis. In other words, it includes not only epithelial malignancies (carcinomas) but also mesenchymal malignant tumors (sarcomas). The cells tend to replicate, thereby invading surrounding tissues and metastasizing to remote parts of the body.

A chemical may be identified as a carcinogen based on observations in humans and supported by tests in laboratory animals. Human data may be derived from clinical observations as noted above. However, the relationship between the development of a cancer and the exposure to a chemical is complex. Firstly, there is a long latency, generally in years or decades, between the exposure and the development of the cancer. Furthermore, humans are exposed to a multiplicity of potentially carcinogenic factors. In view of these facts, very extensive epidemiological studies are needed.

In addition to human data, laboratory tests in animals can provide valuable supporting evidence. An important one involves chronic exposure of animals to the test chemical. However, animals, as humans, develop cancer even without being exposed to a known carcinogen. In view of this, it is generally agreed (e.g., WHO, 1969) that the presence of one or more of the following responses of the test animal be considered as positive for carcinogenesis:

1 An increase in the frequency of one or several types of tumors that also occur in the controls
2 The development of tumors not seen in the controls
3 The occurrence of tumors earlier than in the controls
4 An increase in the number of tumors in individual animals, compared to the controls.

Weight of evidence

Evidence of carcinogenicity consists of human and animal data. However, because of interspecies differences in response to chemicals, sound human data are given much greater weight. In fact, the earliest discoveries of chemical carcinogens were made in humans, as noted above (p. 90). In view of the seriousness of cancer, however, it would be grossly imprudent to wait for relevant results to be generated from long-term human studies to assess each chemical for its carcinogenicity. Consequently, appropriate studies need be carried out in animals. The significance of the results unfortunately varies greatly among different studies. For example, aflatoxin B_1 induced tumors in a variety of animals, with small doses (in ppb), and with a relatively short latent period. On the other hand, saccharin yielded positive results inconsistently, with very large doses (in tens of thousands ppm), and only after very long periods of treatment. Furthermore, the experimental design and conduct of the studies also differ in their adequacy (see pp. 107–108).

To facilitate the evaluation of such diverse findings, a *weight of evidence* scheme has been adopted. The findings may be considered "sufficient" when there are benign and malignant tumors in multiple species or strains or in multiple experiments, or there are large numbers of tumors or at an unusual site or being that of a special type.

"Limited" evidence means positive results in only one species, strain or experiment, or when the experimental design or conduct is inadequate. "Inadequate" evidence applies to results that are difficult to interpret. Similarly, data obtained in humans also vary greatly in their significance. Using these criteria, EPA (1996) and IARC (1987) classified chemical carcinogens in five categories (Table 7.1).

Mode of action

Chemical carcinogenesis, as shown in Figure 7.1, is a multistage process. Carcinogenic chemicals act by initiating certain genetic changes in a cell, promoting the formation of a neoplasm, converting the neoplasm to a cancer, or enhancing the activity of another chemical.

Table 7.1 Classification of carcinogens based on "weight of evidence"

Categories	IARC	EPA	Human data	Animal data
Human carcinogen	I	A	Sufficient	Sufficient or limited
Probable human carcinogen	2A	B1, B2[1]	Limited or inadequate[2]	Sufficient
Possible human carcinogen	2B	C	Absent or inadequate	Sufficient or limited[2]
Not classifiable	3	D	Absent or inadequate	Inadequate or absent
Not carcinogenic	4	E	Absent or extensive negative data	Negative evidence in at least two species

Notes
1 EPA classifies carcinogens with sufficient animal data as "Probable Human Carcinogen" and places them in Category B1 or B2 depending on the weight of the human data.
2 IARC accepts positive genotoxicity in lieu of human data.

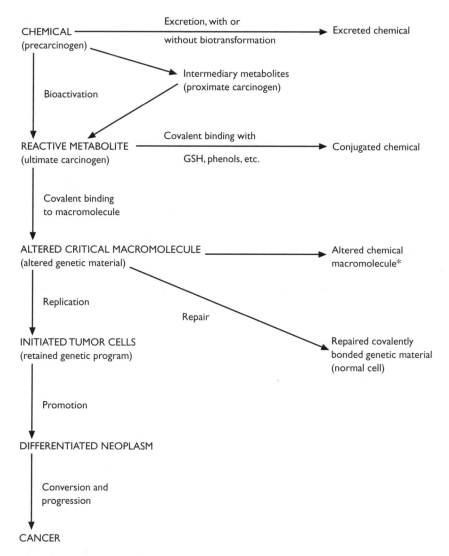

Figure 7.1 Schematic diagram depicting fate of a genotoxic carcinogen and its relation with carcinogenesis. Events in the left-hand column lead to cancer formation, whereas those in the right-hand column are harmless. Asterisk indicates the step may be important during other stages of carcinogenesis.

Bioactivation

Most carcinogenic chemicals per se are inactive. However, they undergo bioactivation in the body to yield reactive metabolites. A common type of reactive metabolite is epoxide. For example, aflatoxin B_1 is converted to

xin-8,9-epoxide. Benzene, vinyl chloride, and a number of polycyclic
ocarbons also form epoxide. Other carcinogens, such as AAF and
certain aminoazo dyes form N-hydroxy derivatives (see Appendix 3.1).
Certain chemicals are bioactivated to ultimate carcinogens via an intermediary step. An example of this is benzo-a-pyrene (BaP) which forms BaP-
7,8-epoxide, the intermediary carcinogen. The latter then transforms to
BaP-7,8-diol-9,10-epoxide, the ultimate carcinogen.

Interaction with macromolecules

The reactive metabolites bind with macromolecules. Some of them, such as
proteins, may not play a critical role in carcinogenesis. However, when
DNA is the target, the reaction may lead to point mutation, frame-shift
mutation and others. These changes may not persist: they may be reversed
by an error-free DNA repair or disappear when the cell dies.

Initiation

If the cell with an altered DNA undergoes mitosis, the alteration will be
retained. The cell with the altered DNA is termed an "initiated" cell.
Depending on the site of the alteration, the cell may be partially or fully
neoplastic. The process generally involves the conversion of proto-
oncogenes to oncogenes.

Proto-oncogenes may be converted to *oncogenes* through translocation
to a different chromosomal site, or other mechanisms such as genetic
amplification, insertions, and gene mutation (Bishop, 1987). In addition,
there are *onco-suppressor genes*; a lack of their expression or an inactiva-
tion of their products may also lead to carcinogenesis (Weinberg, 1989).
One of them, the p53 suppressor gene, is mutated in about half of human
cancers (Greenblatt *et al.*, 1994; Sugimura and Ushijima, 2000).

Promotion

The initiated tumor cell, with altered genotype and phenotype, may remain
dormant for a long period of time before it becomes a tumor through cell
proliferation in the presence of *promoters* (Butterworth and Goldworthy,
1991). The dormancy is probably due to the suppressant influence of the
surrounding normal cells exerted through certain intercellular communication (Trosko and Chang, 1988). The influence can be reduced by programmed cell death (apoptosis), cell killing (e.g., from cytotoxic
chemicals), cell removal (e.g., partial hepatectomy), growth factors (e.g.,
hormones), and other factors.

While initiation is generally considered to be a permanent process,
promotion is not. Furthermore, it is reversible. Therefore, for an initiated

cell to continue to replicate, it must be exposed to a promoter more or less continuously.

Conversion and progression

These are characterized by biochemical and/or morphological changes in the activity or structures of the genome. The mechanism of action is not fully understood, but may involve activation of the initiated cells by exposure to clastogenic agents or complete carcinogens (Pitot *et al.*, 1988). During this period, the neoplasm may convert from benign to malignant tumor which is invasive and metastatic.

Similar to initiation, progression is an irreversible process. Table 7.2 provides a list of the characteristics of initiation, promotion and progression.

Categories of carcinogens

Carcinogens may also be classified according to their *mode of action* into genotoxic and nongenotoxic carcinogens.

Genotoxic carcinogens

Genotoxic carcinogens initiate tumors by producing DNA damage (Figure 7.1). There are two types.

Direct-acting carcinogens

These chemicals are also known as ultimate carcinogens. They are electrophilic and can bind to DNA and other macromolecules. Examples are alkyl and aryl epoxides, lactones, sulfate esters, nitrosamides, nitrosoureas, and platinum amine chelates. Because of their high reactivity, these direct-acting carcinogens are often more active *in vitro* but less so *in vivo*.

Precarcinogens

They are also known as procarcinogens. They require conversion through bioactivation to become ultimate carcinogens, either directly or via an intermediary stage, the proximate carcinogens. Most of the presently known chemical carcinogens fall into this class. These include the polycyclic aromatic hydrocarbons (PAH), aromatic amines, halogenated hydrocarbons, nitrosamines, cycasin, aflatoxin B, pyrrolizidine alkaloids, safrole, and thioamides. Different types of bioactivations (such as formation of epoxides, N-hydroxy derivatives) are involved in their conversion to the direct-acting agents, as discussed in Chapter 3. These chemicals may also

Table 7.2 Morphologic and biologic characteristics of the stages of initiation, promotion, and progression in hepatocarcinogenesis in the rat

Initiation	Promotion	Progression
Irreversible with constant "stem cell" potential. Initiated "stem cell" not morphologically identifiable	Reversible	Irreversible Measurable and/or morphologically discernible alteration in cell genome's structure
Efficacy sensitive to xenobiotic and other chemical factors	Promoted cell population existence dependent on continued administration of the promoting agent	
Spontaneous (fortuitous) occurrence of initiated cells can be quantitated Requires cell division for "fixation"	Efficiency sensitive to dietary and hormonal factors	Growth of altered cells sensitive to environmental factors during early phase
Dose–response does not exhibit a readily measurable threshold	Dose–response exhibits measurable threshold and maximal effect dependent on dose of initiating agent	Benign and/or malignant neoplasms characteristically seen
Relative effect of initiators depends on quantitation of focal lesions following defined period of promotion	Relative effectiveness of promoters depends on time and dose rate to reach maximal effect and dose rate	"Progressor" agents act to advance promoted cells into this stage but may not be initiating agents

Source: Pitot, Beer, and Hendrich, 1988.

activate proto-oncogene to oncogene, and inactivate onco-suppressor genes.

As noted above, timely and error-free DNA repair play an important part in the prevention of neoplastic transformation. An interesting example is dimethylnitrosamine. Its damage to hepatocyte DNA is rapidly repaired in the rat but only slowly in the hamster, and the latter is thus more susceptible than the rat to this carcinogen. Furthermore, in the rat it induces tumors in the brain where the repair mechanism is deficient (see p.45).

Nongenotoxic carcinogens

These substances do not damage DNA but enhance the growth of tumors induced by genotoxic carcinogens or induce tumors through other mechanisms. These are briefly described below.

Cocarcinogens

These substances enhance the effects of genotoxic carcinogens when given simultaneously. They may act by effecting an increase in the concentration of the initiator, the genotoxic carcinogen itself, or that of the reactive metabolite. This can be achieved either by an increase of the absorption of the carcinogen, via the gastrointestinal tract or the skin, or by an increase of the bioactivation. The same result can also be achieved through a decrease of the elimination of the initiator either by inhibiting the detoxification enzymes or by depleting the endogenous substrates involved in phase II reactions, such as glutathione.

Apart from increasing the concentration of the reactive species at the site of action, cocarcinogens may inhibit the rate or fidelity of DNA repair, or they may enhance conversion of DNA lesions to permanent alterations.

Tobacco smoke contains relatively small amounts of genotoxic carcinogens, such as PAH and nitrosamines; its marked carcinogenic effects are perhaps attributed to catechols which act as cocarcinogens.

Promoters

These chemicals increase the effects of initiators when given subsequently. The classic example of this phenomenon was provided by studies demonstrating that an initial application on mouse skin of a carcinogenic PAH did not induce skin cancer until after applying, at the same site, phorbol esters from croton oil (Berenblum and Shubik, 1947, 1949). The application of the promoters could be delayed for months or even a year without losing the effect. These studies clearly demonstrate the *two-stage* process of carcinogenesis as well as the persistence of the effect of the initiator.

Incidentally, croton oil is also cocarcinogenic since it is effective when applied at the same time as the initiator.

The possible mechanisms of action of promoters include:

1 stimulation of cell proliferation through cytotoxicity or hormonal effects;
2 inhibition of intercellular communication, thereby releasing the initiated cells from the restraint exercised by the surrounding normal cells; and
3 immunosuppression.

Cytotoxicants such as nitrilotriacetic acid (NTA), a noneutrophying replacement for phosphate in household detergent, produce tumors through cell proliferation resulting from cell injury and death. Unleaded gasoline and a number of other chemicals have been shown to induce renal tubular necrosis resulting from deposition of $\alpha 2u$-globulin in male rats. The cell death and subsequent regeneration are believed to cause kidney tumors in male rats (Swenberg et al., 1989).

Hormones such as estradiol and diethylstilbestrol have been shown to cause an increase in tumors in animals (e.g., breast cancer in mice) and in humans (e.g., endometrial cancer in menopausal females maintained on estrogen). These substances are not genotoxic but act as promoters. The actual initiators are not known. Androgens have little, if any, carcinogenic effect. The herbicide aminotriazole and certain fungicides induce thyroid tumors also through a hormonal mechanism (McClain, 1989).

Gap junction intercellular communication is an important mechanism in regulating cell growth. A number of chemicals interfere with this mechanism, thereby inducing hyperplasia and acting as promoters in carcinogenesis (Trosko and Chang, 1988). Klaunig (1991) listed, among others, a number of pesticides (e.g., chlordane, DDT, dieldrin, endosulfan, lindane) and pharmaceuticals (phenobarbital and diazepam) as being able to inhibit hepatic gap junctional intercellular communication.

Immunosuppressive drugs such as cyclosporin A and azathioprine are increasingly being used in conjunction with organ transplantation. They have been shown to cause leukemias and sarcomas in some of these patients and in mice and rats. The genotoxic agents are likely to be viruses, and the immunosuppressive drugs promote the development of the tumors through nongenotoxic mechanisms (Ryffel, 1992).

Peroxisome Proliferators consist of a variety of chemicals that have the common property of inducing rodent liver tumors and increasing peroxisomes in liver cells. These chemicals have therefore been considered as a special class of carcinogen (Reddy and Lalwani, 1983). Examples are hypolipidemic drugs such as clofibrate and fenofibrate, certain phthalate plasticizers such as di(2-ethylhexyl) phthalate, and the solvent 1,1,2-

tricholoroethylene. These chemicals are not genotoxic, but by increasing the number of peroxisomes, they may increase the formation of H_2O_2, leading to the formation of reactive oxygen species and thereby enhancing cell replication (Lake, 1995).

Solid state carcinogens

These are exemplified by asbestos and implanted materials such as plastics, metal, and glass. These substances has no genotoxicity, and they produce tumors of mesenchymal origin. While the precise mode of action is not known, the tumors they induce are preceded by an exuberant foreign-body reaction including hyperplastic fibrosis with a high frequency of chromosomal changes in the preneoplastic cells (Weisburger and Williams, 1993).

Metals and metalloids

Arsenic, cadmium, chromium, nickel and their compounds are carcinogenic in humans. A number of others such as beryllium, cobalt and lead are considered to be carcinogens in animals (IARC, 1987). Arsenic was thought to be an exception in that it is carcinogenic in humans but not in animals. Recent data, however, show that intratracheal instillation of As_2O_3 in Syrian hamsters resulted in an increase in pulmonary adenomas, and after intrauterine exposure, apparently caused lung tumors in mice.

The mechanisms of metal carcinogenesis are not fully understood, but may involve genotoxic and/or epigenetic activities. Sunderman (1984) has listed a number of promising avenues for research. Among them are the formation of cross-links between DNA and proteins or between adjacent DNA strands, and impairment of the fidelity of DNA replication by altering the conformation of DNA polymerases. These substances may be classified as genotoxic carcinogens since they alter the gene expression in one way or another. In addition, damages of cytoskeleton by certain metals may contribute to their carcinogenicity (Chou, 1989).

Secondary carcinogens

This term has been used to refer to substances that are not directly carcinogenic but can induce cancer following a distinctly noncarcinogenic effect. For example, polyoxyethylene monostearate (Myrj 45), at very high doses, elicited bladder stones that in turn caused bladder tumors. No tumors were observed in any of the animals that had no bladder stones. On the other hand, this term has also been used in connection with those genotoxic carcinogens that require bioactivation.

Some human carcinogens/target organs

As noted above, the designation of a chemical, or mixture, as a human carcinogen is based on sufficient human data and, as a rule, some animal data. Human carcinogens induce cancers in different organs or systems. Table 7.3 lists the target organs of some human carcinogens, grouped by the "reason"/site of exposure.

Table 7.3 Some human carcinogens and their target organs

Dietary and lifestyle	
Aflatoxin	Liver
Alcoholic beverages	Pharynx, esophagus, liver, larynx, oral cavity
Betal chewing	Mouth, pharynx, larynx
Tobacco smoke	Lung, larynx, oral cavity, pharynx, esophagus, pancreas, kidney
Industrial and environmental	
p-Aminobiphenyl	Bladder
Arsenic	Skin, bronchus, liver
Asbestos	Lung, pleura, peritoneum
Benzene	Bone marrow
Benzidine	Bladder
Cadmium	Lung, prostate
Chromium	Respiratory tract
2-Naphthylamine	Bladder
Nickel	Nasal sinus, bronchus
Polynuclear aromatic hydrocarbons, from coke, coal, tar, etc.	Skin, bronchus
Vinyl chloride monomer	Liver
Wood dust	Nasal sinus
Manufacturing	
Aluminum production	Lung, bladder
Auramine manufacture	Bladder
Boot and shoe manufacture	Nasal cavity, hematopoietic system
Coke production	Skin, lung, kidney
Iron and steel founding	Nasal cavity
Magenda manufacture	Bladder
Painting	Lung
Rubber industry	Bladder, hematopoietic system
Medicinal	
Azathioprine	Lymph node, skin
Cyclophosphamide	Bladder, bone marrow
Estrogens	Cervix, uterus, breast
Methoxypsoralem with UV radiation	Skin
Phenacetin	Renal pelvis
Thorotrast	Liver

In addition to the carcinogens related to diet and lifestyle, it is generally recognized that high intake of fat and/or calories, and deficiencies in vitamins A and E pose risks of increases of certain cancers. However, these factors, in the strict sense, are not carcinogens, but they modify/promote carcinogenesis by certain indirect mechanisms. Caloric restriction reduces carcinogenesis and increases survival time.

As noted above, certain biochemical changes take place in the body after exposure to a carcinogen. Some of these changes can be detected in biological samples. Clinically, they may serve to monitor such exposure or to assess the progress of cancer and progress of treatment. Appendix 7.2 describes a few examples to illustrate their uses.

Tests for carcinogenicity

Short-term tests for mutagenesis/carcinogenesis

In recent years, a number of relatively simple and much shorter tests have been devised and employed to detect the mutagenic activity of chemicals. These tests utilize a variety of systems, including microbes, insects, and mammalian cells, as well as a battery of parameters such as gene mutation, chromosomal effects, and DNA repair. These mutagenesis tests and tests using cell transformation as end points will be described and discussed in the next chapter.

Although not all mutagens are carcinogenic, nor vice versa, the relationship between these two activities is nevertheless so close that mutagenesis tests are performed frequently as a rapid screening of chemicals for their potential carcinogenicity. To improve the reliability of the results, a battery of these tests is usually conducted (e.g., U.S. ISGC, 1986). Weisburger and Williams (1993) recommended the following short-term *in vitro* tests:

1 bacterial mutagenesis,
2 mammalian mutagenesis,
3 mammalian cell DNA repair,
4 chromosome integrity, and
5 cell transformation.

The results of these tests are also useful in defining the mechanism of action. Descriptions of these tests are provided in Chapter 8.

Limited carcinogenicity tests

Limited carcinogenicity tests are superior to the mutagenesis tests in that the end-point is tumor formation. Furthermore, the duration of these tests is much shorter than that of the long-term carcinogenicity studies.

Skin tumors in mice

Mouse skin responds to topical application of chemicals, such as poly-cyclic aromatic hydrocarbons, and crude products, such as tars from coal and petroleum, by the formation of papillomas and carcinomas. This procedure, introduced by Berenblum and Shubik (1947), has been widely used. Mouse skin responds positively apparently because it has the enzymes that convert the substances into active metabolites.

Some chemicals act as initiator and as promoter; they may therefore be referred to as complete carcinogens. Others act mainly or exclusively as initiators. Their carcinogenicity is revealed only after the application of a promoter. Results obtained in the mouse skin test reported in the literature on the effects of chemicals as initiators and as promoters have been compiled by Pereira (1982).

Pulmonary tumors in mice

Strain A mice spontaneously have an essentially 100% lung tumor incidence by 24 months of age. Positive results from carcinogens can be obtained in about 24 weeks when few controls have tumors. With some chemicals, the test can be completed in 12 weeks (Shimkin and Stoner, 1975).

Altered foci in rodent liver

It has been demonstrated that distinct liver foci appear before the development of hepatocarcinoma. These foci are resistant to iron accumulation, a phenomenon that can be identified histochemically. There are also abnormalities in certain enzymes, which can be demonstrated histochemically. The latter alteration occurs in rats but not in mice. These foci can be detected within three weeks of exposure and occur in large numbers in 12–16 weeks (Goldfarb and Pugh, 1982).

Breast cancer in female rats

Polycyclic hydrocarbons can induce breast cancers in young female Sprague-Dawley and Wistar rats. The tumors can develop in less than six months (Huggins *et al.*, 1959). The SD rat lacks progesterone but has very high estrogen levels.

Long-term carcinogenecity studies

These studies are designed to provide definitive information on the carcinogenic effects of chemicals on the test animals. Because of the great expense and time required, they are undertaken usually after a review of other data, such as the chemical structure and results from short-term mutagenesis tests and long-term chronic toxicity studies, which are described, respectively, below and in Chapter 6.

Guidelines on the long-term carcinogenicity studies are outlined in this section. More detailed descriptions and references to some comments are provided in a number of papers (WHO, 1969; OECD, 1981; U.S. ISGC, 1986).

Animals

Rats and mice are generally preferred because of their small size, short life-span, ready availability, and an abundance of information on their response to other carcinogens. Hamsters are also used, especially in studies on cancers of the bladder, breast, gastrointestinal tract, and respiratory tract. Dogs and nonhuman primates are occasionally used for their posit-ive response to 2-naphthylamine, the latter also for their higher phyloge-netic order. But their use is limited because of their large size and relatively long life-span, thereby requiring a 7- to 10-year exposure to the chemical on test.

The characteristics of a preferred strain are:

1 known sensitivity to substances of similar chemical structure,
2 low incidence of spontaneous tumors, and
3 similarity of its rate and pattern of biotransformation and those of humans, if known.

Both sexes should be included in these studies; differences in response to the carcinogenic activity of chemicals are well documented. To provide a sufficient number of animals surviving until the appearance of tumors for statistical analysis, it is a common practice to start the tests with 50 animals of each sex per dose group, including the controls.

Inception and duration

The studies are generally started shortly after weaning the animals to allow maximum duration of exposure. The duration of the studies is generally 24 months in rats and 18 months in mice. If the animals are in good con-dition, the duration may be extended to 30 and 24 months, respectively.

Route of administration

The chemical under test should be given to the animals by the route of human exposure and the usual route is oral. This principle readily applies to food additives and contaminants as well as most drugs. For industrial and environmental chemicals, the main route of entry is inhalation. Alternatively, the test chemical may be instilled intratracheally.

Doses and treatment groups

Usually two or three dose levels are included in such studies. In addition, control groups are also included for comparison. The doses are selected on the basis of the short-term studies and metabolism data, with the aim that the high dose would produce some minor signs of toxicity but not significantly reduce the life-span of the animals. The two lower doses are generally some fractions of the high dose (e.g., $\frac{1}{2}$ and $\frac{1}{4}$) and are expected to permit the animals to survive in good health or until a tumor develops.

The "maximally tolerated dose" (MTD) is generally used as the high dose. It is estimated from 90-day studies and defined as one that would (1) not produce morphologic evidence of toxicity of a severity that interferes with the interpretation of the long-term study, and (2) not comprise so large a fraction of the animal's diet that it might lead to nutritional imbalance (U.S. ISGC, 1986). However, the use of MTD has been criticized, especially when it is much higher than the expected human exposure; there is the possibility of alteration of metabolic pattern by "overloading" the animals (Mermelstein et al., 1994).

An untreated group consisting of the same number, or a larger number, of animals as each dose group is included. In addition to these negative controls, another group of animals is often incorporated that is given a known carcinogen at a dose level that had been shown to be carcinogenic. The positive controls provide more confidence in the results on the test chemical by serving as a check on the sensitivity of the particular lot of animals used as well as the adequacy of the facilities and procedures in the specific laboratory. It will also provide some indication of the relative potency of the test chemical. If a vehicle, such as acetone or dimethyl sulfoxide, is to be used, its possible effect should also be tested in a group of animals as vehicle control.

Observations and examinations

The animals should be examined daily for mortality and morbidity. Dead and moribund animals should be removed from the cage for gross and microscopic examinations whenever the condition of the tissues permit. The onset, location, size, and growth of any unusual tissue masses should be carefully examined and recorded. Signs of toxicity should also be noted. All animals found dead or dying should be subjected to gross autopsy. The survivals at the end of the study should be sacrificed and examined. In addition, a number of organs should be weighed, including the liver, kidneys, heart, testes, ovaries, and brain. Samples of all tissues should be preserved for histologic examination. Microscopic examinations should be done on all tumor growths and all tissues showing gross abnormalities.

Reporting of tumors

As carcinogenesis can manifest in a variety of forms (see "Definition"), it is necessary to record the following:

1 The number of various types of tumors (both benign and malignant), and any unusual tumors
2 The number of tumor-bearing animals
3 The number of tumors in each animal
4 The onset of tumors whenever determinable.

Evaluation

Preliminary assessment

Chemical structure

A number of chemicals are known to be carcinogenic. A list of known and suspected human carcinogens is presented in Table 7.3 and Appendix 7.1 respectively. In addition, a large number of chemicals have been shown to be carcinogenic in animals (see "Genotoxic Carcinogens"). While chemicals that have structures similar to any of these or other carcinogens/ mutagens are not necessarily carcinogens, they should be assigned high priority in carcinogenicity testing programs. In fact, certain chemical structures have been shown to be correlated with carcinogenicity (e.g., Ashby and Tennant, 1988).

Mutagenicity

Mutagenic agents produce heritable genetic changes essentially through their effects on DNA. The mutagenicity tests also provide information on the mode of action as well as on the question as to whether metabolic activation is required for the mutagenicity. While positive results from these tests do not constitute positive evidence that the chemical is carcinogenic, they do indicate that extensive testing is required. Furthermore, the mutagenesis data are useful in the risk assessment of the chemical in question. On the other hand, negative results do not establish the safety of the chemical.

Limited carcinogenicity tests

The end point in these tests is tumor formation. Therefore, certain chemicals, such as cocarcinogens that yield negative results in mutagenesis tests, may be positive in these tests. Positive results from more than one of these limited carcinogenicity tests may be considered unequivocal qualitative evidence of carcinogenicity.

Definitive assessment

Data from well-designed and properly executed long-term carcinogenicity studies generally provide a sound basis for assessment of the carcinogenic potential.

General considerations

Results from these studies are generally more reliable than those from the rapid screening tests. But the conclusiveness of the results depends on a number of factors. For example, too few animals surviving until tumor development may preclude statistical analysis of the data. This event may occur as a result of insufficient animals placed in each dosage group and/or excessive mortality resulting from improper husbandry or from competing toxicity of the chemical given at inordinately high dose levels. The thoroughness of the postmortem examination also plays an important role. This applies to the gross as well as the microscopic examinations.

Tumor incidence

As noted at the beginning of the chapter, carcinogenesis may manifest in one of the four forms or any combination thereof. An appreciable increase in the tumor-bearing animals is the most common form. The occurrence of unusual tumors is an important phenomenon if there are a significant number of them; when one or only a few of them are detected, further critical examination is required. An increase in the number of tumors per animal without a concomitant increase in the tumor-bearing animals usually indicates cocarcinogenicity only. The tumors in the experimental animals may not be at the same stage of development. The stages may include, for example, atypical hyperplasia, benign tumors, carcinomas *in situ*, invasion of adjacent tissues, and metastasis to other parts of the body. Although tumors of the same type but at different stages should be separately tabulated, they should be combined for statistical analysis.

Dose–response relationship

As a rule, a positive dose–response relationship is apparent. However, there may be a lower tumor incidence in the high-dose group. This phenomenon usually results from poor survival among these animals, which succumb to competing toxic effects of the chemical.

Reproducibility of the results

The confidence in a carcinogenicity study is enhanced if the results are produced in another strain of animals. Reproducibility in another species is even more significant. However, if negative results are obtained in another species, this fact may not nullify the positive findings but does justify further investigation.

Evaluation of safety/risk

The various approaches used in the evaluation of the safety/risk of carcinogens are discussed in Chapter 25. The following points, however, are worthy of emphasizing.

First, while the tests enumerated above are a valuable basis for risk/safety assessment, other data relating to the mechanism of action and influences of modifying factors are also essential (U.S. ISGC, 1986). The significant differences between genotoxic and nongenotoxic carcinogens are also considered as valid reasons for assessing their risks differently: it is generally assumed that genotoxic carcinogens exhibit no threshold, whereas nongenotoxic carcinogens induce cancer secondary to other biological effects which are likely to show no-effect dose levels. However, a chemical, such as chloroform, may act as an epigenetic as well as a genotoxic carcinogen.

Furthermore, there are chemicals with carcinogenicity secondary to noncarcinogenic biologic or physical effects that are elicited only at dose levels that could never be approached in realistic human exposure situations. There was general consensus that there are threshold doses for such secondary carcinogens (Lu, 1976; Munro, 1988). The U.S. ISGC (1986) also cautions that extremely high doses of a toxicant may exhibit *qualitatively* different distribution, detoxication, and elimination of the toxicant. The response at such doses therefore may not be applicable to more realistic exposure conditions. Furthermore, evidence of extensive tissue damage, disruption of hormonal function, formation of urinary stones, and saturation of DNA repair function should be carefully reviewed.

Carcinogens also differ in the potency and latent periods. Some carcinogens are active in a particular species, whereas others affect several species and strains of animals. All these factors must be taken into account in evaluating the safety/risk of carcinogens.

Finally, it is important to bear in mind that chemicals differ tremendously in their value to humans. For example, the use of a food color can often be suspended on the basis of suggestive carcinogenicity data. On the other hand, life-saving drugs, even when there is evidence of their carcinogenicity in humans, may still be used clinically. There are also environmental carcinogens, including those in food, that cannot be eliminated with present technology (see also Ames, 1989).

References

Ames, B. N. (1989) What are the major carcinogens in the etiology of human cancer? Environmental pollution, natural carcinogens, and the causes of human cancer: Six errors, in *Important Advances in Oncology, 1989*, V. T. Da Vita, Jr. *et al.* (eds), Philadelphia, PA: J. P. Lippincott.

Ashby, J. and Tennant, R. W. (1988) Chemical structure, *Salmonella* mutagenicity and extent of carcinogenicity among 222 chemicals tested in rodents by the U.S.NCI/NTP. *Mutat. Res.* 204:17–115.

Berenblum, I. and Shubik, P. (1947) A new quantitative approach to the study of the stages of chemical carcinogenesis in the mouse's skin. *Br. J. Cancer* 1:383–391.

Berenblum, I. and Shubik, P. (1949) An experimental study of the initiating stage of carcinogenesis, and a re-examination of the somatic cell mutation theory of cancer. *Br. J. Cancer* 3:109–118.

Bishop, J. M. (1987) The molecular genetics of cancer. *Science* 235:305–311.

Butterworth, B. E. and Goldworthy, T. L. (1991) The role of cell proliferation in multistage carcinogenesis. *Proc. Soc. Exp. Biol. Med.* 198:683–687.

Chou, I. N. (1989) Distinct cytoskeletal injuries induced by As, Cd, Co, Cr, and Ni compounds. *Biomed. Enviro. Sci.* 2:358–365.

Environmental Protection Agency (EPA) (1996) *Guidelines for Arcinogen Risk Assessment.* Fed. Reg. 61:17957–18010.

Fritsche, H. A. (1982) Tumor marker tests in patient monitoring. *Lab. Med.* 13:528–533.

Goldfarb, S. and Pugh, M. B. (1982) The origin and significance of hyperplastic hepatocellular islands and nodules in hepatic carcinogenesis. *J. Am. Coll. Toxicol.* 1:119–144.

Greenblatt, M. S., Bennett, N. P., Hollstein, M., and Harris, C. C. (1994) Mutations in the p53 tumor suppressor gene: Clues to cancer etiology and molecular pathogenesis. *Cancer Res.* 55:4855–5878.

Huggins, C., Briziarelli, G., and Sutton, H., Jr. (1959) Rapid induction of mammary carcinoma in the rat and the influence of hormones on the tumors. *J. Exp. Med.* 109:25–41.

IARC (1987) *Monographs for Carcinogenic Chemicals: Overall Evaluation of Carcinogenicity: An Updating of IARC Monographs*, vols. 1–42, Suppl. 7. Lyon, France: International Agency for Research on Cancer.

Kadlubar, F. F., Butler, M. A., Kaderlick, K. R. *et al.* (1992) Polymorphisms for aromatic amine metabolism in humans: Relevance for human carcinogenesis. *Environ. Health Perspect.* 98:69–74.

Klaunig, J. E. (1991) Alterations in intercellular communication during the stage of promotion. *Proc. Soc. Exp. Biol. Med.* 198:688–692.

Lake, B. G. (1995) Mechanisms of hepatocarcinogenicity of peroxisome-proliferating drugs and chemicals. *Ann. Rev. Pharmacol. Toxicol.* 35:483–507.

Lu, F. C. (1976) Threshold doses in chemical carcinogenesis: Introductory remarks. *Oncology* 33:50.

McClain, R. M. (1989) The significance of hepatic microsomal enzyme induction and altered thyroid function in rats: Implications for thyroid gland neoplasia. *Toxicol. Pathol.* 17: 294–306.

Marks, F. and Furstenberger, G. (1988) Multistage carcinogenesis in animal skin: The reductionist's approach in cancer research, in *Theories of Carcinogenesis*, O. H. Iverson (ed.), Washington, DC: Hemisphere.

Mermelstein, R., Marrow, P. E., and Christian, M. S. (1994) Organ or system overload and its regulatory implications. *J. Am. Col. Toxicol.* 13:143–147.

Munro, I. C. (1988) Risk assessment of carcinogens: Present status and future directions. *Biomed. Environ. Sci.* 1:51–58.

OECD (1981) *OECD Guidelines for Testing of Chemicals.* Paris, France: Organization for Economic Cooperation and Development.

Pereira, M. A. (1982) Mouse skin bioassay for chemical carcinogens. *J. Am. Coll. Toxicol.* 1:47–82.

Pereira, M. A. (ed.) (1983) International Symposium on Tumor Promotion. *Environ. Health Perspect.* 50:3–330.

Pitot, H. C. (1986) Oncogenes and human neoplasia. *Clin. Lab. Med.* 6:167–179.

Pitot, H. C., Beer, D., and Hendrich, S. (1988) Multistage carcinogenesis: The phenomenon underlying the theories, in *Theories of Carcinogenesis*, O. H. Iversen (ed.), Washington, DC: Hemisphere.

Qian, G. S., Ross, R. K., Yu, M. C., Yuan, J. M., Gao, Y. T., Henderson, B. E., Wogan, G. N., and Groopman, J. D. (1994) A follow-up study of urinary markers of aflatoxin exposure and liver cancer risk in Shanghai, China. *Cancer Epid. Biomarkers, Prevention* 3:3–10.

Rachko, D. and Brand, G. (1983) Chromosomal aberrations in foreign body tumorigenesis of mice. *Proc. Soc. Exp. Biol. Med.* 172:382–388.

Reddy, J. K. and Lalwani, N. D. (1983) Carcinogenesis by hepatic peroxisome proliferators: Evaluation of the risk of hyperlipidemic drugs and industrial plasticizers to humans. *CRC Crit. Rev. Toxicol.* 12:1–58.

Ryffel, B. (1992) The carcinogenicity of cyclosporin. *Toxicol.* 73:1–22.

Seidegard, J., Pero, R. W., Markowitz, M. M. *et al.* (1990) Isoenzyme(s) of gluthhione transferase (class mu) as a marker for susceptibility to lung cancer: A follow-up study. *Carcinogenesis* 11:33–36.

Shimkin, M. B. and Stoner, G. D. (1975) Lung tumors in mice: Application to carcinogenesis bioassay. *Adv. Cancer Res.* 21:2–58.

Sugimura, T. and Ushijima (2000) Genetic and epigenetic alterations in carcinogenesis. *Mutat. Res.* 462:235–246.

Sunderman, F. W., Jr. (1984) Recent advances in metal carcinogenesis. *Am. Clin. Lab. Sci.* 14:93–122.

Swenberg, J. A., Short, B., Borghoff, S., Strasser, J., and Charbonneau, M. (1989) The comparative pathobiology of $\alpha_{2\mu}$-globulin nephropathy. *Toxicol. Appl. Pharmacol.* 97:35–46.

Trosko, J. E. and Chang, C. C. (1988) Chemical and oncogene modulation of gap junctional intercellular communication, in *Tumor Promoters: Biological Approaches for Mechanistic Studies and Assay Systems*, R. Langenbach *et al.* (eds), New York, NY: Raven Press.

U.S. EPA (1996) Guidelines for carcinogen risk assessment. *Fed. Reg.* 61:17951.

U.S. ISGC (1986) Chemical carcinogens: A review of the science and its associated principles. U.S. Interagency Staff on Carcinogens. *Environ. Health Perspect.* 67:201–282.

Weinberg, R. A. (1989) Oncogenes, antioncogenes, and the molecular bases of multistep carcinogenesis. *Cancer Res.* 49:3713–3721.

Weisburger, J. H. and Williams, G. M. (1981) Basic requirements of health risk analysis: The decision point approach for systematic carcinogen testing, in *Proceedings of the Third Life Sciences Symposium on Health Risk Analysis*. Philadelphia, PA: Franklin Press.

Weisburger, J. H. and Williams, G. M. (1993) Chemical carcinogenesis, in *Casarett and Doull's Toxicology*, M. O. Amdur, J. Doull, and C. D. Klaassen (eds), New York, NY: McGraw-Hill, pp. 127–200.

WHO (1969) *Principles for the Testing and Evaluation of Drugs for Carcinogenicity*. WHO Tech. Rep. Ser. 426.

Additional reading

WHO (1993) Biomarkers and Risk Assessment: Concepts and Principles. *Envir. Health Criteria* 155, Geneva: World Health Organization.

Appendix 7.1 Probable carcinogenic chemicals

An IARC Working Group (IARC, 1987) concluded that the following are probably carcinogenic to humans:

Acrylonitrile
Adriamycin
Androgenic (anabolic) steroids
Benz[a]anthracene
Benzidine-based dyes
Benzo[a]pyrene
Beryllium and beryllium compounds
Bischloroethyl nitrosourea (BCNU)
1-(2-Chloroethyl)-3-cyclohexyl-1-nitrosourea (CCNU)
Cisplatin
Creosotes
Dibenz[a,h]anthracene
Diethyl sulfate
Dimethylcarbamoyl chloride
Dimethyl sulfate
Epichlorohydrin

Ethylene dibromide
Ethylene oxide
N-ethyl-N-nitrosourea
Formaldehyde
5-Methoxypsoralen
4,4'-Methylene bis(2-chloroaniline) (MOCA)
N-methyl-N'-nitro-N-nitrosoguanidine (MNNG)
N-methyl-N-nitrosourea
Nitrogen mustard
N-nitrosodiethylamine
Nitrosodimethylamine
Phenacetin
Polychlorinated biphenyls
Procarbazine hydrochloride
Propylene oxide
Silica, crystalline
Styrene oxide
Tris(1-aziridinyl)phosphine sulfide (Thiotepa)
Tris(2,3-dibromopropyl) phosphate
Vinyl bromide

Some 200 other chemicals have been recognized by IARC as possible human carcinogens.

Appendix 7.2 Biomarkers of carcinogenesis/human cancers

Biomarkers of exposure and initiation

Initiation is associated with covalent binding of electrophilic carcinogens or their reactive metabolites to DNA. The carcinogen–DNA adduct can be demonstrated and quantified to indicate exposure and effect of the carcinogen. This procedure has been applied to situations wherein human exposure to a particular carcinogen is suspected, for example in the determination of exposure to aflatoxin B_1 and its relationship to hepatocellular carcinoma (Qian et al., 1994).

Biomarker of promotion

Promotion has been most extensively studied in *skin* carcinogenesis. A variety of biochemical changes have been noted in initiated as well as normal cells on treatment with promoters, the most active of which is TPA (12-o-tetradecanoy1 phorbol 13-acetate). The changes include accumulation of plasminogen activator and increased prostaglandin synthesis.

Growth factors, protein kinase C, TPA-and dioxin-responsive elements in genes, interaction of promoters with oncogenes and/or suppressor genes are being studied to determine their role as markers of preneoplasia in the liver.

Tumor markers

α-Fetoprotein (AFP) is a product of fetal liver and hepatocarcinoma. AFP had therefore been used to screen large populations for hepatocellular carcinomas, allowing early detection and treatment. However, it has been shown to be non-specific. Human chorionic gonadotropin (HCG) is a sensitive marker and can be used to detect cancers of male and female sex organs at a subclinical phase. Carcinoembryonic antigen (CEA) is found in patients with carcinoma of the colon and rectum. PSA (prostate-specific antigen) has been shown to be a useful biomarker of tumor and other lesions of the prostate. CA 125 is useful in diagnosing and monitoring treatment of ovarian cancer.

Biomarkers of susceptibility

Individuals with certain genetic disposition may be more susceptible to carcinogenesis. For example, those with xeroderma pigmentosa are prone to skin cancer. Polymorphism of x-oxidation has been linked to susceptibility to colon cancer (Kadlubar et al., 1992) and polymorphism in glutathione S-transferase to increased lung cancer (Seidegard et al., 1990).

Chapter 8

Mutagenesis

CONTENTS

Introduction

Mutagenesis can occur as a result of interaction between mutagenic agents and the genetic materials of organisms. While spontaneous mutation and natural selection are the major means of evolution, a number of toxicants, in recent decades, have been found to be mutagenic to a variety of organisms.

Health hazards

The hereditary effects of human exposure to these mutagenic substances cannot be ascertained at present. However, some spontaneous abortions, stillbirths, and heritable diseases have been shown to be related to changes in DNA molecules and to chromosomal aberrations. There are approximately 1,000 dominant gene mutations responsible for various illnesses, including the hereditary neoplasms such as bilateral retinoblastoma, and about the same number of recessive gene disorders such as sickle-cell anemia, cystic fibrosis, and Tay-Sachs disease. In addition, abnormal chromosomal numbers are associated with such diseases as Down's syndrome, Klinefelter's syndrome, and Edward's syndrome. These have been estimated to occur with an incidence of 0.5% among the live births in the United States. The true effects of any additional mutagen in the environment can only manifest after a lapse of several generations. The seriousness of this matter therefore warrants the extensive investigations in the various fields of mutagenesis.

A number of human diseases are the result of defects of the DNA repair systems. For example, patients with xeroderma pigmentosa are deficient in excision repair in the skin; they are susceptible to ultraviolet light and many chemical carcinogens and thus are prone to developing skin tumors. Those with ataxia telangiectasia have such deficiencies in the lymphoid system and are susceptible to X-rays and the carcinogen methyl nitronitrosoguanidine. Fanconi's anemia is associated with defective DNA repair in the blood and skeleton. The afflicted persons are susceptible to mitomycin C and psoralens.

On the other hand, tests for mutagenicity in recent years have become more widely used because of their value as a rapid screening for carcino-

Table 8.1 Examples of chromosomal abnormalities associated with human cancers

Neoplasm	Abnormality of chromosome
Chronic myelogenous leukemia	Translocation of chromosomes 9 and 22
Acute monocytic leukemia	Loss of long arm of chromosome 11
Small cell lung cancer	Loss of short arm of chromosome 6
Myeloproliferative diseases	Extra chromosome 1
Retinoblastoma	Deletion of chromosome 13

genicity (see Chapter 7). This development stems mainly from the fact that most mutagens have been found to be carcinogens. Furthermore, these tests, with a variety of end points, are useful in the elaboration of the mode of action of carcinogens. It is also worth noting that various gene mutation and chromosomal abnormalities have been detected in human tumors. Some examples are listed in Table 8.1. For a more extensive review on this topic, see Rabbitts' review (1994).

Categories of mutagenesis and their tests

It is well known that DNA, consisting of nucleotide bases, plays a key role in genetics. First, it transmits the genetic information from one generation of cells to the next through self-replication. This is done by the separation of the double strands of the DNA molecule and the synthesis of new daughter strands. Second, the genetic information coded in the DNA molecule is expressed through the transcription of a complementary RNA strand from one strand of DNA, which serves as a template, and the subsequent translation of the information from the RNA to the amino acids in proteins. Every set of three nucleotide bases, a codon, specifies an amino acid. Derangement of the bases therefore alters the amino acid content of the protein synthesized.

In earlier studies, the mutagenic activity was demonstrated mainly in fruit flies and onion root tips because of the simpler techniques involved. More recently, many new test systems have been developed. They range in complexity from microorganisms to intact mammals. The use of such widely different organisms is based on the fact that all double-stranded DNA share the same biochemical characteristics, which are listed in Table 8.2.

At present, there are more than 100 test systems. A number of exemplary tests are outlined in this chapter under four major categories, namely, gene mutation, chromosomal effects, DNA repair and recombination, and others, which are designed to confirm carcinogenicity. Because of the brevity of their description, at least one reference is cited for each test. Additional references and more details are given elsewhere on these and other tests (EPA, 1994; OECD, 1987; Hoffmann, 1996).

Table 8.2 Basic biochemical characteristics of all double-stranded DNA

1	DNA consists of two different purines (guanine, adenine) and two different pyrimidines (thymine and cytosine).
2	A nucleotide pair consists of one purine and one pyrimidine[adenine/thymine (A-T) or guanine/cytosine (G-C)].
3	Nucleotide pairs are connected into a double helix molecule by sugar-phosphate backbone linkages and hydrogen bonding.
4	The A-T base pair is held by two hydrogen bonds, while the G-C is held by three.
5	The distance between each base pair in a molecule is 3.4Å, producing 10 nucleotide pairs per turn of the DNA helix.
6	The number of adenine molecules must equal the number of thymine molecules in a DNA molecule. The same relationship exists for guanine and cytosine molecules. However, the ratio of A-T to G-C base pairs may vary in DNA from species to species.
7	The two strands of the double helix are complementary and antiparallel with respect to the polarity of the two sugar-phosphate backbones, one strand being 3'-5' and the other being 5'-3' with respect to the terminal OH group on the ribose sugar.
8	DNA replicates by a semiconservative method in which the two strands separate and each is used as a template for the synthesis of a new complementary strand.
9	The rate of DNA nucleotide polymerization during replication is approximately 600 nucleotides per second. The helix must unwind to form templates at a rate of 3600 rpm to accommodate this replication rate.
10	The DNA content of cells is variable (1.8×10^9 daltons for *Escherichia coli* to 1.9×10^{11} daltons for human cells).

Source: Brusick, 1987, p. 15.

It is worth noting that gene mutation may be detected in all organisms including bacteria. On the other hand, effects related to chromosomes (aberration, aneuploidy and DNA repair) can only be detected in higher organisms, that is those with chromosomes.

Gene mutation

Gene mutations involve additions or deletions of base pairs or substitution of a wrong base pair in the DNA molecules. Substitutions consist of trans-itions and transversions. The former involve the replacement of a purine (adenine, guanine) by another or a pyrimidine (cytosine, thymine) by another. With transversion, a purine is replaced by a pyrimidine, or vice versa. When the number of base pairs added or deleted is not a multiple of three, the amino acid sequence of the protein coded distal to the addition or deletion will be altered. This phenomenon is called frame-shift mutation and is likely to affect the biologic property of the protein. Figure 8.1 clearly illustrates the effects of a deletion and an addition of a nucleotide base.

In addition, a mutagenic chemical, or a part of it, may be incorporated

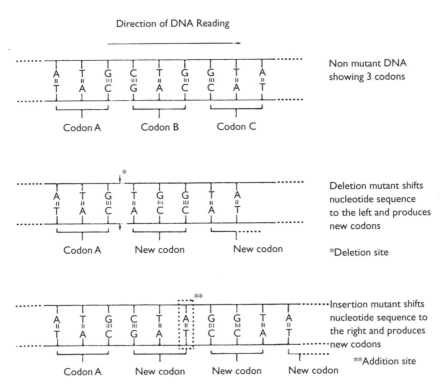

Figure 8.1 Frame-shift mutation resulting from deletion or insertion of a nucleotide base. A series of new codons is formed distal to the deletion or insertion, and hence new amino acids in the protein synthesized.

Source: Brusick, 1987.

into the DNA molecule. For example, a number of electrophilic compounds react with DNA forming covalent addition products, known as "DNA adducts." Thus acetylaminofluorene (AAF) binds specifically to the carbon at the 8-position of guanine. For a partial list of such chemicals, see discussions on procarcinogens in *Categories of carcinogens* in Chapter 7. Alkylating agents, such as ethylnitrosourea and diethyl sulfate, donate an alkyl group to DNA.

These various changes in the DNA molecule may cause the substitution of a new amino acid in the subsequently coded protein molecule or result in a different sequence of amino acids in the protein synthesized. Furthermore, a protein synthesis termination codon may be formed, giving rise to a shortened protein. While the first type of effect may or may not result in a modification of the biologic property of the protein molecule, the latter two types almost invariably do.

Microbial tests in vitro

These involve prokaryotic and eukaryotic microorganisms.

Prokaryotic microorganisms

Such microorganisms consist of various strains of bacteria. For the detection of point mutations the commonly used bacteria are *Salmonella typhimurium* and *Escherichia coli*. Most bacterial systems are intended to detect reverse mutation. For example, the Ames test (Ames, 1971) measures the reversion of histidine-dependent mutants of *S. typhimurium* to the histidine-independent wild type. The mutants are incubated in a medium that contains insufficient histidine to permit visible growth. If the toxicant added to the culture medium is capable of inducing reverse mutation, then the bacteria can become histidine-independent and grow appreciably in the histidine-deficient medium. It is customary to use several strains because of their specificity. Their mutation to histidine independency results from either frame-shift or base-pair substitution; different mutagens may affect one strain but not the other.

A number of strains of *S. typhimurium* have been rendered more sensitive to the effects of mutagens through alterations in the permeability of their cell walls (deficient in lipopolysaccharide) and in their DNA excision repair capabilities (through a specific deletion in the DNA molecule) and through the bearing of an ampicillin-resistance factor (Ames *et al.*, 1975; McCann *et al.*, 1975). These various strains (e.g., TA 98, 100, 1537) may be susceptible to different mutagens.

Since many mutagens are inactive before bioactivation, the test can be carried out with a bioactivating system included in the *in vitro* procedure. The bioactivating system usually consists of the microsomal fraction (containing the mixed-function oxidase system) of the liver of the rat or other animals, although the human liver is also used for special purposes. The activity of the microsomal enzyme is usually enhanced by pretreating the animal with an inducing agent, such as 3-methylcholanthrene, phenobarbital, or polychlorinated biphenyls (PCB). Appropriate cofactors are also added to the mixture prior to incubation.

Strains of *E. coli* that are tryptophan-dependent are also used to detect reverse mutation. Mutagenic changes will result in tryptophan-independent strain (Ames *et al.*, 1975).

Eukaryotic microorganisms

Certain strains of *Saccharomyces*, *Schizosaccharomyces*, *Neurospora*, and *Aspergillus* have been developed to detect mainly reverse mutations and, to a limited extent, forward mutations. Like the bacterial systems, these systems in general also include bioactivating enzymes and cofactors. For example, a type of mutant of *Saccharomyces cerevisiae* requires adenine and produces red-pigmented colonies, whereas the wild type microorganisms are adenine-independent and produce white colonies. Thus the reverse mutation can be determined by the prevalence of white colonies (Brusick and Mayer, 1973).

Microbial tests in vivo (host-mediated assay)

In this type of test, the microorganisms are injected into the peritoneal cavity of the host mammal (usually the mouse). They can also be injected into the circulatory system or the testes. The toxicant is injected into the host, usually prior to the introduction of the microorganisms. After a few hours elapse, the host is sacrificed. The microorganisms are then collected and examined for manifestations of mutation. These assays have the advantage of incorporating the biotransformation of the toxicant in the host mammal but have the drawback that the microorganisms can only be kept in the host for a relatively short time. Apart from microorganisms, cells from multicellular animals can also be used in the host-mediated assay (Gabridge and Legator, 1969). Despite its theoretical advantage, the procedure has been found to be insensitive to certain types of carcinogens and hence is unsuitable as a routine screening procedure (Simmons *et al.*, 1979).

A modified procedure involves pretreatment of the host with a toxicant, collecting the urine from the host, and injecting the urine, which may contain a high concentration of the metabolite(s) of the toxicant, back into the host. This modified procedure demonstrates positive mutagenicity with 2-acetylaminofluorene, which yields negative results with the regular host-mediated assay (Durston and Ames, 1974).

Insects

The fruit fly *Drosophila melanogaster* is the most commonly used insect. It is well characterized genetically. It has the advantage over microorganisms in that it metabolizes toxicants in a manner that is similar to mammals. Furthermore, it is superior to mammals in two respects, namely, its generation time is only 12–14 days, and it can be tested in sufficient numbers at much lower cost.

The sex-linked recessive lethal test measures the lethal effect on the F_2 males after exposing the males of the parental generation. It is the preferred procedure because the X chromosome represents about 20% of the total genome, and it is capable of screening for point mutation and short deletions at about 800 loci on the X chromosome (Lee *et al.*, 1983).

Mammalian cells in culture

The commonly used systems include cells from mouse lymphoma, human lymphoblasts and cells from the lung, ovary, and other tissues of Chinese hamsters. These cells usually maintain a near-diploid chromosome number, grow actively, and have high cloning efficiency. Both forward and reverse mutations can occur, and the mutants respond selectively to nutritional, biochemical, serologic, and drug-resistant growth manipulations.

For example, cells from mouse lymphoma, which are heterozygous at the thymidine kinase locus (TK+/−), may undergo forward mutation, for example, via the action of a mutagen, and become TK−/−. Both genotype TK+/− and TK−/− can grow in a normal medium, but TK−/− can also grow in a medium containing 5-bromo-2′-deoxyuridine (BrdU). The mutagenicity of a toxicant can thus be determined by comparing the growth of the lymphoma cells in the presence and absence of the toxicant both in a medium containing BrdU and in a normal medium (DeMarini et al., 1989).

In Chinese hamsters, as in humans, the use of preformed hypoxanthine and guanine is controlled by an X-linked gene. Mutant cells at these loci are deficient in the enzyme hypoxanthine-guanine phosphoribosyl transferase and can be identified by their resistance to toxic purine analogs, such as 8-azaguanine or 6-thioguanine, that kill the cells that utilize these analogs (DeMarini et al., 1989).

These cell lines are generally deficient in metabolizing enzymes. Therefore, such enzyme systems are often added (microsome-mediated). Alternatively, these cells can be cocultivated with other cells that possess greater ability to biotransform toxicants. Such a cell-mediated system involves the use of freshly isolated hepatocytes as a feeder system (Williams, 1979). It offers an additional advantage of having capabilities to conjugate as well as to degrade toxicants.

Gene mutation tests in mice

The mouse spot test

This test is designed to detect gene mutation in somatic cells. Basically it involves treating pregnant mice whose embryos are heterozygous at specific coat color loci and examining the newborn for any mosaic patches in the fur. Such patches indicate the formation of clones of mutant cells that are responsible for the color of the fur. This test is relatively inexpensive and takes only a few weeks to complete. Although it may yield false-positive results, it has not yet yielded false-negative results. The spot test is therefore a useful prescreen for heritable germinal mutations in mammals (Russell, 1978).

The specific locus test

The specific locus test was developed for determining the mutagenicity of ionizing radiation in the germ cells. This procedure was later adapted to assess the mutagenicity of chemicals (Searle, 1975). It has the advantage of directly detecting in intact mammals the mutagenic effects of toxicants in the germ cells, but it usually requires a very large number of animals.

It involves exposing nonmutant mice to the chemical and subsequently mating them to a multiple-recessive stock. Mutant offspring have altered phenotypes expressed in hair color, hair structure, eye color, ear length, and other traits. Some mutants are mosaic rather than whole animal. Mutation can also be detected by the rejection or acceptance of skin grafts made between first-generation offspring. It can be further characterized immunogenetically (Russell and Shelby, 1985).

Chromosomal effects

The effect of a toxicant on chromosomes may be large enough to be visible microscopically, and manifest as structural aberrations or as changes in number. The former, *aberrations*, include deletions, duplications, and translocations. The latter, *aneuploidy*, involve a decrease or increase in the number of the chromosomes. Some of the effects are heritable.

The mode of action underlying these effects may involve molecular cross-linkage, which may cause an arrest of the synthesis of DNA, thereby leaving a gap in the chromosome. An unsuccessful repair of the DNA damage may also be responsible. Nondisjunction (failure of a pair of chromosomes to separate during mitotic division) can lead to mosaicism. A nondisjunction during gametogenesis (meiotic nondisjunction) gives rise to daughter cells that contain either one extra chromosome or one less than normal. The former is known as *trisomy* and the latter *monosomy*.

A number of test systems have been developed to determine the chromosomal effects. The following are the major systems.

Insects

Drosophila melanogaster has the advantage in that the chromosomes of some of its cells are superior in size and morphology. In addition, the chromosomal effects can be readily confirmed genetically, such as the sex-linked recessive lethalilty. The chromosomal effects include loss of X and Y chromosomes, and translocations of fragments between second and third chromosomes.

Effects on the sex chromosome can also be detected by phenotypic changes, such as body color, and color and shape of the eye (National Research Council, 1983).

Cytogenetic studies with mammalian cells

In vitro tests

For cytogenetic tests, the commonly used cells are derived from Chinese hamster ovaries and human lymphocytes. These cells are cultured in suitable media. They are then exposed to different concentrations of the test chemical in the presence or absence of a bioactivator system (usually the microsomal fraction of the rat liver homogenate). The test generally includes two positive control mutagens, namely, ethylmethane sulfonate, which is direct-acting, and dimethylnitrosamine, which requires bioactivation. After an appropriate incubation period, the cell division is arrested by the addition of colchicine. The cells are then mounted, stained, and scored (Preston et al., 1981).

An example of scoring of *aberrations* is shown below: chromatid gap, chromatid break, chromosome gap, chromatid deletion, fragment, acentric fragment, translocation, triradial, quadriradial, pulverized chromosome, pulverized chromosomes, pulverized cells, ring chromosome, dicentric chromosome, minute chromosome, greater than 10 aberrations, polyploid, and hyperploid (Brusick, 1987).

In vivo tests

Mammalian cells used in the *in vivo* study of chromosomal effects include germ cells and somatic tissues. The chemical to be tested is administered to intact animals, such as rodents and humans. The somatic tissues commonly used are bone marrow and peripheral lymphocytes. A classic protocol using bone marrow from mice, rats, or hamsters has been provided by the Ad Hoc Committee of the Environmental Mutagen Society and the Institute for Medical Research (1972). The scoring is the same as in the *in vitro* test.

The *micronucleus* test is a somewhat simpler *in vivo* procedure. It involves the use of polychromatic erythrocyte stem cells of CD-1 mice. Six hours after two treatments with the test chemical, given 24 hours apart, the animals are killed and the bone marrow is collected from both femurs. An increase in micronucleated cells over the controls (about 0.5%) is considered positive (Schmid, 1976). Many other types of cells may also be used. These micronuclei represent fragments of chromosome and chromatid resulting from spindle/centromere dysfunction.

For tests on *germ cells,* the male animal is usually used. In order to allow cells of different stages of spermatogenesis to be exposed, the chemical is given daily for five days and the animals sacrificed one, three, and five weeks following the last dose. The sperm is collected surgically from the caudae epididymides. After mounting and staining, the incidence of abnormal spermheads is determined, and it is compared with the negative and positive controls (Wyrobek and Bruce, 1975).

Sister Chromatid Exchange (SCE)

This test measures a reciprocal exchange of DNA between two sister chromatids of a duplicating chromosome. The exchange takes place because of a breakage and reunion of DNA during its replication. The test can be done with mouse lymphoma cells, Chinese hamster ovary cells, and human lymphocytes. It may also be done *in vivo*, by collecting cells from treated animals. The procedure involves labeling of cells with 5-BrdU (5-bromo-deoxyuridine), and after two cycles of replication, the cells are stained with a fluorescent-plus-Giemsa technique. The frequency of sister chromatid exchanges per cell and per chromosome is scored and compared. The exchange is visible because, in one chromatid, the semiconservative replication of DNA results in a substitution of BrdU in *one* polynucleotide strand, and in the other chromatid the BrdU is substituted in *both* polynucleotide strands (Wolff, 1977).

While the mechanism underlying SCE is not fully understood, it shows that a chemical has attacked the chromosomes or impaired their replication. The test has the advantage of being simple to perform. Furthermore, its endpoint is often observed at concentrations much lower than those required with other tests (NRC, 1983).

Dominant lethal test in rodents

This test is designed to demonstrate toxic effects on germ cells in the intact male animal, usually the mouse or rat. The effects can manifest in the mated females as dead implantations and/or preimplantation losses (the difference between the number of corpora lutea and the number of implantations). These effects are generally due to chromosomal damages, which lead to developmental errors that are fatal to the zygote. However, other cytotoxic effects can also cause early fetal death (see also Chapter 18).

Heritable translocation test in mice

This test is intended to detect the heritability of chromosomal damages. The damages, consisting of reciprocal translocation in the germ line cells of the treated male mice, are transmitted to the offspring. By mating the male F_1 progeny with untreated female mice, the chromosomal effects are revealed by a reduction of viable fetuses. The presence of these reciprocal translocations can be verified by the presence of translocation figures among the double tetrads at meiosis (Adler, 1980).

DNA repair and recombination

These biologic processes are not mutations per se, but they occur after DNA damage. These phenomena therefore indicate existence of DNA damages, which are caused essentially by mutagens. There are three main types of DNA damages that can be repaired: missing, incorrect, or altered bases; interstrand cross-links; and strand breaks.

Bacteria

Among *E. coli* there are those with normal DNA polymerase I enzyme, which is capable of repairing DNA damage, and those deficient in this enzyme. Mutagens induce DNA damage and thereby impair the growth of the *E. coli* that is deficient in the repair enzyme, whereas the growth of those with this enzyme is not affected. The DNA repair-efficient strain is included to rule out the effect of cytotoxicity (Rosenkranz *et al.*, 1976).

Similarly, there are also recombination efficient and deficient strains of *Bacillus subtilis*. Damage to DNA is repaired in the former strain through recombination but not in the latter. Mutagens will thus inhibit the growth of the latter but not the former.

Yeasts

Various eukaryotic microorganisms, such as *Saccharomyces cerevisiae*, have been used to test the mutagenicity of chemicals by the induced mitotic crossing-over and mitotic gene conversion. These effects on DNA result in the growth of colonies with different colors (Zimmermann *et al.*, 1984).

Mammalian cells/UDS

Unscheduled DNA synthesis (UDS) is an indication of DNA repair. It can be detected in human cells in culture. The synthesis is determined by the amount of radioactive thymidine incorporated per unit weight of DNA over the control value. This is done both in the presence and absence of an added activator system (Stich and Laishes, 1973). Such synthesis can also be determined in primary rat liver cells. The extent of DNA synthesis is determined using an autoradiographic method. Since these cells have sufficient metabolic activity, there is no need to add an activator system (Williams, 1979).

Because of their greater relevance to genetic risk, germ cells have also been used in UDS tests: male mice are treated with a suspected mutagen, and [³H]-thymidine ([³H]-dT) is injected intratesticularly. Any incorporation of [³H]-dT into the DNA of meiotic and post-meiotic germ cells (see

p. 252) indicates the production of repairable damage to the DNA (Russell and Shelby, 1985).

Other tests

As noted in Chapter 7, a number of related mutagenesis tests are used to determine carcinogenicity.

In vitro transformation of mammalian cells

Cells from the BALB/3T3 mouse are commonly used in this test. Others include Syrian hamster embryo cells, mouse 10T1/2 cells, and human cells. Normally these cells will grow in the culture medium to form a monolayer. Those treated with a carcinogen, however, will reproduce without being attached to a solid surface and grow over the monolayer. The appearance of such multilayered colonies indicates malignant transformation. This end point can be confirmed by injecting these cells into syngeneic animals. In general, malignant tumors will develop if the cells have undergone transformation (Kakunaga, 1973). Therefore, in general, positive results from this test are especially significant.

Nuclear enlargement test

HeLa cells are grown in culture medium and treated with different concentrations of the chemical on test. After an appropriate duration, the cells are harvested and counted. They are then stripped of their cytoplasmic material and the size of the nucleus is determined with a particle counter. An increase in the nuclear size indicates carcinogenicity of the chemical (Finch et al., 1980).

Evaluation

Selection of test systems

Since mutagens affect the genetic material in different ways, they may yield negative results in one test but positive in others. To rule out false-negatives (and false-positives), it is advisable to conduct several tests, preferably of different categories. OECD (1987) recommended a series of tests for screening, confirmation, and risk assessment (Table 8.3).

The Committee on Chemical Environmental Mutagens of the National Research Council recommended a mutagen assessment program (National Research Council, 1983). It suggests that the mutagenesis tests be placed in three tiers. Tier I consists of (1) the Salmonella/microsome gene-mutation test, (2) a mammalian cell gene-mutation test, and (3) a mammalian cell chromosomal breakage test. If all tests are negative, the chemical is considered

Table 8.3 Utility and application of assays

A	Assays that may be used for mutagen and carcinogen screening
	Salmonella typhimurium reverse mutation assay
	Escherichia coli reverse mutation assay
	Gene mutation in mammalian cells in culture
	Gene mutation in *Saccharomyces cerevisiae*
	In vitro cytogenetics assay
	Unscheduled DNA synthesis *in vitro*
	In vitro sister chromatid exchange assay
	Mitotic recombination in *Saccharomyces cerevisiae*
	In vivo cytogenetics assay
	Micronucleus test
	Drosophila sex-linked recessive lethal test
B	Assays that confirm *in vitro* activity
	In vivo cytogenetics assay
	Micronucleus test
	Mouse spot test
	Drosophila sex-linked recessive lethal test
C	Assays that assess effects on germ cells and that are applicable for estimating genetic risk
	Dominant lethal assay
	Heritable translocation assay
	Mammalian germ cell cytogenetic assay

Source: OECD, 1987.

a presumed mammalian nonmutagen. If two of these tests are positive, it is classified as a presumed mammalian mutagen. If only one is positive, then the Tier II test (*Drosophila* sex-linked lethal-mutation) is conducted. For further screening of the most crucial chemicals, supplemental tests are done. A specific-locus test is recommended for chemicals with a potential mutagenicity in mammalian germ cells, and a dominant lethal test should be done for those having chromosomal effects. See also WHO (1990).

Many chemicals have been tested for genotoxicity (mutagenicity, carcinogenicity and developmental toxicity) using a multiplicity of tests. To facilitate the task of a "weight-of-evidence" analysis of the genotoxicity of the chemicals and an analysis of the merit of the tests used in generating the data, a method has been proposed by the International Commission for Protection Against Environmental Mutagens and Carcinogens (ICPEMC, 1992).

Significance of results

Relation between mutagenicity and carcinogenicity

A number of investigators have shown the relation between carcinogens and mutagens. For example, McCann *et al.* (1975) reported on their study of 300 substances for mutagenicity in the *Salmonella*/microsome test. The results were compared with the reported carcinogenicity or noncarcinogenicity of these substances. The authors demonstrated a high correlation between these toxic effects: 90% (156/175) of carcinogens are mutagenic in the test. Few noncarcinogens showed any degree of mutagenicity.

More recently, Mason *et al.* (1990) compiled information on the correlation between carcinogenicity in rodents and mutagenicity as determined by *S. typhimurium*. The correlations varied between 55% and 93%.

It is of interest to note that many recent studies demonstrate that certain human leukemias, lymphomas, and solid tumors are associated with specific chromosomal alterations, some of which are listed in Table 8.1. Furthermore, gene mutations and chromosomal damages can convert proto-oncogenes to active oncogenes (Bishop, 1991; Barrett, 1993). For further discussions on the effects of such conversion, see the section on "Mode of action" of carcinogenesis, Chapter 7.

Heritable effects

At present there is no direct correlation between laboratory tests for heritable mutations induced by chemical toxicants and human experience. Nevertheless, if a substance has been shown to be mutagenic in a variety of test systems including heritable mutations in intact mammals, it must be considered as a mutagen in humans unless there is convincing evidence to the contrary. Fortunately, for many chemicals, such as food additives, pesticides, cosmetics, and most drugs, where human exposure can be avoided, any incidence of mutagenicity will be sufficient to warrant suspension of their use (see Flamm, 1977). For environmental pollutants and occupational toxicants that are mutagenic, all efforts should be made to reduce human exposure to them.

As mentioned above, the study of mutagenesis is a new discipline. The rapidly accumulating knowledge in this field will, in all probability, improve the interpretation of the significance of the mutagenicity testing results.

References

Ad Hoc Committee of the Environmental Mutagen Society and the Institute of Medical Research (1972) Chromosome methodologies in mutagen testing. *Toxicol. Appl. Pharmacol.* 22:269–275.

Adler, I. D. (1980) New approaches to mutagenicity studies in animals for carcinogenic and mutagenic agents. I. Modification of heritable translocation test. *Teratogen. Carcinogen. Mutagen* 1:75–86.

Ames, B. N. (1971) The detection of chemical mutagens with enteric bacteria, in *Chemical Mutagens: Principles and Methods for Their Detection*, vol. 1, A. Hollander (ed.), New York, NY: Plenum Press, pp. 267–282.

Ames, B. N., McCann, J., and Yamasaki, E. (1975) Methods for detecting carcinogens and mutagens with the *Salmonella*/mammalian-microsome mutagenicity test. *Mutat. Res.* 31:347–364.

Bailey, D. W. and Kohn, H. I. (1965) Inherited histocompatibility changes in progeny of irradiated and unirradiated inbred mice. *Genet. Res.* 6:330–340.

Barrett, J. C. (1993) Mechanisms of multistep carcinogenesis and carcinogen risk assessment. *Environ. Health Persp.* 100:9–20.

Bishop, J. M. (1991) Molecular themes in oncogenesis. *Cell* 64:235–248.

Brusick, D. J. (1994) Genetic toxicology, in *Principles and Methods of Genetic Toxicology, 3rd edn*, A. W. Hayes (ed.), New York, NY: Raven Press.

Brusick, D. J. (1987) *Principles of Genetic Toxicology*, 2nd edn. New York, NY: Plenum Press.

Brusick, D. J. and Mayer, V. W. (1973) New developments in mutagenicity screening techniques with yeast. *Environ. Health Perspect.* 6:83–96.

DeMarini, D. M., Brockman, H. E., deSerres, F. J. *et al.* (1989) Specific-locus induced in eukaryotes (especially mammalian cells) by radiation and chemicals: A perspective. *Mutation Res.* 220:11–29.

Durston, W. E. and Ames, B. N. (1974) Simple method for the detection of mutagens in urine: Studies with the carcinogen 2-acetylaminofluorene. *Proc. Natl. Acad. Sci. (USA)* 71:737–741.

EPA (1994) *Health Effects Test Guidelines, Title 40, Part 798*. Washington, DC: U.S. Environmental Protection Agency.

Finch, R. A., Evans, I. M., and Bosmann, H. B. (1980) Chemical carcinogen *in vitro* testing: A method for sizing cell nuclei in the nuclear enlargement assay. *Toxicology* 15:145–154.

Flamm, W. G. (Chairman, DHEW Working Group on Mutagenicity Testing) (1977) Approaches to determining the mutagenic properties of chemicals: Risk to future generations. *J. Environ. Pathol. Toxicol.* 1:301–352.

Gabridge, M. G. and Legator, M. S. (1969) A host-mediated microbial assay for the detection of mutagenic compounds. *Proc. Soc. Exp. Biol. Med.* 130:831–834.

Hoffmann, G. R. (1996) Genetic toxicology, in *Casarett and Doull's Toxicology*, C. D. Klaassen (ed.), New York, NY: McGraw-Hill.

ICPEMC (1992) A method for combining and comparing short-term genotoxicity test data. The basic system. *Mutat. Res.* 266:7–25.

Kakunaga, T. (1973) A quantitative system for assay of malignant transformation by chemical carcinogens using a clone derived from BALB/3T3. *Int. J. Cancer* 12:463–473.

Lee, W. R., Abrahamson, S., Valencia, R. *et al.* (1983) The sex-linked recessive lethal test for mutagenesis in *Drosophila melanogaster*: A report of the U.S. EPA Gene-Tox Program. *Mutat. Res.* 123:183–279.

Leifer, Z., Kada, T., Mandel, M. *et al.* (1981) An evaluation of tests using DNA repair-deficient bacteria for predicting genotoxicity and carcinogenicity: A report of the U.S. EPA Gen-Tox Program. *Mutation Res.* 87:211–297.

McCann, J., Choi, E., Yamasaki, E., and Ames, B. N. (1975) Detection of carcinogens as mutagens in the *Salmonella*/microsome tests assay of 300 chemicals. *Proc. Natl. Acad. Sci. (USA)* 72:5135–5139.

Mason, J. M., Langenbach, R., Sheldby, M. D., Zeigler, E., and Tennant, R. W.

(1990) Ability of short term tests to predict carcinogenesis in rodents. *Annu. Rev. Pharmacol. Toxicol.* 30:149–268.

National Research Council (NRC) (1983) *Identifying and Estimating the Genetic Impact of Chemical Mutagens.* A report of the Committee on Chemical Environmental Mutagens, National Research Council. Washington, DC: National Academy Press.

OECD (Organization for Economic Cooperation and Development) (1987) *OECD Guidelines for Testing Chemicals.* Washington, DC: OECD Publications and Information Center.

Preston, R. J., Au, W., Bender, M. A. *et al.* (1981) Mammalian *in vivo* and *in vitro* cytogenetic assays: A report of the U.S. EPA Gene-Tox Program. *Mutat. Res.* 87:143–188.

Rabbitts, T. H. (1994) Translocations in human cancer. *Nature* 372:143–149.

Rosenkranz, H. S., Gutter, G., and Spek, W. J. (1976) Mutagenicity and DNA-modifying activity: A comparison of two microbial assays. *Mutat. Res.* 41:61–70.

Russell, L. B. (1978) Somatic cells as indictors of germinal mutations in the mouse. *Environ. Health Perspect.* 24:113–116.

Russell, L. B. and Shelby, M. D. (1985) Tests for heritable genetic damage and for evidence of gonadal exposure in mammals. *Mutat. Res.* 154:69–84.

Schmid, W. (1976) The micronucleus test. *Mutat. Res.* 31:9–15.

Searle, A. G. (1975) The specific locus test in the mouse. *Mutat. Res.* 31:277–290.

Simmons, V. F., Rozenkranz, H. S., Zeiger, E., and Poirier, L. A. (1979) Mutagenic activity of chemical carcinogens and related compounds in the intraperitoneal host-mediated assay. *J. Natl. Cancer Inst.* 62:911–918.

Stich, H. F. and Laishes, B. A. (1973) DNA repair and chemical carcinogens. *Pathobiol. Annu.* 3:341–376.

WHO (1990) *Summary Report on the Evaluation of Short-term Tests for Carcinogenesis.* WHO Environ. Health Criteria 109.

Williams, G. M. (1979) The status of *in vitro* test systems utilizing DNA damage and repair for the screening of chemical carcinogens. *J. Assoc. Off. Anal. Chem.* 63:857–863.

Wolff, S. (1977) Sister chromatid exchange. *Annu. Rev. Genet.* 11:183–201.

Wyrobek, A. J. and Bruce, W. R. (1975) Chemical induction of sperm abnormalities in mice. *Proc. Natl. Acad. Sci. (USA)* 72:4425–4429.

Zimmermann, F. K., von Borstel, R. C., von Halle, E. S. *et al.* (1984) Testing of chemicals for genetic activity with *Saccharomyces cerevisiae*: A report of the U.S. EPA Gene-Tox Program. *Mutation Res.* 133:199–244.

Chapter 9

Developmental toxicology

CONTENTS

Introduction

Historical background

Congenital malformations have been observed for centuries without knowing their etiology. It was only early last century that a variety of malformations were reported among the offspring of mothers who had been exposed to radiation, nutritional deficiencies, or certain viral infections. A connection was not suspected to exist between congenital malformation and chemicals because there was a tendency among toxicologists to assume that the natural protective mechanisms, such as detoxication, elimination, and placental barrier, were sufficient to shield the embryo from maternal exposure to chemicals. On the other hand, it was not unexpected that the natural protective mechanisms were ineffective against ionizing radiation, viruses, and nutritional deficiencies.

A new era in teratology was initiated as a result of the clinical use of thalidomide, a sedative-hypnotic. This drug, first introduced in the late 1950s in Germany, was found to be relatively nontoxic in experimental animals and in humans. It was used, among other indications, for the relief of morning sickness during pregnancy. In 1960, a few cases of phocomelia were reported. In the following year, there were many more cases. Phocomelia is a very rare type of congenital malformation, with shortening or absence of limbs. The causative agent in these cases was soon traced to the ingestion of thalidomide by the mothers, mainly between the third and eighth week of pregnancy. The use of the drug was promptly prohibited. In spite of that action, more than 10,000 such malformed babies were born in a number of countries (Lenz and Knapp, 1962). The profound, tragic effect on the malformed individuals and the traumatic impact on the families and society were so great that all feasible steps were instituted in an attempt to prevent the occurrence of such a man-made teratogenesis. One of these steps was to subject numerous drugs, food additives, pesticides, environmental contaminants, and other chemicals to various types of testing to determine their potential teratogenicity.

Some toxic effects on the fetus are not observable at birth. They may manifest as delayed developmental toxicity. An outstanding example is diethylstilbestrol (DES). The offspring of mothers who had taken this drug to prevent premature birth showed adverse effects in their sex organs only many years later. To embrace such delayed effects, the science "teratology" is now more commonly referred to as "developmental toxicology."

Embryology

After fertilization, the ovum undergoes a precise sequence of cell proliferation, differentiation, migration, and organogenesis. The embryo then passes through a set of metamorphoses and a period of fetal development before birth.

Predifferentiation stage

During this stage the embryo is not susceptible to teratogenic agents. These agents either cause death of the embryo by killing all or most of the cells, or have no apparent effect on the embryo. Even when some mildly harmful effects have been produced, the surviving cells can compensate and form a normal embryo. This resistant stage varies from five to nine days depending on the species.

Embryonic stage

This is the period when the cells undergo intensive differentiation, mobilization, and organization. It is during this period that most of the organogenesis takes place. As a result, the embryo is most susceptible to the effects of teratogens. This period generally ends some time from the tenth to the fourteenth day in rodents and in the fourteenth week of the gestation period in humans. Furthermore, not all organs are susceptible at the same time of the pregnancy. Figure 9.1 shows that the rat embryo is most

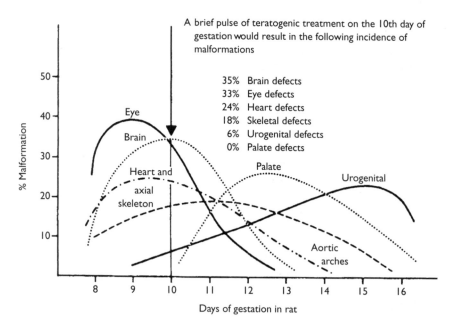

Figure 9.1 Expected incidences of malformation of different organs and systems the susceptibilities of which vary according to the days of gestation. A brief exposure to a teratogen on the tenth day of gestation is expected to induce a variety of malformations, with their incidences shown here.

Source: Reprinted from *Teratology: Principles and Techniques* by J. G. Wilson; by permission of the University of Chicago Press.

susceptible between days 8 and 12 for most organs, but the palate and urogenital organs are more susceptible at a later stage.

Fetal stage

This stage is characterized by growth and functional maturation. Teratogens are thus unlikely to cause morphologic defects during this stage, but they may induce functional abnormalities. Whereas morphologic defects are in general readily detected at birth or shortly thereafter, functional abnormalities, such as CNS deficiencies, may not be diagnosed for some time after birth.

The effects of developmental toxicants may precede the fertilization as well as after the delivery. A summary of the relationship between the stage of exposure and the effects on development are summarized in Table 9.1.

Teratogens (developmental toxicants) and their effects

Many chemical and physical agents may affect the conceptus. The effect may result in one or more of the following manifestations: death and/or various types of malformations. In addition, growth retardation, functional

Table 9.1 Relationship between developmental stage and fetal outcome

Development stage	Target system	Observed effect
Spermatozoa	Whole body	Decreased birth weight
		Neonatal mortality
Oocyte	Whole organism	Cell death
		Congenital anomalies
Placenta	Cardiovascular	Interference with active transport
		Alterations in maternal–fetal circulation
	Metabolism	Changes in biosynthesis of nutrients
		Changes in biotransformation of xenobiotics
Embryo	Whole organism	Intrauterine growth retardation
		Congenital anomalies
Fetus	Whole body	Growth retardation
	Reproductive and kidney	Genitourinary abnormalities
	Bone	Skeletal anomalies
Neonate	CNS	Neurobehavioral abnormalities
		Withdrawal symptoms
		Altered mental ability
	Reproductive	Altered fertility
	Respiratory	Respiratory depression
	Musculature	Hypotonia
	Whole organism	Neonatal death

Source: Adapted from Lock and Kacew (1988), Kacew and Lock (1990), and Kacew (1995).

disorders and certain other effects are observed shortly or much later after birth. They are generally referred to as developmental toxicity.

A variety of agents are known to be teratogenic in humans. These include radiation, certain infections, nutritional imbalance, and certain drugs and chemicals. The more important agents and their effects are outlined below. Additional information may be found in Shepard (1992) and Beckman *et al.* (1997).

Radiation for diagnostic or therapeutic purposes may cause embryonic death, leukemia, microcephaly, and skeletal and genital anomalies.

Infections that can cause congenital anomalies include German measles, herpes simplex, syphilis and toxoplasmosis. A variety of congenital anomalies have been reported, e.g., microcephaly, glaucoma, cataract and hemolytic anemia.

Metabolic imbalance, such as folic acid deficiency, diabetes, phenylketonuria may cause spina bifida, anencephaly, mental retardation, etc.

Drugs and other chemicals that are known for their developmental toxicity are listed below with their major effects:

Alcohol: microcephaly, mental retardation
Androgens: masculinization of female offsprings
Cocaine: fetal loss, microcephaly, neuro-behavioral abnormalities
Diethylstilbestrol (DES):
  1 *At birth*: clitoromegaly in female newborns (Bongiovanni *et al.*, 1959)
  2 *Years later*: adenocarcinoma of the vagina and cervix of the female offspring (Poskanzer and Herbst, 1977); abnormal structural and functional disorders of the genital organs of male offspring (Bibbo *et al.*, 1977)
Diphenylhydantoin: microcephaly, mental retardation, cleft plate
Methyl mercury: cerebral palsy, microcephaly, blindness, cerebellar hypoplasia
Retinoids (including vitamin A): malformations of the face, limbs, CNS, heart and skeletal system
Thalidomide: phocomelia (short or absent limbs)
Valproic acid: spina bifida

Mode of action

A variety of chemicals have been shown to be teratogenic in humans and/or animals. In view of the great diversity of the properties of these agents, it is not surprising that many different mechanisms are involved in their teratogenic effects.

Interference with nucleic acids

Many agents interfere with nucleic acid replication, transcription, or RNA translation. Their effects may result in cell death or somatic mutation in the embryo. Structural or functional defects may occur where enough cells are so affected. Ionizing radiation and genotoxic carcinogens are likely to act through this mechanism. Although some chemicals, such as carbon tetrachloride and nitrosamines, also yield metabolites that react with nucleic acids, their reactive metabolites are too unstable to reach the embryo. Therefore, these toxicants are carcinogenic but not potent teratogens.

Deficiency of energy supply and osmolarity

Certain teratogens can affect the energy supply for the metabolism of the organism by restricting the availability of substrates either directly (e.g., dietary deficiencies) or through the presence of analogs or antagonists of vitamins, essential amino acids, and others such as 6-amino-nicotinamide, which also interfere with glycolysis. In addition, hypoxia and agents inducing hypoxia (CO, CO_2) can be teratogenic by depriving the metabolic process of the required oxygen and probably also by the production of osmolar imbalances. These can induce edema and hematomas, which in turn can cause mechanical distortion and tissue ischemia.

Inhibition of enzymes

Inhibitors of enzymes, such as 5-fluorouracil, can induce malformation through interference with differentiation or growth, by inhibiting thymidylate synthetase. 6-Aminonicotinamide, which inhibits glucose-6-phosphate dehydrogenase, is also a potent teratogen.

Oxidative stress

Teratogens such as phenytoin undergo bioactivation and induce lipid peroxidation, protein oxidation and protein degradation in both maternal and embryonic tissues. These biochemical changes may be responsible for the teratogenesis (Liu and Wells, 1995).

Others

It should be noted that the mode of action of many teratogens is as yet unknown. Furthermore, a potential teratogen may or may not exert teratogenic effects depending on such factors as bioactivating mechanism, stability of the reactive metabolites, ability to cross the placental barrier,

Table 9.2 Factors associated with ability of chemicals to reach target fetus site

Physico-chemical properties	The ability of chemicals to reach the fetus are dependent on water solubility, lipid solubility and molecular weight
Pharmacokinetics	Fetus effects observed are dependent on chemical concentration in maternal circulation in fetal blood supply, placental and fetal chemicals metabolism, changing volume distribution and elimination (fetal renal function)
Chemical structure	Two chemicals of similar structure will cross the placenta yet only the one with a specific structural form will produce an effect
Duration of exposure	A single administration of a high dose can produce damage to the same extent as chronic, low-dose treatment
Implantation site	Improper implantation can result in malformation
Mechanical	Deformations in structures of uterine tissue affect circulation to placenta and fetus
Nutrition	Nutritional deficiency in the mother can influence placental transfer of essential nutrients to fetus. Excess nutrients can also cause adverse fetal effects
Physiological status	The absence of maternal hormones can alter the ability of fetus to cope with chemicals
Developmental state	Teratogenic agents act selectively on developing cells
Infection (disease)	Change in maternal body temperature can prolong half-life of drugs, predisposing the fetus to enhanced toxicity
Genetic	Inborn errors of metabolism can predispose a fetus to enhanced toxicity
Drug interactions	The presence of more than one drug and/or chemical can increase susceptibility of the fetus
Environment	Various factors in outdoor or indoor environment can modify toxico kinetics and thereby affect placental transfer
Multifactorial (gene– environment interactions)	Various factors in environment in specific, susceptible population can modify toxico kinetics and placental transfer

Source: Adapted from Lock and Kacew (1988), Kacew and Lock (1990), and Kacew (1995, 1997).

and detoxifying capability of the embryonic tissues. These and other factors are listed in Table 9.2.

Teratogens of special interest

Thalidomide, as noted earlier, is otherwise a relatively safe drug but induced an episode of unprecedented tragic congenital malformation. This episode broadened the scope of teratology. Unfortunately, after some 25 years of intensive study, the mechanism underlying its teratogenicity remains to be confirmed. The proposed mechanisms include interference with folic acid or glutamic acid metabolism, depurination of DNA, and acylation of polyamines. In addition to these biochemical investigations, a number of target tissues have been studied without definitive answer. These are limb mesenchyme tissue, mesonephric-limb tissue, and the developing neural crest tissue (Manson and Wise, 1993). A detailed account of the 24 different approaches that have been explored is provided by Stephens (1988).

Diethylstilbestrol (DES) was used in the 1940s to 1970s to prevent threatened abortion. Unfortunately, a few of the young adult female offspring (usually at age 19–22 yr) of these mothers developed adenocarcinoma of the vagina and cervix; more of them developed other disorders of the vagina and cervix (Pskanzer and Herbst, 1977). In addition, abnormal structural and functional disorders of the genital organs were observed in some male offspring (Bibbo *et al.*, 1977).

Testing procedures

Animals

Rats, rabbits, mice, and hamsters are the commonly used animals, because of their ready availability, easy handling, larger litter size, and short gestational period. The use of nonhuman primates has also been suggested because of their phylogenetic proximity to humans. There are advantages and disadvantages of various species of animals for use in teratology. On balance, it would appear that rabbits and nonhuman primates offer more advantages.

Administration of the chemical

At least three dosage levels are used. The higher dosage should include some maternal (and/or fetal) toxicity, such as reduction in body weight. The lowest dosage should induce no observable ill effect. One or more doses should be appropriately interspersed between the two extremes. Two control groups are included. One of these is given the vehicle or physiologic saline, and the other receives a substance of known teratogenic activity. These groups will provide information on the incidence of spontaneous malformations and the sensitivity of the specific lot of animals under the existing experimental conditions. In addition to these contemporary controls, data from historical controls are also useful. The test substances should be administered by the route that simulates the human exposure situations. The timing of administering the chemical is important. For routine teratologic studies, it is customary to administer the chemical during the entire period of organogenesis when the embryo is most susceptible.

Observations

The pregnant animals are examined daily for gross signs of maternal toxicity which may adversely affect the fetus. Fetuses are usually surgically removed from the mother about one day prior to the expected delivery to avoid cannibalism and permit counting of resorption sites and dead fetuses. The following observations are to be made and recorded: number of corpora lutea, implantations, resorptions, dead fetuses, and live fetuses. Other observations include sex of each live fetus, weight of each live fetus, length (crown–rump) of each live fetus, and abnormalities of each fetus.

Detailed examinations are performed to determine the different types of abnormalities. Each fetus is examined for external defects. In addition, about two-thirds of the fetuses are examined for skeletal abnormalities after staining with alizarin red. The remaining one-third of the fetuses are examined for visceral defects after fixation in Bouin's fluid and sectioned with a razor blade.

Delayed effects of toxicants are generally observed on the fetal central nervous, genitourinary or respiratory system. In testing toxicants suspected of having such potentials, a sufficient number of pregnant females are allowed to deliver their pups. These pups are nursed either by their biologic mothers or by foster mothers. In the latter case, the potential effects of postnatal exposure are eliminated.

Neuromotor and behavioral tests may be used to detect CNS effects. In evaluating two known teratogens, Goldey *et al.* (1994) measured motor activity, acoustic startle, T-maze delayed alternation, and measurement of total and regional brain weight as well as glial fibrillary acidic protein. Male rats exposed to TCDD *in utero* and lactationally may exhibit altered androgenic status, including reduced sperm count and testosterone levels (Mably *et al.* (1992). You *et al.* (1998) observed impaired male sexual development in rats exposed *in utero* and lactationally to p,p'-DDE.

More detailed information may be found in EPA (1994).

Evaluation of teratogenic effects

Categories and relative significance

Resorption is a manifestation of death of the conceptus, and is determined by the difference in the number of corpora lutea and implantations.

Fetal Toxicity may manifest as reduced body weight on the nonviable fetus. This type of data is often useful as corroborating evidence in assessing the teratogenicity of the toxicant in question.

Malformations may involve external and/or internal structures. Minor abnormalities, or deviations, generally do not affect the survival of the fetus. Examples are supernumary ribs and decreased or abnormal sternal ossification.

Major malformations, such as spina bifida or hydrocephalus, are incompatible with survival, growth and fertility.

Minor anomalies are of doubtful significance. Examples are curly tail, straight legs, malrotated limbs and paws, wristdrop, protruding tongue, enlarged atria and/or ventricles, abnormal pelvic development, and translucent skin.

Extrapolation to humans

The results obtained in teratogenesis studies in animals cannot be readily extrapolated to humans. However, the value of animal teratogenicity studies to the assessment of human health hazards was shown by Frankos (1985). Analyzing the FDA data, he noted that 37 of the 38 known human teratogens were positive in at least one laboratory animal test species, and that 130 of the 165 chemicals showing no teratologic findings were negative in at least one laboratory animal test species. In view of the above, it is prudent to carry out appropriate animal tests on all chemicals to which women of child-bearing age may be exposed. If positive results are obtained with a substance, especially when this is so in more than one species of animal, exposure of women of child-bearing age to this substance should be avoided, if possible.

References

Beckman, D. A., Fawcett, L. B., and Brent, R. L. (1997) Developmental toxicity, in *Handbook of Human Toxicology*, E. J. Massaro (ed.), Boca Raton, FL: CRC Press, pp. 1022–1029.

Bibbo, M., Gill, W., Azizi, F., Blough, R., Fnag, V., Rosenfield, R., Schumacher, G., Sleeper, K., Sonek, M., and Wild, G. (1977) Follow-up study of male and female offspring of DES-exposed mothers. *Obstet. Gynacol.* 49:1–8.

Bongiovanni, A. M., DiGeorge, A. M., and Grumbach, M. M. (1959) Masculinization of the female infant associated with estrogenic therapy alone during gestation: four cases. *J. Clin. Endocrinal. Metab.* 19:1004–1011.

EPA (1994) *Health Effects Test Guidelines/Code of Federal Regulations, Title 40, Part 789*. Washington, DC: Environmental Protection Agency.

Frankos, V. H. (1985) FDA perspectives on the use of teratology data for human risk assessment. *Fundam. Appl. Toxicol.* 5:615–625.

Goldey, E. S., O'Callaghan, J. P., Stanton, M. E., Barone, S., Jr., and Crofton, K. M. (1994) Developmental neurotoxicity: Evaluation of testing procedures with methylagomethanol and methylmercury. *Fundam. Appl. Toxicol.* 23:447–464.

Herbst, A. L., Ulfelder, H., and Poskanzer, D. C. (1971) Adenocarcinoma of the vagina: association of maternal stilbestrol therapy with tumor appearance in young women. *N. Engl. J. Med.* 284:878–881.

Kacew, S. (1995) Neonatal toxicology, in *General and Applied Toxicology*, B. Ballantyne, T. Marrs and P. Turner (eds), London: Macmillan.

Kacew, S. (1997) General principles in pediatric pharmacology and toxicology, in *Environmental Toxicology and Pharmacology of Human Development*, S. Kacew and G. H. Lambert (eds), Washington, DC: Taylor and Francis.

Kacew, S. and Lock, S. (1990) Developmental aspects of pediatric pharmacology and toxicology, in *Drug Toxicity and Metabolism in Pediatrics*, S. Kacew (ed.), Boca Raton, FL: CRC Press.

Lenz, W. and Knapp, K. (1962) Thalidomide embryopathy. *Arch. Environ. Health* 5:100–105.

Liu, L. and Wells, P. G. (1995) Potential molecular targets mediating chemical teratogenesis: *In vitro* peroxidase-catalyzed phenytoin metabolism and oxidative damage to proteins and lipids in marine maternal hepatic microsomes and embryonic 9000 g supernatant. *Toxicol. Appl. Pharmacol.* 34:71–80.

Lock, S. and Kacew, S. (1988) General principles in pediatric pharmacology and toxicology, in *Toxicologic and Pharmacologic Principles in Pediatrics*, S. Kacew and S. Lock (eds), Washington, DC: Hemisphere Publishing.

Mably, T. A., Moore, R. W., and Peterson, R. E. (1992) *In utero* and lactational exposure of male rats to 2, 3, 7, 8-tetrachlorodibenzo-*p*-dioxin: 1. Effects on androgenic status. *Toxicol. Appl. Pharmacol.* 114:97–107.

Manson, J. M. and Wise, L. D. (1993) Teratogens, in *Casarett and Doull's Toxicology*, M. O. Amdur, J. Doull, and C. D. Klaassen (eds) New York, NY: McGraw-Hill, pp. 226–254.

Poskanzer, D. and Herbst, A. (1977) Epidemiology of vaginal adenosis and adenocarcinoma associated with exposure to stilbestrol *in utero*. *Cancer* 39:1892–1895.

Shepard, T. H. (1992) *Catalog of Teratogenic Agents*, 7th edn. Baltimore, MD: Johns Hopkins University Press.

Stephens, T. D. (1988) Proposed mechanisms of action in thalidomide embryopathy. *Teratology* 38:229–239.

You, L., Casanova, M., Archibeque-Engle, S., Sar, M., Fan, L. Q., and Heck, H. d'A. (1998) Impaired male sexual development in perinatal Sprague-Dawley and Long-Evans hooded rats exposed in utero and lactationally to p,p'-DDE. *Toxicol. Sci.* 45:162–173.

Appendix 9.1 Teratogens in animal models

1 Physical agents: hypothermia and hyperthermia, hypoxia, radiation.
2 Agents producing hypoxia: carbon monoxide, carbon dioxide.
3 Infections: rubella viruses, syphilis.
4 Dietary deficiency or excess: vitamins A, D, and E, ascorbic acid, nicotinamide, trace metals (Zn, Mn, Mg, Co).
5 Vitamin antagonists: antifolic drugs, 6-aminonicotinamide.
6 Hormone deficiency or excess: cortisone, hydrocortisone, thyroxine, vasopressin, insulin, androgens, estrogens.
7 Natural toxins: aflatoxin B_1, ochratoxin A, ergotamine, nicotine.
8 Heavy metals: methyl mercury, phenylmercuric acetate, lead, thallium, strontium, selenium.

9 Solvents: benzene, carbon tetrachloride, 1,1-dichloroethane, dimethyl sulfoxide, propylene glycol, xylene.
10 Insecticides, herbicides, fungicides.
11 Azo dyes: trypan blue, Evans blue, Niagara blue.
12 Antibiotics: dactinomycin, penicillin, streptomycin, tetracyclines.
13 Sulfonamides: sulfanilamide, hypoglycemic sulfonamides.
14 Drugs and chemicals: caffeine, carbutamide, chlorcyclizine, chlorpromazine and derivatives, diphenylhydantoin, hydroxyurea, imipramine, meclizine, nitrosamines, pilocarpine, quinine, rauwolfia, thalidomide, triparanol, veratrum alkaloids, vinca alkaloids.

Chapter 10

Lactation

CONTENTS

General remarks

Following birth, the fetal stage develops into the neonate or infant. Exposure to drugs and environmental agents can either be direct through inhalation, ingestion, etc., or indirectly via the mother's milk. The importance and necessity of breast milk in the developing neonate has been clearly shown (Kacew, 1994; Berlin and Kacew, 1997). Table 10.1 lists some of the disease conditions where the frequency of occurrences of these disorders was clearly diminished in breast-fed infants. Breast-feeding has distinct advantages nutritionally, immunologically and psychologically, and despite the presence of environmental toxins, should be encouraged. At present, it should be stressed that human milk remains the best nutrient source for the healthy term infant (Redel and Shulman, 1994). This is clearly seen in the emphasis on promotion of breast-feeding by both pro-

Table 10.1 Adverse infant conditions protected by breast-feeding

Infant mortality
Sudden infant death syndrome
Respiratory tract disease
Food allergies
Atopic dermatitis
Otitis media
Asthma
Immune system disorders
    a   Lymphomas
    b   Celiac disease
    c   Insulin-dependent diabetes mellitis
    d   Inflammatory bowel disease
    e   Crohn's disease
    f   HIV-related mortality
Cholera
Giardia lamblia diarrhea
Rotavirus diarrhea
Shigellosis
Bacteremia and meningitis
Chronic liver disease

Source: Adapted from Kacew (1994, 2000).

fessionals and lay persons. The incidence of breast-feeding in North America has varied over the years from 25% (1970) to 56% (1981), and most recent studies show that about 54% of women discharged from hospital to home are breast-feeding (Berlin, 1989; Lawrence, 1989; Buttar, 1994). The resurgence in the number of women breast-feeding will increase even further as the educational awareness of benefits of lactation is promoted amongst men of expectant mothers. Wilson *et al.* (1986) estimated that a figure of 70% of breast-feeding mothers in the USA was equivalent to approximately 2.5 million women. Even at 50%, in 1994, there were 4 million new mothers in the USA, so more than 2 million infants went home receiving breast milk. A health goal established by a workshop sponsored by Human Health Services was that, by the year 2000, 75% of newborns would be breast-fed and 50% would still be breast-fed by six months of age. The breast-feeding mother is subjected to exposure from environmental contaminants, and these pollutants may be present in human milk. In the majority of cases, it is still more beneficial to breast-feed despite the presence of such contaminants.

Benefits of breast-feeding

Breast-feeding confers to the infant certain benefits which are summarized in Table 10.1 and discussed in the following sections.

Immune system

The beneficial effects of breast-feeding against immune system disorders are well-established (Davis *et al.*, 1988; Mayer *et al.*, 1988; Kramer, 1988). The finding that lead interferes with the immune system indicates that the presence of this metal in milk may not confer protection in lead-exposed mothers. It should also be noted that in the presence of environmental toxicants and a condition of malnourishment, the immune system is further compromised as there is an increased sensitivity to viral infection. The transmission of human immunodeficiency virus (HIV) during breast-feeding from infected mothers to suckling infants is well-documented (Oxtoby, 1988). Based on this knowledge the question arises as to the advantages of bottle-feeding in HIV-infected mothers. In an extensive study Lederman (1992) demonstrated that exclusive breast-feeding, even in situations where mothers were HIV-infected, there was a decrease in the estimated infant mortality rate especially in population areas where HIV prevalence was low. Although lactation does not protect against HIV transmission, breast-feeding is clearly beneficial in reducing infant mortality. In a population where HIV infection is exceedingly high, bottle-feeding is preferable. Bearing this in mind the benefits of breast-feeding substantially outweigh HIV transmission as one must consider infant mortality. Clearly, breast-feeding protects against infant mortality regardless of cause and this physiologic process should not be discontinued.

Cancer

The beneficial effects of protecting breast-fed infants against lymphoidal hypertrophy and lymphomas have been documented (Davis *et al.*, 1988). This protective antineoplastic effect was found to extend to the mother where lactation for prolonged periods was correlated with a reduction in breast cancer (McTiernan and Thomas, 1986). Although Kvale and Heuch (1988) failed to demonstrate any association in a large cohort study, in the more extensive and recent finding of Newcomb *et al.* (1994), a positive inverse correlation between lactation and risk of breast cancer was noted in premenopausal women. However, no reduction in the risk of breast cancer was found in postmenopausal women with a history of lactation. Regardless of the fact that breast cancer occurs in less than one quarter of all cases reported and that lactation provides a slight protective effect, it was concluded that any factor which reduces the incidence of breast cancer should be encouraged.

Avoidance of food allergies

In the case of food allergies or atopic dermatitis it is generally accepted that breast-feeding delays the development of these disorders (Lucas *et al.*,

1990). While Kramer (1988) suggested that breast-feeding provided protection against allergic diseases, these manifestations occurred in exclusively breast-fed infants. However, it should be noted that the incidence of food allergies decreased dramatically in exclusive breast-fed infants. In recent studies the maternal diet was found to be a critical factor in the development of allergic manifestations in lactating infants. Ingestion of a maternal hypoallergenic diet devoid of cow's milk, eggs and fish during lactation decreased the cumulative incidence and current prevalence of atopic dermatitis during the first six months of age with continuation to the age of four (Chandra et al., 1989; Sigurs et al., 1992). Breast-feeding per se is effective in protecting against allergic disorders provided the offending stimulus is not ingested by the mother for transmission to the infant via the milk.

Psychological bonding

Breast-feeding is known to create a special psychological bond between infant and mother that ultimately leads to a socially healthier child. In addition, lactation enhances maternal postpartum recovery and body weight returns to prepartum levels more rapidly. The physiological process of breast-feeding plays a critical role in human growth and development. The use of bottles to feed nursing infants with milk formula in developing countries was found to enhance morbidity and mortality. In affluent nations, inadequate knowledge on growth patterns between breast-fed and bottle-fed infants resulted in inappropriate counseling against lactation. In an extensive study, Dewey et al. (1992) demonstrated that the growth pattern was equivalent between breast-fed and formula-fed infants from birth to the first three months. However, breast-fed infants gained significantly less weight from three to 12 months without any deleterious effects on nutrition, morbidity, motor activity level or behavioral development. It is evident that breast-fed infants are leaner and do not display a faltering growth pattern; women should be encouraged to continue the lactational process beyond three months. With the knowledge that growth in breast-fed infants is generally less than formula-fed, growth per se as an index of toxicity in the first year of life is not appropriate.

Maternal nutrient intake is an important factor in the growth pattern of the infant. If a deficiency of zinc exists, there may be a delay in infant growth. Thus, in conditions of adequate maternal zinc concentrations, lactation should be encouraged despite a decreased infant growth pattern. A maternal diet deficient in essential nutrients such as iron or calcium results in a greater bioavailability of mammary lead, with consequent developmental delay.

Toxicants

The nursing mother can serve as a source of neonatal exposure to drugs or chemicals. No matter whether the agent is an OTC medication or prescribed by a physician, most drugs are detectable in breast milk. The presence of a drug in maternal milk may be construed as a potential hazard to the infant even though only 1–2% of total intake is likely to be found there. Hence the primary consideration in maternal drug therapy is the risk to the nursing infant rather than the mere presence of xenobiotic in the milk. Based on the numerous advantages of breast-feeding, the benefit of this physiological process in the majority of cases far exceeds the potential risk. Although it may be inadvertent, the suckling infant also derives environmental chemicals from the mother. These chemicals are excreted in breast milk and pose a serious potential hazard to the infant (see Table 10.2). Unlike drug therapy, which can be voluntarily terminated, environmental exposure may be chronic and, consequently, more toxic. In addition, environmental chemicals and drugs both present in milk can enter the infant to exert a synergistic adverse effect. Some of these are discussed in the following sections.

Silicone

Silicone is a polymeric substance which is inert and is unlikely to produce a toxic manifestation. Based on these properties the use of silicone for breast implantation was considered ideal; however, retrospective studies revealed an increased incidence of rheumatologic disorders, in particular, scleroderma and arthritis. Levin and Ilowite (1994) reported that in infants of breast-fed mothers with silicone implants there was a decreased lower sphincter pressure and abnormal esophageal wave propagation. Clearly

Table 10.2 Toxicants identified in human breast milk and adverse infant effects

Chemical	Effect
Silicone	Esophageal dysfunction
Hexachlorobenzene	Porphyria cutanea tarda
Polychlorinated biphenyls	Abnormal skin pigmentation, bone defects, growth retardation, hypotonia
Perchlorethylene	Obstructive jaundice
Methyl mercury	Developmental delay, abnormal muscle tone, mental retardation, decrease suckling response
Lead	Poor mental performance, central nervous system toxicosis
Nicotine	Decreased weight gain
Cadmium	Lower birth weight

Source: Adapted from Kacew (1994), Berlin and Kacew (1997).

the inert material silicone was associated with infant esophageal disease as a result of lactational exposure. It has been suggested that leakage from the implant produces immunologic substances that lead to scleroderma development. Normally human milk contains immunological components which provide protection against diseases. In the presence of silicone the breast milk would contain components which may immunologically-compromise the infant not only with esophageal dysfunction but also with increased susceptibility to other immune-related diseases.

Mercury

Lactational exposure of human infants to metals is a concern and raises the issue of risk vs. benefit in the maintenance of the breast-feeding process. Mercury levels in milk are usually low (<1 ng/ml) but in environmental disasters as in Minimata, Japan, the levels reached 50 ng/ml. Numerous studies exist on the effects of either prenatal or during both pregnancy and postnatal exposure to metals on developing infants, but few reports are available on the consequences of the presence of metals exclusively in breast milk on children. Bearing in mind the consequences of methyl mercury poisoning, especially in Minimata, Japan, consideration should be given to the contribution of lactational exposure to the observed neuronal disturbances where nursing mothers ingesting mercury-contaminated fish resulted in severe neurological disorders in human infants (Matsumoto et al., 1965). Takeuchi (1968) clearly demonstrated the effects of epidemic methyl mercury exposure on fetal and newborn development. Industrial release of methyl mercury into Minamata Bay followed by accumulation in edible fish and ingestion by lactating females resulted in the transfer of metal to the suckling human infant. Similarly, Amin-Zaki et al. (1974) demonstrated that ingestion of homemade bread prepared from wheat treated with the fungicide methyl mercury by lactating mothers produced a significant rise is human infant metal levels. In fish-eating populations in Canada, maternal ingestion of mercury-contaminated food during pregnancy and lactation resulted in abnormal muscle tone and reflexes in boys but not girls (McKeown-Eyssen et al., 1983). In a New Zealand study, Kjellstrom et al. (1989) reported developmental retardation in four-year old children of mothers eating mercury-contaminated fish during pregnancy and lactation. Although emphasis was placed on the consequences of prenatal exposure in the Canadian and New Zealand studies, the contribution of milk mercury to toxic outcome was neglected. It should be noted that in some patients with Minamata disease the neurological symptoms developed not at the time of exposure but years later. Further, the reported number of cases where children born in a mercury-contaminated area in Japan were healthy yet developed neuropathy in childhood. The contribution of breast milk mercury to late-onset

Minamata disease remains to be resolved. Mammary transfer of methyl mercury to suckling infants has been reported to produce neurological lesions. This finding clearly indicates a positive correlation between exposure to high concentrations of metal in mammary tissue and toxicity in suckling infants.

Although the precise contribution of mammary-derived methyl mercury to the observed adverse effects on neurologic and behavioral changes in suckling pups is not known. It was found that postnatal exposure directly to newborns of this metal produced ocular defects. In contrast, there was a lack of an ocular effect in fetuses of prenatal exposed dams suggesting that lactation methyl mercury may in part contribute to the observed toxicity. It is well-known that methyl mercury is secreted more readily in the maternal colostrum, the period at which eye defects were reported, and crosses into the suckling infant. Mercury itself decreases the suckling response in human infants. Since milk contains essential nutrients for neurological and behavioral development, it is conceivable that less suckling and feeding would contribute to the mercury-induced nervous disorders as there is less nutritional supply and this is associated with delayed growth processes.

Lead

In a number of studies conducted in the United States and Europe, the content of lead in human milk ranged from 5–68 ng/ml (Rabinowitz *et al.*, 1985). Levels in Boston averaged 1.7 ng/ml in 1979. Dillon (1974) found lead levels of approximately 26 ng/ml in seven different U.S. cities. In Mexico City, milk lead levels reached 45 ng/ml (Berlin and Kacew, 1997). It is not surprising that upon examination of the source of infant lead intoxication, breast milk contained far less lead than either formula or environmental sources such as ceramic-leachable kitchenware, paint chips, etc. (Rabinowitz *et al.*, 1985). There is evidence to suggest a correlation between poor mental performance as evidenced by the Bayley Infants Assessment Test and increased lead level (Needleman *et al.*, 1983). These findings prompted Newman (1993) to recommend the promotion of breast-feeding, as human milk was a less suitable transmission vehicle for lead contamination compared to formula feeding. Further it should be stressed that the best source for daily nutrition amongst infants is human milk.

Although the contribution of exclusive mammary lead exposure to the observed CNS toxic consequences remains undefined, there is evidence to suggest that the presence of lactational metal results in newborn toxicity. Direct application of topical lead ointment on the breast was reported to produce central nervous system toxicosis in the human infant (Dillon, 1974). The presence of lead in mammary tissue alters the nutritional value of milk as reflected by decreases in the essential elements copper, zinc and iron, which are required for mammalian metabolism and CNS function. The absorption of calcium, iron and vitamin D is affected by lead. In conditions of diets deficient in essential elements, lead absorption and toxicity is enhanced in infants. As breast milk is a source of lead for suckling infants, it is conceivable that during iron-deficiency anemia or calcium-deficient dietary intake in mothers, the bioavailability of milk lead would be increased, resulting in greater toxicity. Evidence suggested that lead exposure may interfere with maternal metabolic pathways resulting in decreased utilization of nutrients in the diet, and thus an absence of nutritional components present in milk. This altered milk composition would consequently adversely affect newborn development.

Halogenated hydrocarbons

Chemical exposure via accidents and hazardous waste sites has resulted in toxicant accumulation in breast milk. The human maternal ingestion of a fungicide, hexachlorobenzene-treated wheat resulted in chemical accumulation in breast milk. Suckling infants subsequently developed symptoms of a disease, pembe yara, and a condition of prophyria cutanea tarda (Peters et al., 1982). Exposure to organophosphate pesticides such as chlorpyrifos, malathion, etc., is worthy of mention, as these compounds have been identified in breast milk (Berlin and Kacew, 1997). Ingestion of chlorpyrifos by a three-year old infant resulted in delayed polyneuropathy with transient bilateral vocal paralysis (Aiuto et al., 1993). Although lactation per se was not involved in this specific case, the importance lies in the fact that the manifestations of exposure did not occur until one to three weeks later. One should be aware that the consequences of lactational exposure to toxicants can also be delayed. This is supported by the findings where a mother was exposed to 2,4-diphenoxyacetic acid (2,4-D) spray during pregnancy and lactation. Examination of the infant at five and 24 months of age revealed multiple malformations and severe mental retardation. Although the mammary tissue content of 2,4-D was not determined, prolonged maternal exposure with consequent transmission to the infant was suggested to result in the observed toxicity. The fact that lactational derived organophosphate pesticides alter suckling infant metabolism and that toxicity may be delayed suggest that breast-feeding in severe exposure conditions should be minimized.

Ingestion of polychlorinated biphenyl-contaminated rice oil by nursing mothers was attributed to produce low birth weight human infants, growth retardation, abnormal skin pigmentation as well as bone and tooth defects (Yamaguchi et al., 1971). In extensive studies in North Carolina, Rogan et al. (1986) measured the levels of polychlorinated biphenyls in human milk and found an associated hypotonicity and hyporeflexia in nursing infants. Organochlorine pesticides including, DDT, aldrin and dieldrin have been identified in human milk (Berlin and Kacew, 1997). However, it is surprising that manifestations of toxicity in suckling infants following maternal organochlorine exposure have not been reported. This should not be deemed that the presence of organochlorine contaminants in breast milk lacks an effect on the infant, as these environmental toxicants induce mammary carcinoma and may act as co-carcinogens. It is well-known that suckling infants of cigarette smoking mothers are more prone to respiratory irritation and infections. However, cigarette smoking in the presence of atmospheric pollutants exerted an additive toxic effect on the mother. Conceivably, the presence of organochlorine compounds and nicotine in breast milk would increase infant toxicity with the hydrocarbons acting as cocarcinogens. Hence in susceptible suckling infants these compounds may precipitate autoimmune diseases, lymphomas, etc.

Solvents

The aromatic hydrocarbon toluene is utilized as a solvent or thinner in numerous industrial products including paints, glue, and resins. The lipophilic property of toluene is of interest in light of the physicochemical properties of breast tissue. Hersh et al. (1985) demonstrated that in infants of approximately four years of age maternal exposure to toluene throughout pregnancy via glue sniffing produced embryopathy, mental deficiency and postnatal growth delay. There is no doubt that in utero exposure to toluene was manifested in teratogenesis. However, as there was evidence of postnatal growth deficiency and toluene has a high affinity for fat, it is also possible that these infants were exposed to this solvent via the mother's milk. This is supported by the finding that obstructive jaundice developed in lactating infants of mothers exposed to the dry-cleaning solvent, perchloroethylene (Bagnell and Ellenberg, 1977). It is well-established that exposure to the organic solvents during pregnancy results in toxemia and anemia. Unfortunately, infants born to these mothers were not followed during lactation. However, as these environmental chemicals accumulate in breast milk and produce metabolic maternal alterations, it is conceivable that solvents may alter infant development. The release of organic solvents from breast milk fat needs to be considered amongst solvent abusers in light of adverse consequent effects reported in children (Schreiber, 1997).

References

Aiuto, L. A., Pavlakis, S. G., and Boxer, R. A. (1993) Life-threatening organophosphate-induced delayed polyneuropathy in a child after accidental chlorpyrifos. J. Pediatr. 122:658–660.
Amin-Zaki, L., Elhassini, S., Majeed, M. A., Clarkson, T. W., Doherty, R. A., and

Greenwood, M. R. (1974) Studies of infants postnatally exposed to methylmercury. *J. Pediatr.* 85:81–84.

Bagnell, P. C. and Ellenberg, H. A. (1977) Obstructive jaundice due to a chlorinated hydrocarbon in breast milk. *Can. Med. Assoc. J.* 117:1047–1048.

Berlin, C. M., Jr. (1989) Drugs and chemicals: exposure of the nursing mother. *Pediatr. Clin. North Am.* 36:1089–1097.

Berlin, C. M., Jr. and Kacew, S. (1997) Environmental contamination human milk, in *Environmental Toxicology and Pharmacology of Human Development*, S. Kacew and G. H. Lambert (eds), Washington, DC: Taylor & Francis.

Buttar, H. S. (1994) Neonatal risks of drugs excreted in breast milk. *Can. Pharm. J.* 127:14–19.

Chandra, R. K., Puri, S., and Hamed, A. (1989) Influence of maternal diet during lactation and use of formula feeds on development of atopic eczema in high risk infants. *Br. Med. J.* 299:228–230.

Davis, M. K., Savitz, D. A., and Graubard, B. I. (1988) Infant feeding and childhood cancer. *Lancet* 2:365–368.

Dewey, K. G., Heining, M. J., Nommsen, L. A., Peerson, J. M., and Lonnerdal, B. (1992) Growth of breast-fed and formula-fed infants from 0 to 18 months: the DARLING study. *Pediatrics* 89:1035–1041.

Dillon, H. K. (1974) Lead concentration in human milk. *Am. J. Dis. Child.* 128:491–492.

Hersh, J. H., Podruch, P. E., Rogers, G., and Weisskopf, B. (1985) Toluene embryopathy. *J. Pediatr.* 106:922–927.

Kacew, S. (1994) Current issues in lactation: advantages, environment, silicone. *Biomed. Environ. Sci.* 7:307–319.

Kacew, S. (2000) Neonatal toxicology, in *General and Applied Toxicology*, B. Ballantyne, T. Marrs and T. Syversen (eds), New York, NY: Macmillan.

Kjellstrom, T., Kennedy, P., Wallis, S., Stewart, A., Friberg, L., Lind, B., Wutherspoon, P., and Mantell, C. (1989) *Physical and mental development of children with prenatal exposure to mercury from fish. Stage 2. Interviews and psychological tests at age 6*, Solna, National Swedish Environmental Board, p. 112 (Report no. 3642).

Kramer, M. S. (1988) Does breast feeding help protect against atopic disease? Biology, methodology and a golden jubilee of controversy. *J. Pediatr.* 112:181–190.

Kvale, G. and Heuch, I. (1988) Lactation and cancer risk: Is there a relation specific to breast cancer? *J. Epidemiol. Community Health* 42:30–37.

Lawrence, R. A. (1989) Breastfeeding and medical disease. *Med. Clin. North Am.* 73:583–603.

Lederman, S. A. (1992) Estimating infant mortality from human immunodeficiency virus and other causes in breast-feeding and bottle-feeding populations. *Pediatrics* 89:290–296.

Levine, J. J. and Ilowite, N. T. (1994) Sclerodermalike esophageal disease in children breast-fed by mothers with silicone breast implants. *J. Am. Med. Assoc.* 271:213–216.

Lucas, A., Brooke, O. G., Morley, R., Cole, J. T., and Bamford, M. F. (1990) Early diet of preterm infants and development of allergic or atopic disease: randomized prospective study. *Br. Med. J.* 300:837–840.

McKeown-Eyssen, G. E., Ruedy, J., and Neims, A. (1983) Methylmercury exposure in Northern Quebec. II. Neurological finding in children. *Am. J. Epidemiol.* 118:470–479.

McTiernan, A. and Thomas, D. B. (1986) Evidence for a protective effect of lactation on risk of breast cancer in young women: results from a case-control study. *Am. J. Epidemiol.* 124:353–358.

Matsumoto, M., Koya, G., and Takeuchi, T. (1965) Fetal Minimata Disease. *J. Neuropathol. Exp. Neurol.* 24:563–574.

Mayer, E. J., Hamman, R. F., Gay, E. C., Lezotte, D. C., Savitz, D. A., and Klingensmith, G. J. (1988) Reduced risk of IDDM among breast-fed children. *Diabetes* 37:1625–1632.

Needleman, H., Bellinger, D., Leviton, A., Rabinowitz, M., and Nichols, M. (1983) Umbilical cord blood lead levels and neuropsychological performance at 12 months of age. *Pediatr. Res.* 17:179A.

Newcomb, P. A., Storer, B. F., Longnecker, M. P., Mittendorf, R., Greenberg, E. R., Clapp, R. W., Burke, K. P., Willett, W. C., and MacMahon, B. (1994) Lactation and reduced risk of premenopausal breast cancer. *New Engl. J. Med.* 330:81–87.

Newman, J. (1993) Would breast-feeding decrease risks of lead intoxication? *Pediatrics* 90:131.

Oxtoby, M. J. (1988) Human immunodeficiency virus and other viruses in human milk: placing the issues in broader perspective. *Pediatr. Infect. Dis. J.* 7:825–835.

Peters, H. A., Gocmen, A., Gripps, D. J., Bryan, G. T., and Dogramaci, I. (1982) Epidemiology of hexachlorobenzene-induced porphyria in Turkey. *Arch. Neurol.* 39:744–749.

Rabinowitz, M., Leviton, A., and Needleman, H. (1985) Lead in milk and infant blood: a dose–response mode. *Arch. Environ. Health* 40:283–286.

Redel, C. A. and Shulman, R. G. (1994) Controversies in the composition of infant formulas. *Pediatr. Clin. N.A.* 41:909–924.

Rogan, W. J., Gladen, B. C., McKinney, J. D., Carreras, N., Hardy, P., Thullen, J., Tinglestad, J., and Tully, M. (1986) Neonatal effects of transplacental exposure to PCBs and DDE. *J. Pediatr.* 109:335–341.

Schreiber, J. S. (1997) Transport of organic chemicals to breast milk: tetrachlorothene case study, in *Environmental Toxicology and Pharmacology of Human Development*, S. Kacew and G. H. Lambert (eds), Washington, DC: Taylor & Francis.

Sigurs, N., Hattevig, G., and Kjellman, B. (1992) Maternal avoidance of eggs, cow's milk and fish during lactation: effect on allergic manifestation, skin-prick test, and specific 1gE antibodies in children at age 4 years. *Pediatrics* 89:735–739.

Takeuchi, T. (1968) Pathology of Minimata Disease, in *Minimata Disease*, M. Kutsune (ed.), Japan: Kunamoto University.

Wilson, J. T., Hinson, J. L., Brown, R. D., and Smith, I. J. (1986) A comprehensive assessment of drugs and chemical toxins excreted in breast milk, in *Human Lactation*, vol. 2, M. Hamosh, A. D. Goldman, (eds), New York, NY: Plenum Publishing Corporation.

Yamaguchi, A., Yoshimura, T., and Kuratsune, M. (1971) A survey of pregnant women having consumed rice oil contaminated with chlorobiphenyls and their babies. *Fukuoka Acta. Med.* 62:117–122.

Part III

Target organs and systems

Chapter 11

Toxicology of the immune system

General considerations

The function of the immune system is to protect the host against foreign organisms (virus, bacteria, fungus), "foreign cells" (neoplasm), and other foreign substances. Its importance is evidenced by the seriousness of immunodeficiency: patients with this disorder are prone to be affected by infection and tumors. Immunodeficiency can be congenital or acquired; the latter is also known as AIDS (acquired immunodeficiency syndrome).

The immune system is composed of several types of organs, cells, and noncellular components. The functions of the individual components are in general interrelated. Thus, upon encountering a foreign substance, a cascade of reactions usually appears between different types of cellular and humoral components. These reactions involve the recognition, memory, and response to the foreign substance, and are designed for its elimination or control.

A variety of toxicants are known to suppress immune function. This effect will lead to lowered host resistance to bacterial and viral infections, and to parasitic infestation, as well as lowered control of neoplasm. In addition, certain toxicants may provoke exaggerated immune reactions leading to local or systemic reactions. Furthermore, it may even result in "autoimmune reactions."

This chapter briefly describes the components of the immune system and their functions, major immunotoxicants, and appropriate testing procedures.

Components of the system

The immune system consists of a network of organs including the bone marrow, thymus, spleen, and lymph nodes. From these organs, various lymphocytes and other cells with different immune functions are derived.

Some of the components are involved in specific immune responses, and others in nonspecific responses. Both types of cells are derived from the pluripotent cells in the bone marrow. From these cells are generated the lymphoid stem cells. Some of these cells are processed through the thymus and become T cells (T lymphocytes); others go through the "bursal equivalent" tissues (including bone marrow, lymph nodes, lymphoid

Table 11.1 The cells and primary soluble mediators: innate vs. acquired immunity

Characteristic	Innate immunity	Acquired immunity
Cells involved	Polymorphonuclear cells (PMN)	T Cells
		B Cells
	Monocyte/macrophage	Macrophages
	NK cells	NK Cells
Primary soluble mediators	Complement	Antibody
	Lysozyme	Cytokines
	Acute phase proteins	
	Interferon α/β	
	Cytokines	

Source: Adapted from Burns, Meade and Munson (1996).

tissues in the gut such as appendix, cecum, and Peyer's patches) to become B cells (B lymphocytes). Still others are released from the bone marrow without further processing. These are known as natural killer (NK) cells. Unlike the T cells and B cells, NK cells are also involved in nonspecific defense against neoplasms, and certain other foreign substances.

Other pluripotent stem cells give rise to myeloid stem cells, from which are derived monocytes, mast cells, and polymorphonuclear (PMN) cells. Monocytes then become macrophages, which are involved in specific (acquired) and nonspecific (innate) immune reactions. In addition, there are three types of PMN cells, namely, neutrophils, eosinophils, and basophils. These cells are involved in nonspecific defense mechanisms.

T cells

As noted above, the T cells, after passing through the thymus, enter the blood and constitute 70% of the circulating lymphocytes. Some settle in thymus-dependent areas of the spleen and lymph nodes. On contact with antigens processed by antigen-presenting cells (APCs, such as macrophages and B cells), the T cells undergo proliferation and differentiation. Some of these cells become "activated" and responsible for mediating cellular immunity. Others become T memory cells, which can be activated by combining with antigens; still others by becoming *helper* cells. Once activated, helper T cells will proliferate and secrete lymphokines. The lymphokines will cause the B cells to become plasma cells.

The activated T cells react either directly with cell-membrane-associated antigens or by releasing various soluble factors known as lymphokines. There are a large number of lymphokines (see next section).

B cells

Other stem cells undergo changes in certain tissues as noted above to become B cells (B lymphocytes). They enter the blood to constitute 30% of the lymphocytes. The primary immune response is initiated by the contact of antigen with B cells, which then differentiate and proliferate. Some of these become *memory* cells, which retain the surface immunoglobulin receptors, whereas others become *plasma* cells. The latter type of cells bear on cell surface IgM and IgD immunoglobulins. Exposure of the memory cells to the same antigen at a later time results in the secondary immune response.

Other types of cells

Other lymphocytes lack the characteristic surface markers of the T cells and the B cells, but they participate in the nonspecific immune system functions. These are the null cells. Some of these, the *natural killer* (NK) cells, have spontaneous (without prior sensitization) cytolytic activity against other cells, especially leukemia and carcinoma cells.

Macrophages are also derived from the stem-cell pool in the bone marrow. After their release, they appear in the bloodstream as monocytes and in the tissues as histiocytes. On contact with a foreign body, they engulf the foreign body and become activated macrophages. These cells are rich in cytoplasmic hydrolytic enzymes. Most bacterial cells are readily digested by these enzymes. Macrophages can also be activated to become APCs.

Langerhans cells, located in the skin, are also derived from bone marrow and act as APCs. They serve to process dermal antigens and initiate contact allergy and rejection of skin graft.

Among the *polymorphonuclear cells*, neutrophil PMNs have phagocytic activity. The eosinophils possess cytotoxic function, and basophils (which become mast cells in tissues) release histamine and other substances, thereby initiating local reactions to a foreign substance inducing immediate hypersensitivity.

Soluble mediators

Immunoglobins are proteins produced by plasma cells (derived from B cells). They have specific antibody activities. Their specificity is determined by the amino acid sequence and the tertiary surface configuration. There are five major types of immunoglobins. Their characteristics and functions are outlined in Table 11.2.

Table 11.2 Characteristics of immunoglobulins

Class	Mol. wt.	Mean survival $T_{1/2}$ (days)	Mean serum conc. (mg/dl)	Major function
IgG	150,000	20	720–1,500	Most prevalent; major antibody for toxins, viruses, and bacteria
IgA	170,000	6	90–325	In secretions from mucosa; for early antibacterial and antiviral defense
IgM	900,000	10	45–150	Major antibody after exposure to most antigens
IgD	180,000	3	3	Present on B cell surface, function as an antigen receptor
IgE	200,000	2	0.03	Fixed on mast cells, responsible for immediate type hypersensitivity

Interleukins (cytokines) are proteins produced by activated T cells (lymphokines) or monocytes/macrophages (monokines) in response to antigenic or mitogenic stimulation. They promote the proliferation of T cells, B cells, and hematopoietic stem cells.

The complement system consists of more than 30 plasma and body fluid proteins. These proteins complement a variety of immune functions, such as adherence of antibody-coated bacteria to macrophages, modulation of immune response, and lysis of cells. Immunotoxicants can activate or inhibit the complements. Macrophages and certain lymphocytes are capable of synthesizing certain important cytokines, such as tumor necrosis factor (Ruddle, 1994), and growth factors; the latter play a central role in the fibrotic lung lesions in humans exposed to asbestos and silica (see Chapter 12).

Immunotoxicants

Major immunotoxicants

A variety of substances have been found to affect the immune system. They may be placed in five categories as follows:

1   Medicinal products: among those, the antineoplastic drugs cyclophosphamide, nitrogen mustards, 6-mercaptopurine, azathioprine, methotrexate, 5-fluorouracil, actinomycin, doxorubicin are more frequently implicated. A number of other drugs that induced autoimmune reactions are listed in Table 11.3.
2   Heavy metals, organometals: beryllium, nickel, chromium, gold, methyl mercury, platinum, organic tin compounds, sodium arsenite and arsenate, and arsenic trioxide.
3   Pesticides: pyrethroids, chlordane, DDT, dieldrin, methylparathion,

Table 11.3 Examples of drugs that induce autoimmune syndromes

Autoimmune syndrome	Examples of drugs
Hepatitis	Erythromycin, floxacilin, halothane, methyldopa
Hemolytic anemia	Amoxacillin, nomifensine, probenecid, tolbutamide
Lupus erythematosus	Hydralazine, procainamide
Nephritis	Captopril
Neutropenia	Methyldopa, penicillamine
Oculo-cutaneous snydrome	Practolol
Thrombocytopenia	Acetaminophen, quinine

Source: Adapted from Pohl *et al.* (1988) and Behan *et al.* (1976).

carbofuran, maneb, hexachlorobenzene (HCB), carbaryl, 2,4-D, paraquat, diquat.

4   Halogenated hydrocarbons: TCDD, PCB, polybrominated biphenyls (PBB), trichloroethylene, chloroform, pentachlorophenol.

5   Miscellaneous compounds: benzo[a]pyrene, methylcholanthrene, diethylstilbestrol, 2-methoxyethanol, benzene, corticosteroids, TPA, penicillin, sulfites, substilisin, formaldehyde, toluene diisocyanates.

The effects of toxicants on the immune system are complex; some suppress the cell-mediated immunity, others the humoral immunity, and still others may even stimulate certain immune functions (Table 11.4).

Effects on immune functions

The function of the immune system is, as noted above, to protect the host against foreign organisms (viruses, bacteria, etc.), "foreign" cells (tumors), and other foreign substances. When the system functions properly, the foreign agents are eliminated promptly and efficiently. However, with certain agents, in some individuals, the immune system may respond in

Table 11.4 Effects of in vivo exposure to chemicals on immune functions and host resistance

Parameters	DES	BaP	TPA
Resistance to [A8]Listeria[A7] challenge	D	NE	I
Resistance to tumor challenge	D	NE	D
Trichinella expulsion	D	D	NE
Thymus weight	D	NE	D
Delayed hypersensitivity	D	NE	NE
Lymphocyte responses*	D	D†	D
T-cell quantification	D	–	D
Spontaneous lymphocyte cytotoxicity	NE	NE	D
Antibody plaque response	D	D	D
Immunoglobulins, M, G, and A levels	NE	NE	D
Macrophage phagocytosis	I	NE	I
Macrophage cytostasis	I	NE	I
RES clearance time	I	NE	I
Bone marrow cellularity‡	D	D	NE

Source: Data from Dean et al., 1982. (Copyright, 1982, American Society for Pharmacology and Experimental Therapeutics.)

Notes
DES, diethylstilbestrol; BaP (benzo[a]pyrene); TPA (12-o-tetradecanoylphorbol 13-o-acetate); D, decreased; I, increased; NE, no effect; –, not tested.
*Lymphocyte responses to phytohemagglutinin, concanavalin A, lipopolysaccharide and mixed lymphocyte culture.
†Decreased, except the response to mixed lymphocyte culture.
‡Colony-forming units multipotent cells and granulocyte/macrophage progenitors.

adverse manners. These may manifest as (1) immunosuppression and immunodeficiency, (2) hypersensitivity and allergy, and (3) autoimmunity. These are outlined below.

Hypersensitivity and allergy

There are four types of such reactions. With Type I, the reactions are immediate (usually within 15 minutes), resulting from a second or subsequent exposure to an antigen. The first exposure to that antigen induces the production of IgE antibodies. Subsequent exposure to the same antigen triggers the release of existing histamine, heparin, serotonin, prostaglandins, etc. These substances induce a variety of clinical manifestations, such as asthma, rhinitis, urticaria, and anaphylaxis. Allergenic agents are diverse in nature. Notable examples are metals (nickel, beryllium, platinum compounds), therapeutic agents (penicillin), food additives (sulfites, MSG, tartrazine, benzoates), food (chocolate, peanuts), pesticides (pyrethrum), and industrial chemicals such as toluene diisocyanate (TDI).

Type II and Type III hypersensitivity reactions are less common. Type II is characterized by cytolysis through IgG and/or IgM. The targets are usually erythrocytes, leucocytes, platelets and their progenitors. The result of the cytolysis is hemolytic anemia, leucopenia or thrombocytopenia. The offending agents include gold salts, chlorpromazine, phenytoin, sulfonamides and TDI. Type III, also known as Arthus reactions, are mediated mainly by IgG. The antigen–antibody complexes are deposited in the vascular endothelium. Depending on the site, the damaged blood vessels may cause lupus erythematosus (e.g., procainamide), and glomerular nephritis (e.g., gold).

Type IV is a delayed hypersensitivity reaction. The latent period is usually between 12 and 48 hours. The reaction is mediated by T cells (rather than antibodies) and characterized by perivascular infiltration of monocytes, lymphocytes, and lymphoblasts (resulting from local transformation of lymphocytes). Clinically, this is seen with contact dermatitis and granulomatous reactions. A commonly encountered hypersensitivity inducer is nickel, which also induces immediate immune reaction. Others include beryllium, chromium, formaldehyde, thimerosol (a mercurial compound widely used as an antimicrobial agent), and TDI.

Autoimmunity

With autoimmune diseases, the immune system produces antibodies to endogenous antigens, thus damaging normal tissues. Hemolytic anemia is an example of such disorders with phagocytosis of antibody-sensitized erythrocytes leading to hemolysis and anemia. Certain chemicals and metals have been reported to induce such diseases. For example, the pesticide dieldrin has been shown to cause hemolytic anemia. Exposure to gold and mercury has been associated with a type of glomerular nephritis that is considered an autoimmune disease (Dean *et al.*, 1982).

In addition, a number of drugs are known to be toxic through their effects on the cellular or humoral immunity, inducing autoimmune diseases. Clinically these conditions manifest as hepatitis, nephritis, hemolytic anemia, neutropenia, thrombocytopenia, etc. (see also Chapters 12–15). Table 11.3 is a compilation of such drugs.

The mode of action of these drugs appears to be mediated through covalent binding of the drug or its metabolite to tissue macromolecules. The target specificity may be related to differences in tissue distribution of the conjugates. In general, the incidence of these side effects is low. The low incidence might be due to complex genetic makeup, which determines the levels of activating and detoxicating enzymes (Pohl *et al.*, 1988; Park and Kiteringham, 1990).

Immunosuppression and immunodeficiencies

Many immunotoxicants suppress immune functions. An extensively studied immunotoxicant is TCDD. Its effect on the immune system is one of the most sensitive targets for toxicity. It suppresses all the specific immune functions tested, while sparing the nonspecific functions, such as the NK cell activity and macrophage functions. Its immunotoxicity is apparently mediated through binding to the *Ah* receptors on lymphoid cells (Luster *et al.*, 1989).

Other immunosuppressants have more restricted activities. For example, antineoplastic drugs such as cyclosporin adversely affect B cells; T cells that have undergone antigenic differentiation may also be affected. Metals such as lead and mercury impair both humoral and cell-mediated host resistance. In addition, gold may also induce glomerular nephritis through an autoimmune mechanism resulting in deposits in the glomeruli. Nickel may suppress immune functions through a variety of mechanisms; however, its major clinical effect is hypersensitivity. Organochlorine pesticides impair immune functions mainly in neonatal animals. Carbaryl depresses antibody response and phagocytosis by granulocytes. Corticosteroids depress immune functions as well as inflammatory responses.

Immunotoxicities: testing procedures

As noted above, the immune system is composed of a variety of cellular and humoral components and has numerous activities. An immunotoxicant can affect any one or more of these components and activities. It is therefore necessary to have an array of tests to demonstrate the various types of effects.

Immunocompetence tests in intact animals

These tests are designed to study the effects of chemicals on host resistance/susceptibility to bacterial, viral, and parasitic diseases as well as to bacterial endotoxins and tumor cells. In general, mice are used because of the large number of animals required.

The test chemical is given to the animals by an appropriate route, preferably mimicking the human exposure. Usually three dose groups plus a control group are included in the test. The duration of the dosing is generally 14 or 90 days. After this pretreatment, the animals are given a suitable quantity of the challenging agent. The quantity of the agent is selected on the basis that 10–20% of the mortality or morbidity is induced in the control animals. Increased mortality or morbidity indicates decreased host resistance. A list of various infectious agents has been compiled by Bradley and Morahan (1982).

Cell-mediated immunity

This can be studied in intact animals or with cells *in vitro*. In the intact animals, usually mice, the commonly used procedure is to determine the *delayed hypersensitivity* response to a specific antigen. The antigen, such as sheep erythrocytes or keyhole limpet hemocyanin, is injected into a footpad or an ear of the animal. Four days later, a challenging dose of the antigen is given at the sensitized site. The extent of the swelling or the amount of localized radioactivity from a radiolabeled substance, such as ^{125}I-labeled human serum albumin or tritiated thymidine, is measured (Luster *et al.*, 1982; Munson *et al.*, 1982; Sanders *et al.*, 1982).

In vitro tests are conducted on cells collected from animals pretreated with the test chemical. Such tests include lymphocyte proliferation and lymphocyte subpopulation. The *lymphocyte proliferation* assay is done by culturing, in the presence of mitogens, lymphocytes collected from the spleen of pretreated animals. Mitogens such as phytohemagglutinin and concanavalin A are capable of inducing proliferation of normal T lymphocytes, whereas lipopolysaccharides, such as the cell membrane of gram-negative bacteria, affect B lymphocytes. Immunosuppressive agents inhibit lymphocyte proliferation. The extent of proliferation can be determined by the incorporation of tritiated thymidine into DNA (Luster *et al.*, 1982).

Lymphocytes, as noted above, consist of T cells, B cells, and null cells, and the T-cell population is composed of T-memory, T-helper, and T-killer cells. Techniques for their enumeration include the use of immunofluorescence, rosette formation, histochemistry, cell electrophoresis, cytolysis, and fluorescence-activated cell sorting (Norbury, 1982).

Humoral immunity

A commonly used procedure, the plaque assay, involves quantitative determination of plaque-forming cells (PFC) of the IgM class: four days after the mouse has been sensitized to an antigen (e.g., sheep erythrocytes), the spleen is removed and a cell suspension is made. A quantity of the antigen, along with a suitable complement, is added to the suspension. The mixture is then spread on a slide and the number of plaques is counted. This represents the primary humoral immune response. To determine the secondary immune response, the mouse is given on day 10 a second dose of the antigen. On day 15 the spleen is removed and the above procedure is repeated with an additional step of incubation with rabbit anti-mouse IgG to develop the IgG-producing plaques. Reduced plaques indicate immunosuppression (Spyker-Cranmer et al., 1982). Instead of sheep erythrocytes, which are T-dependent antigens, lipopolysaccharides, which are T-independent antigens, may be used.

The levels of various immunoglobulins (IgG, IgM, IgA) in the serum may be directly measured. The techniques for their measurement have been reviewed by Davis and Ho (1976). The number of B cells in the spleen also provides information on the status of humoral immunity (Dean et al., 1982). The procedures and advantages of the enzyme-linked immunosorbent assay (ELISA) in testing chemicals for immunotoxicity have been elaborated by Vos et al. (1982).

Macrophage and bone marrow

The functions of macrophages can be tested in a number of ways: (1) the number of resident peritoneal cells, (2) phagocytosis, (3) lysosomal enzymes, (4) cytostasis of tumor target cells, and (5) reticuloendothelial system uptake of ^{132}I-triolein. Parameters of bone marrow activity include (1) cellularity, (2) colony-forming units of pluripotent cells, (3) colony-forming units of granulocyte/macrophage progenitors, and (4) iron incorporation in the bone marrow and spleen (Dean et al., 1982).

Others

A variety of pathotoxicologic data are also useful indicators of immune function: (1) hematology profile: erythrocyte count, leukocyte count, differential cell count; (2) serum proteins: albumin, globulin, albumin/globulin ratio; (3) weights: body, spleen, thymus, and adrenals; and (4) histology: thymus, adrenal, lung, kidney, heart, spleen, and cellularity of spleen and bone marrow. For example, thymic atrophy appears to be a very sensitive indicator of immunotoxicity. A paucity of lymphoid follicles and germinal centers in the spleen is indicative of B-cell deficiency, whereas

Table 11.5 NTP tier testing for chemical-induced immunotoxicity in mice

Parameter	Testing
Tier 1	
Hematology	White blood cell count and differential count
Weights	Body, spleen, thymus, kidney, liver
Histology	Spleen, thymus, lymph node cellularity
Humoral immunity	PFC to T-cell-dependent and -independent antigens
Cell-mediated immunity	Lymphocyte transformation with concanavalin A
Nonspecific immunity	Natural killer cell function
Tier 2	
T and B cells	Enumeration of these cells in spleen
Humoral immunity	Quantitation of IgG response to sheep red blood cells (RBCs)
Cellular immunity	T-cell cytolysis of tumors
Nonspecific immunity	Macrophage function
Host resistance	Syngeneic tumors: PYB6 sarcoma, B16 F10 melanoma
	Bacterial models: listeria, streptococci
	Virus: influenza
	Parasite: plasmodium yoelii

Source: Adapted from Luster *et al.* (1988).

T-cell deficiency is characterized by lymphoid hypoplasia in the paracortical areas (Dean *et al.*, 1982).

Because of the multiplicity of the tests, "tier approaches" have been proposed. The National Toxicology Program's tier testing is summarized in Table 11.5. Toxicants testing positive in Tier 1 tests can be further evaluated with tests selected from Tier 2.

Evaluation

A number of immunotoxicants have been investigated with the tests listed in Table 10.3. Analysis of the results demonstrated that:

1 No single test per se was adequate in predicting impaired host resistance,
2 On the other hand, whenever the host resistance was impaired, one or more immune function tests were affected,
3 Most immune tests yielded useful results; total white blood cell count and PFC response to lipopolysaccharide, however, were relatively poor indicators of host resistance,
4 Host resistance depended not only on the extent of immunosuppression but also on the concentration of infectious agents administered (Luster *et al.*, 1993).

References

Behan, P. O., Behan, W. M. H., Zacharias, F. J., and Nicholls, J. T. (1976) Immunological abnormalities in patients who had the oculomueocutaneous syndrome associated with practol therapy. *Lancer* ii:984–987.

Bradley, S. G. and Morahan, P. S. (1982) Approaches to assessing host resistance. *Environ. Health Perspect.* 43:65–71.

Burns, L. A., Meade, B. J., and Munson, A. E. (1996) Toxic responses of the immune system, in *Casarett and Doull's Toxicology*, C. D. Klaassen (ed.), New York, NY: McGraw-Hill, pp. 335–402.

Davis, N. C. and Ho, M. (1976) Quantitation of immunoglobulins, in *Manual of Clinical Immunology*, N. R. Rose and H. Friedman (eds), Washington, DC: American Society of Microbiology.

Dean, J. H., Luster, M. I., Boorman, G. A., and Lauer, L. D. (1982) Procedure available to examine the immunotoxicity of chemicals and drugs. *Pharmacol. Rev.* 34:137–148.

Loose, L. D. (1982) Macrophage induction of T-suppressor cells in pesticide-exposed and protozoan-infected mice. *Environ. Health Perspect.* 43:89–97.

Luster, M. I., Ackermann, M. F., Germolec, D. R., and Rosenthal, G. J. (1989) Perturbations of the immune system by xenobiotics. *Environ. Health Perspect.* 81:157–162.

Luster, M. I., Dean, J. H., and Boorman, G. A. (1982) Cell-mediated immunity and its application in toxicology. *Environ. Health Perspect.* 43:31–36.

Luster, M. I., Munson, A. E., Thomas. P. T., Hosapple, M. P., Fenters, J. D. *et al.* (1988) Development of a testing battery to assess chemical-induced immunotoxicity: National Toxicology Program's guidelines for immunotoxicity evaluation in mice. *Fundam. Appl. Toxicol.* 10:2–19.

Luster, M. I., Portier, C., Pait, D. G., Rosenthal, G. J. *et al.* (1993) Risk assessment in immunotoxicology. II. Relationship between immune and host resistance tests. *Fundam. Appl. Toxicol.* 21:71–82.

Munson, A. E., Sanders, V. M., Douglas, K. A., Sain, L. E., Kauffmann, B. M., and White, K. L. (1982) *In vivo* assessment of immunotoxicity. *Environ. Health Perspect.* 43:41–52.

Norbury, K. C. (1982) Immunotoxicology in the pharmaceutical industry. *Environ. Health Perspect.* 43:53–59.

Park, B. K. and Kiteringham, N. (1990) Drug-protein conjugation and its immunological consequences. *Drug Metab. Rev.* 22:87–144.

Pohl, L. R., Satoh, H., Christ, D. D., and Kenna, J. G. (1988) The immunologic and metabolic basis of drug hypersensitivities. *Annu. Rev. Pharmacol.* 28:367–387.

Ruddle, N. H. (1994) Tumor necrosis factor (TNFα) and lymphotoxin (TNFβ). *Curr. Opin. Immunol.* 4:327–332.

Sanders, V. M. *et al.* (1982) Humoral and cell-mediated immune status in mice exposed to trichloroethylene in the drinking water. *Toxicol. Appl. Pharmacol.* 62:358–368.

Sharma, R. P. and Reddy, R. V. (1987) Toxic effects of chemicals on the immune system, in *Handbook of Toxicology*, T. J. Haley and W. O. Berndt (eds), Washington, DC: Hemisphere, pp. 559–591.

Spyker-Cranmer, J. M., Barnett, J. B., Avery, D. L., and Cranmer, M. F. (1982) Immunoteratology of chlordane: Cell-mediated and humoral immune responses in adult mice exposed in utero. *Toxicol. Appl. Pharmacol.* 62:402–408.

Temple, L., Kawabata, T. T., Munson, A. E., and White, K. L. (1993) Comparison of ELISA and plaque-forming cell assays for measuring the humoral immune response to SRBC in rats and mice treated with benzo[a]pyrene or cyclophosphamide. *Fund. Appl. Toxicol.* 21:412–419.

Vos, J. G., Krajnac, E. I., and Beekhof, P. (1982) Use of the enzyme-linked immunosorbent assay (ELISA) in immunotoxicity testing. *Environ. Health Perspect.* 43:115–121.

Additional reading

Descates, J. (1999) *An Introduction to Immunotoxicology.* Randon, U.K. and Philadelphia, PA: Taylor & Francis.

WHO (1996) Principles and methods for assessing direct immunotoxicity associated with exposure to chemicals. *Environ. Health Criteria* 180. Geneva: World Health Organization.

Chapter 12

Respiratory system

Inhalation toxicology

CONTENTS

Introduction

With industrialization, the respiratory system of humans is increasingly exposed to airborne toxicants. Human health effects and a number of testing procedures are briefly described in this chapter.

Structure

The respiratory tract is a complex system, both in structure and function. It consists of the nasopharnx, the tracheal and bronchial tract, and the pulmonary acini, which are composed of respiratory bronchioles, alveolar ducts, and alveoli. The nasopharynx serves to remove large particles from the inhaled air, add moisture, and moderate the temperature. The tracheal and bronchial tract serves as the conducting airway to the alveoli.

Functions

The pulmonary acini are the sites where oxygen and carbon dioxide are exchanged between the blood and the air, and are the main sites of absorption of toxicants that exist in the form of gases and vapors. The alveoli are lined with epithelial cells, especially those of type I. These cells have a very thin cytoplasm (0.1–$0.2\,\mu m$), but each covers a relatively large surface ($2,290\,\mu m^2$). The cuboidal ($63\,\mu m^2$) type II cells can undergo mitosis and, in time, mature to type I cells. In addition, there are endothelial cells, macrophages, and fibroblasts.

Apart from its vital function in the exchange of oxygen and carbon dioxide, the respiratory system also regulates the blood concentrations of angiotensin, biogenic amines, and prostaglandins. Furthermore, it can excrete toxicants that have been absorbed from the lungs or via other routes. Although liver is the primary site, pulmonary tissue possesses cytochrome p450 enzymes involved in xenobiotic detoxication.

Defense mechanisms

The trachea and bronchi are lined with ciliated epithelium and covered with a thin layer of mucus secreted by certain cells in the epithelial lining. This lining, with the cilia and mucus, can move particles deposited on the surface up to the mouth. The particle-containing mucus can then be eliminated from the respiratory tract by spitting or swallowing.

The respiratory tract has various cytochrome P-450 enzyme systems, which may detoxify certain toxicants. However, many toxicants may be activated by these enzyme systems. They are concentrated in the Clara cells and, to a lesser extent, in the type II cells (Dormons and Van Bree, 1995). The Clara cells are located at the boundary where alveolar ducts branch from bronchioles.

Apart from clearance and detoxication, the respiratory tract also possesses mechanisms to phagocytize and engulf toxicants, notably solid particles. The main effector is the macrophage. Similar to the enzyme systems, the macrophage may also aggravate the toxic effects (Brain, 1992).

Toxicants and their effects

Many toxicants are known to adversely affect the respiratory system in humans and animals. Those that pose serious occupational hazards are listed in Appendix 12.1.

Inhalable toxicants exist in the form of gases, vapors, liquid droplets, and solid particulate matters. Gases and vapors are readily absorbed. The droplets and particulate matters may also be absorbed. However, they vary in size, and their sizes have marked effects on the extent of absorption. In general, large particles ($>10\,\mu$m) do not enter the respiratory tract. Very small particles ($<0.01\,\mu$m) are likely to be exhaled. The optimal size of particle for retention is between 1 and 3 μm. See also Chapter 2.

A toxicant may exert systemic effects after its absorption from the respiratory tract and distribution to other tissues, or it may induce local effects on the respiratory tract, or both. A toxicant may also affect the respiratory tract after exposure from other routes.

Systemic effects

Many chemicals can be absorbed from the inspired air. After absorption, they are carried by the circulating blood to various parts of the body and exert their effects, such as general anesthesia.

Toxic gases can be absorbed from various parts of the respiratory tract including the nasopharynx. The main site of absorption, however, is the alveoli, and the principle mechanism of absorption is simple diffusion. In addition, liquid aerosols and solid particulate matter can also be absorbed via different mechanisms. Further details regarding the uptake of toxicants are given in Chapter 2.

Pulmonary effects

A variety of pulmonary effects have been observed. These are briefly described under five categories. Additional details and references have been provided by Gordon and Amdur (1994).

Local irritation

Ammonia and chlorine are classic examples of irritant gases. They cause bronchial constriction and edema, which result in dyspnea, but chronic effects are rare. Arsenicals induce irritation on acute exposure; after prolonged exposure they can cause formation of lung cancer.

Cellular damage and edema

Toxic *gases*, such as ozone and oxides of nitrogen, can cause cellular damage, perhaps through peroxidation of cellular membranes. Edema ensues as a result of the increased permeability through the damaged membrane. The edematous fluid, however, accumulates in the airway instead of in the interstitial space, as is the case with other tissues. Such effects are also observed after inhalation of toxicants that exist in small particles, such as nickel carbonyl and certain beryllium and boron compounds.

Cellular damage usually affects type I cells in the alveoli. Death of these cells leads to proliferation of type II cells, which then flatten and become type I cells. However, more extensive damage will result in the exudation of fibrin-rich protein, neutrophils and debris into the alveoli. These eventually become fibrous tissue.

Certain organic *solvents*, such as perchloroethylene and xylene, are rapidly absorbed after inhalation and distributed to various parts of the body including the liver, which is the major site of biotransformation. Part of the solvent reenters the lung through circulation and may form reactive metabolites, leading to covalent binding with macromolecules there. This process in turn produces pulmonary cellular damage and edema.

Ipomeanol is a toxin produced by the mold *Fusarium solani*, grown on sweet potatoes. This toxin is interesting in that it causes necrosis of one type of cell only, namely, the Clara cells. These cells bioactivate the toxin to a reactive metabolite that binds to the macromolecules and causes cellular necrosis. This is followed by edema, congestion and hemorrhage in the lungs. Death may ensue (Timbrell, 1991).

Fibrosis (pneumoconiosis)

Pulmonary fibrosis is a serious, debilitating disease. *Silicosis*, with a history that goes back for thousands of years, is caused by crystalline forms of silica (silicon dioxide). Of the crystalline forms, quartz is the most stable. On heating, such as in volcanic eruption and mining, quartz may become tridymite or cristobalite. Both of these forms are more fibrogenic than quartz. The toxic effect stems from the rupture of the lysosomal membrane in a macrophage. The released lysosomal enzymes digest the macrophage, and this process, in turn, releases the silica from the lysed macrophage. And thus the process is repeated. It has been suggested that the damaged macrophage releases factors that stimulate the fibroblasts and the formation of collagen (Brain, 1980). Other cells, such as fibroblasts and epithelial cells, in response to macrophage inflammatory proteins, may also play a role in the fibrotic changes (Driscoll *et al.*, 1993). Kuhn *et al.* (1995) suggest that cytokine is involved in the fibrosis and its increase precedes deterioration of pulmonary function, hence may serve as a biomarker for initiating intervention in exposed workers.

Another major cause of pulmonary fibrosis is *asbestos*. Asbestos refers to a large number of fibrous hydrated silicates of magnesium, calcium, and others. In addition, some of these mineral fibers, such as the blue asbestos (crocidolites), can cause bronchogenic carcinoma and mesothelioma. The white variety (chrysotile) appears to have no effect on the incidence of mesothelioma. The potency of asbestos seems related to the chemical and physical properties. Fibers of $5\,\mu$m in length and $0.3\,\mu$m in diameter appear to be most potent. Various types of man-made refractory ceramic fibers have been used in place of asbestos. In the rat, they also induce fibrosis and carcinoma; but appear to be less carcinogenic than asbestos (Mast *et al.*, 1995).

Other fibrogenic substances include coal dust, kaolin, talc, aluminum, beryllium, and carbides of tungsten, titanium, and tantalum (see Appendix 12.1).

Emphysema is also a debilitating disease. It may be induced by cigarette smoking or exposure to aluminum, cadmium oxide, or oxides of nitrogen, ozone, and others. It has been suggested that the elastic fibers surrounding and supporting the alveoli and bronchi may be damaged by the elastase released from polymorphonuclear granulocytes under certain conditions (Spitznagel *et al.*, 1980).

Allergic response

This type of response is usually induced by pollens, spores of molds, bacterial contaminants, cotton dust, and so forth. Detergents containing enzymes derived from *Bacillus subtilis* have been reported to cause asthma among workers. A common chemical used in plastic industry, toluene diisocyanate (TDI), as other isocyanates, also produces hypersensitivity reaction. It is probable that this reactive chemical binds with proteins in the blood or lungs to form antigen, which stimulates antibody formation. The major response is bronchoconstriction triggered by the reaction between the antigens and circulating or fixed antibodies (Karol and Jin, 1991). Long-term exposure may result in other pulmonary effects such as chronic bronchitis and fibrosis.

Lung cancer

Cigarette smoke contains a number of carcinogens, cocarcinogens and irritants. These substances initiate and promote carcinogenesis. Furthermore, many other substances may induce oxidative stress, thereby adversely affecting health (Appendix 12.2). Some details of this topic have been outlined by Halliwell and Cross (1994). It is well established that cigarette smoking is the leading cause of lung cancer in many countries and that it greatly increases the incidence of lung cancers among asbestos workers (Chapter 5). Other causes of lung cancer include arsenic, chromates, nickel, uranium and coke oven emissions.

Asbestos has been well known for its carcinogenicity in the respiratory tract in humans and animals. Man-made refractory ceramic fibers appear to be carcinogenic also, but only at maximum tolerated doses. Much investigation is in progress to determine their health hazards, if any, in humans. One important approach is to assess their persistence, which is a determinant of their toxicity (Bignon *et al.*, 1994).

Effects on upper respiratory tract

Large airborne particles in the inhaled air are mainly deposited in the nasal passages. They may cause hyperemia, squamous- or transitional-cell metaplasia, hyperplasia, ulceration, and, in certain cases, carcinoma. For example, nickel subsulfide, nickel oxide, and nickel usually exist in large particles during their production and mining; therefore, their effects are mainly on the nasal passage (NAS, 1975). The larynx is also a site of chemical carcinogenesis, for example, with asbestos and chromium. Inhalation of gases and vapors such as sulfur dioxide and toluene may cause irritation of trachea and bronchi. Other toxic effects include deciliation, goblet-cell hyperplasia, and squamous metaplasia.

Effects after other routes of exposure

Paraquat, a herbicide, causes lung damage not only after exposure by inhalation but also after ingestion (Clark *et al.*, 1966). Its storage in the lungs and its inherent toxicity are apparently the reasons for its pulmonary effects after noninhalation routes. In contrast, a closely related herbicide, diquat, although also toxic to cultured lung cells, is not toxic to the lungs either after inhalation or after ingestion. It is interesting that diquat is not retained by the lungs (see also p. 293).

A number of drugs are known to induce pulmonary fibrosis in humans. These include bleomycin, busulfan, cyclophosphamide, gold salts, melphalan, methotrexate, and mitomycin. In these cases, there is an increase in interstitial collagen and in the number of type II cells. Methotrexate and streptomycin have been reported to cause pulmonary eosinophilia (Davies, 1987). Phenylbutazone and oxyphenylbutazone may cause pulmonary edema.

In addition, a number of amphiphilic drugs, such as chloroquine and triparanol, are known to interact with the phospholipids in certain cells to form myeloid bodies and pulmonary foam cells in humans and animals. These bodies and cells lead to alteration of cell activities and later to impairment of respiratory functions (Hruban, 1984).

Testing procedures

The local and systemic effects of toxicants resulting from their exposure via the respiratory tract are usually studied by mixing or suspending the toxicants in the air to be inhaled by the test subject. In exceptional cases the material on test is deposited, in liquid or solid form, in the respiratory tract.

Exposure facilities

The systemic and local effects of toxicants administered to animals through the respiratory tract generally require elaborate facilities. The test animal may be placed in whole-body exposure chambers or exposed through the head or the nose only. Other systems have been designed to study the effects of toxicants through lung-only or partial lung exposure.

A Whole-Body System typically consists of a chamber wherein the test animal is kept. The chamber is equipped with windows for observation of the test animal, and is connected to an air inlet and an air outlet. The toxicant, in the form of vapor or aerosol, is mixed with clean air and introduced into the chamber through the inlet. The outlet is usually connected to a filtering system to remove the toxicant from the exhaust before being released to the atmosphere. Typical systems have been described by Drew and Laskin (1973), and Phalen (1976). More recently, the design, operation, and characterization of a large, chronic inhalation exposure facility, with four $12.6 \, m^3$ exposure chambers, have been described (Schreck et al., 1981). Equipment for generating and controlling atmospheres in inhalation chambers has been described and compared by Rampy (1981) and Davies et al. (1987).

The Head-and-Nose-Exposure Systems have the advantages of (1) avoiding absorption of the toxicant deposited on the fur, thus avoiding absorption through the skin or through the gastrointestinal tract when the animal grooms itself, and (2) requiring a more limited quantity of the test material. However, fitting the head or nostrils of the animals to the apparatus requires some skill and time. A number of such systems have been developed and the references to their descriptions are also given in a WHO document (1978).

Animals, doses, and duration

The commonly used experimental animals are rats, dogs, and monkeys. Others include mice, hamsters, guinea pigs, rabbits, miniature pigs, and donkeys. The choice should be based on a number of criteria. It may be noted that monkeys are distinctly different from humans in spite of their phylogenetic proximity. Horses and donkeys are very similar to humans in this respect. Other factors, which may be more important, are the similarity of their biochemical and physiologic responses to those of humans and an abundance of experimental results, which permits comparison between the toxicities of various chemicals. It has been well documented in epidemiologic studies that people with preexisting cardiopulmonary diseases are at special risk during air pollution episodes (see Chapter 22). To simulate this condition, papain-induced emphysematous animals have been used (Gross *et al.*, 1965).

In general, the dose is the amount of a substance that is administered to an organism. The amount is readily ascertained when the substance is given by a route such as oral, subcutaneous, intravenous, or intraperitoneal. This definition is not applicable to exposure by inhalation, because the amount that is retained in the animal depends on the concentration of the toxicant in the inhaled air as well as the duration of the exposure. In other words, the dose might be *expressed* as the product of the concentration (C) and the time (t). It has been recognized that for a fixed $C \times t$ product the response will be the same. However, this rule is not valid when either C or t is an extreme value. For example, if C is too small, generally no response will be elicited no matter how long the animal is exposed to it.

In most inhalation studies the retained doses are not estimated. Instead, the duration of exposure is kept constant whereas the test animals are exposed to different concentrations of a toxicant. For example, in acute median lethality studies, the animals are exposed, as a rule for four hours. In longer-term studies either a *continuous* (23 hours/day) or an *intermittent* (eight hours/day, five days/week) exposure scheme is adopted, the former being designed to simulate the exposure to environmental pollutants and the latter, industrial situations.

For acute LC_{50} determinations (LC_{50} is the concentration that will cause the death of 50% of the animals at a specified duration of exposure), the duration of exposure is usually between one and four hours. In short-term studies the duration is usually 30 or 90 days, and in long-term studies it is one year or more. The repeated exposures are either on a continuous or intermittent basis, as discussed above.

Observations and examinations

General

These include body weight and food consumption, general observations, laboratory tests, and postmortem examinations. Some details on these are given in Chapter 6.

Respiratory functions

Tests on these functions are often carried out because of their greater sensitivity than morphologic changes and because of their ability to detect reversible effects. As a result, these tests are often used in studies in humans. Similar tests in animals would therefore allow a more valid comparison between humans and the experimental animals with respect to their relative susceptibility to the toxic effects of the substance being tested.

Respiratory frequency is a sensitive indicator of local irritation and is often concentration-related. Certain gases, such as ozone and nitrogen dioxide, increase the frequency, whereas others, such as sulfur dioxide and formaldehyde, decrease it.

Mechanics of respiration can be measured in terms of pulmonary flow resistance and pulmonary compliance. An increase in pulmonary flow resistance can result from bronchoconstriction, swelling of the respiratory mucosa, or an increase in mucus secretion. Pulmonary compliance is decreased by fibrosis, and it is increased in emphysema because of loss of supportive connective tissue. References to their measurements are given in a WHO document (1978).

Respiratory efficiency can be estimated by measuring oxygen and carbon dioxide in the blood or by measuring the rate at which inhaled carbon monoxide is taken into the blood (O'Neil and Raub, 1984).

Morphologic and biochemical changes

As described above, various morphologic changes can result from inhalation exposure to toxicants. These include local irritation, cellular damage, edema, fibrosis, and neoplasms. In addition, toxicants can cause a number of other types of morphologic changes such as inflammation, hyperplasia, and emphysema, as shown in Appendix 12.1.

Some examinations are especially useful. For example, lung-weight increases are indicators of vascular congestion, edema, or increase in connective tissue. Bronchoalveolar lavage (BAL) can provide information on the cell number, type, and morphology as well as on noncellular components, especially the enzyme content. Furthermore, the collagen content can be estimated by determining hydroxyproline or prolylhydroxylase in lung tissues (see Tyler *et al.*, 1985). See also EPA's guide on inhalation toxicity (1994).

In vitro tests

In order to conduct more definitive studies on the effects of toxicants on the respiratory system, various *in vitro* systems have been developed.

Isolated perfused lung

Lungs isolated from rabbits or rats are perfused with heparinized blood at a constant pressure and ventilated with positive pressure through the trachea or negative pressure from outside of the lung. A constant blood flow can be maintained over a period of several hours. The system is especially useful in determining nonrespiratory functions of the lung. For example, the levels of the endogenous hormones and vasoactive amines can be readily determined in the exudate. Furthermore, the pulmonary metabolism of a toxicant can be ascertained by adding it to the perfusate and analyzing the exudate for the toxicant and its metabolite. Some details and references are provided by Anderson and Eling (1976), and Roth (1980).

Tracheal explants and lung organ culture

The effects of toxic gases and vapors can be assessed on the trachea removed from animals, such as rats, that have been exposed to toxicants. When incubated in a tissue culture medium the trachea will continue to secrete mucus glycoproteins. The rate of secretion can be affected by exposure to toxicants. For example, tracheal explants taken from rats exposed to ozone at 0.8 ppm showed an increased rate of secretion, but those from rats exposed to 0.5 ppm ozone or 1.1 mg/m^3 sulfuric acid did not. Exposure to the combination, however, induced significantly greater rates of secretion (Last and Kaizer, 1980).

Isolated cells

Various types of cells from the respiratory system have been isolated and cultured. These include the epithelial cells of the trachea and the lung tissue as well as the endothelial cells. Isolated cultured cells show promise of becoming useful tools in toxicology of the respiratory system. Reiser and Last (1979), for example, pointed out the importance of pulmonary alveolar macrophages and fibroblasts in the development of fibrosis in chronic silicosis. They also noted the likelihood of involvement of other cell types, the precise role of which awaits further studies with isolated cells.

Evaluation

Analyses of the data relating to the effects and the dose are essentially the same as those following other routes of administration, with the exception that the dose is generally handled differently.

As noted above, while the retained dose after exposure by inhalation can be estimated, the common practice is to use the concentration instead. Thus, the results of acute median lethality studies are expressed as LC_{50}. The LC_{50} values of various compounds can be compared, provided the same duration of exposure was used in the inhalation studies.

The determination of the dose–effect and the dose–response relationships can also be done in the conventional manner, using concentrations instead of doses. The procedure employed in the estimation of the *no-effect level*, as described in Chapter 6, can also be adopted in inhalation studies.

Whereas the concentration can be readily expressed with gases and vapors, the *effective* concentration of aerosols is influenced by the particle size, which can greatly influence the deposition, penetration, and absorption of the material. Thus, when reporting inhalation studies, it is necessary to provide information on the median particle size and their geometric standard deviations (Chapter 2).

References

Anderson, M. W. and Eling, T. E. (1976) Studies on the uptake, metabolism, and release of endogenous and exogenous chemicals by the use of the isolated perfused lung. *Environ. Health Perspect.* 16:77–81.

Bignon, J., Saracci, R., and Touray, J. C. (1994) Biopersistence of respirable synthetic fibers and minerals. *Environ. Health Persp.* vol. 102, suppl. 5.

Brain, J. D. (1980) Macrophage damage in relation to the pathogenesis of lung diseases. *Environ. Health Perspect.* 35:21–28.

Brain, J. D. (1992) Mechanisms, measurement and significance of lung macrophage function. *Envir. Health Persp.* 97:5–10.

Clark, D. G., McElligott, T. F., and Hurst, E. W. (1966) The toxicity of paraquat. *Br. J. Ind. Med.* 23:126–132.

Davies, D. W., Walsh, L. C. III, Hiteshaw, M. E., Ménache, M. G., Miller, F. J., and Grose, E. C. (1987) Evaluating the toxicity of urban pattern of oxidant gases. I. An automated chronic gaseous animal inhalation exposure facility. *J. Toxicol. Environ. Health* 21:89–97.

Dormans, J. A. M. A. and Van Bree, L. (1995) Function and response of type II cells to inhaled toxicants. *Inhal. Toxicol.* 7:319–342.

Drew, R. T. and Laskin, S. (1973) Environmental inhalation chambers, in *Methods of Animal Experimentation*, W. I. Day (ed.), New York, NY: Academic Press.

Driscoll, K. E., Hassenbein, D. G., Carter, J. *et al.* (1993) Macrophage inflammatory proteins 1 and 2: Expression by rat alveolar macrophages, fibroblasts, and epithelial cells and in rat lung after minimal dust exposure. *Am. J. Respir. Cell Mol. Biol.* 8:311–318.

EPA (1994) Health effect testing guidelines. *Code of Federal Regulations*, Title 40, Part 798.

Gordon, T. and Amdur, M. O. (1994) Responses of the respiratory system to toxic agents, in *Casarett and Doull's Toxicology: The Basic Science of Poisons*, 4th edn, M. O. Amdur, J. Doull and C. D. Klaassen (eds), New York, NY: McGraw-Hill, pp. 443–462.

Gross, P., Pfitzer, E. A., Tolker, E., Babyak, M. A., and Kaschak, M. (1965) Experimental emphysema: Its production with papain in normal and silicotic rats. *Arch. Environ. Health* 11:50–58.

Halliwell, B. and Cross, C. E. (1994) Oxygen-derived species: Their relation to human disease and environmental stress. *Environ. Health Persp.* vol. 102(Suppl. 10):5–12.

Hruban, Z. (1984) Pulmonary and generalized lysosomal storage induced by amphiphilic drugs. *Environ. Health Perspect.* 55:53–76.

Karol, M. H. and Jin, R. (1991) Mechanism of immunotoxicity to isocyanates. *Chem. Res. Toxicol.* 4:503–509.

Kuhn, D. C., Stauffer, J. L., Gaydos, L. J., and Demers, L. M. (1995) Inflammatory and fibrotic mediator release by alveoli macrophages from coal miners. *J. Toxicol. Environ. Health* 45:9–21.

Last, J. A. and Kaizer, T. (1980) Mucus glycoprotein secretion by tracheal explants: Effect of pollutants. *Environ. Health Perspect.* 35:131–137.

Mast, R. W., McConnell, E. E., Anderson, R. *et al.* (1995) Studies on the chronic toxicity (inhalation) of four types of refractory ceramic fiber in male Fischer 344 rats. *Inhal. Toxicol.* 7:425–467.

National Academy of Sciences (NAS) (1975) *Nickel.* Washington, DC: National Academy of Sciences.

O'Neil, J. J. and Raub, J. A. (1984) Pulmonary function testing in small laboratory animals. *Environ. Health Perspect.* 56:11–22.

Phalen, R. F. (1976) Inhalation exposure of animals. *Environ. Health Perspect.* 16:17–24.

Rampy, L. W. (1981) Generating and controlling atmospheres in inhalation chambers, in *Scientific Considerations in Monitoring and Evaluating Toxicological Research*, E. J. Gralla (ed.), Washington, DC: Hemisphere.

Reiser, K. M. and Last, J. A. (1979) Silicosis and fibrogenesis: Fact and artifact. *Toxicology* 13:51–72.

Roth, J. A. (1980) Use of perfused lung in biochemical toxicology. *Rev. Biochem. Toxicol.* 1:287–309.

Schreck, R. M., Chan, T. L., and Soderholm, S. C. (1981) Design operation and characterization of large volume exposure chambers, in *Proceedings of the Inhalation Toxicology and Technology Symposium*, B. K. J. Leong (ed.), Ann Arbor, MI: Ann Arbor Science.

Spitznagel, J. K., Moderzakowski, M. C., Pryzwansky, K. B., and MacRae, E. K. (1980) Neutral proteases of human polymorphonuclear granulocytes: Putative mediators of pulmonary damage. *Environ. Health Perspect.* 35:29–38.

Timbrell, J. A. (1991) *Principles of Biochemical Toxicology.* London: Taylor & Francis.

Tyler, W. S., Dungworth, D. L., Plopper, C. G., Hyde, D. M., and Tyler, N. K. (1985) Structural evaluation of the respiratory system. *Fundam. Appl. Toxicol.* 5:405–422.

WHO (1978) Inhalation exposure, in *Principles and Methods for Evaluating the Toxicity of Chemicals. Part I.* Environmental Health Criteria 6. Geneva: World Health Organization.

Appendix 12.1 Site of action and pulmonary disease produced by selected occupationally inhaled toxicants

Toxicant	Common name of disease	Acute effect	Chronic effect
Aluminum dust	Aluminosis	Cough, shortness of breath	Interstitial fibrosis
Aluminum abrasives	Shaver's disease, corundum smelter's lung, bauxite lung	Alveolar edema	Fibrotic thickening of alveolar walls, interstitial fibrosis, and emphysema
Ammonia		Immediate upper and lower respiratory tract irritation, edema	Chronic bronchitis
Arsenic		Bronchitis	Lung cancer, bronchitis, laryngitis
Asbestos	Asbestosis		Pulmonary fibrosis, pleural calcification, lung cancer, pleural mesothelioma
Beryllium	Berylliosis	Edema, pneumonia	Pulmonary fibrosis, progressive dyspnea, interstitial granulomatosis, cor pulmonale
Cadmium oxide		Cough, pneumonia	Emphysema, cor pulmonale
Carbides of tungsten, titanium, tantalum	Hard metal disease	Hyperplasia and metaplasia of bronchial epithelium	Fibrosis, peribronchial and perivascular fibrosis
Chlorine		Cough, hemoptysis, dyspnea, tracheo-bronchitis, broncho-pneumonia	
Chromium (VI)		Nasal irritation, bronchitis	Lung tumors and cancers
Coal dust	Pneumoconiosis		Pulmonary fibrosis
Coke oven emissions			Tracheobronchial cancers
Cotton dust	Byssinosis	Tightness in chest, wheezing, dyspnea	Reduced pulmonary function, chronic bronchitis
Hydrogen fluoride		Respiratory irritation, hemorrhagic pulmonary edema	
Iron oxides	Siderotic lung disease	Cough	
	Silver finisher's lung		Subpleural and perivascular aggregations of macrophages

Appendix 12.1 (continued)

Toxicant	Common name of disease	Acute effect	Chronic effect
	Hematite miner's lung		Diffuse fibrosis-like pneumoconiosis
	Arc welder's lung		Bronchitis
Isocyanates		Cough, dyspnea	Asthma, reduced pulmonary function
Kaolin	Kaolinosis		Pulmonary fibrosis
Nickel		Pulmonary edema, delayed by two days (NiCO)	Squamous-cell carcinoma of nasal cavity and lung
Oxides of nitrogen		Pulmonary congestion and edema	Emphysema
Ozone		Pulmonary edema	Emphysema
Phosgene		Edema	Bronchitis
Perchloroethylene		Pulmonary edema	
Silica	Silicosis, pneumoconiosis		Pulmonary fibrosis
Sulfur dioxide		Bronchoconstriction, cough, tightness in chest	
Talc	Talcosis		Pulmonary fibrosis
Tin	Stanosis		Widespread mottling of X-ray without clinical signs
Vanadium		Upper airway irritation and mucus production	Chronic bronchitis

Source: Adapted from Gordon and Amdur, 1994.

Appendix 12.2 Mechanisms underlying the oxidative stress induced by cigarette smoke

1 Smoke contains many free radicals, especially peroxyl radicals, that might attack biological molecules and deplete antioxidants, such as vitamin C and α-tocopherol.
2 Smoke contains oxides of nitrogen, including the unpleasant nitrogen dioxide ($NO_2^{\cdot-}$).
3 The tar phase of smoke contains hydroquinones. These are lipid-soluble and can redox-cycle to form $O_2^{\cdot-}$ and H_2O_2. They can enter cells and may even reach the nucleus to cause oxidative DNA damage. Some hydroquinones may release iron from the iron-storage protein ferritin in lung cells and respiratory tract lining fluids.
4 Smoking may irritate lung macrophages, activating them to make $O_2^{\cdot-}$.[a]
5 Smokers' lungs contain more neutrophils than the lungs of nonsmokers, and smoke might activate these cells to make $O_2^{\cdot-}$.[a]
6 Smokers often eat poorly and drink more alcohol than nonsmokers and have a low intake of nutrient antioxidants.

Source: Halliwell and Cross, 1994.

Note
a The effects of cigarette smoke on phagocytes are dose-related. Low levels may stimulate them, but high levels may poison them and so depress their activity.

Chapter 13

Toxicology of the liver

CONTENTS

General considerations

The liver is the largest and metabolically the most complex organ in the body. It is involved in the metabolism of nutrients as well as most drugs and toxicants. The latter type of substances can usually be detoxified, but many of them can be bioactivated and become more toxic.

Hepatocytes (hepatic parenchymal cells) comprise the bulk of the organ. They are responsible for the liver's central role in metabolism. These cells lie between the blood-filled sinusoids and the biliary passages. Kupffer cells line the hepatic sinusoids and constitute an important part of the reticuloendothelial system of the body. The blood is supplied through the portal vein and hepatic artery, and it is drained through the central veins and then the hepatic vein into the vena cava. The biliary passages begin as tiny bile canaliculi formed by adjacent parenchymal cells. The canaliculi coalesce into ductules, interlobular bile ducts, and larger hepatic ducts (Figure 13.1). The main hepatic duct joins the cystic duct from the gallbladder to form the common bile duct, which drains into the duodenum.

The toxicology of liver is complicated by the variety of liver injuries and by the different mechanisms through which the injuries are induced. The types of injury, the underlying mechanisms, and the morphologic and biochemical changes are described and discussed.

The liver is often the target organ for a number of reasons. Most toxicants enter the body via the gastrointestinal tract, and after absorption

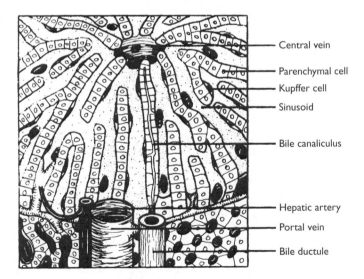

Central vein
Parenchymal cell
Kupffer cell
Sinusoid
Bile canaliculus
Hepatic artery
Portal vein
Bile ductule

Figure 13.1 Schematic structure of the liver indicating the relation between parenchymal cells and vascular and ductal systems.

Source: Klaassen and Watkins, 1984.

they are carried by the hepatic portal vein to the liver. The liver has a high concentration of binding sites. It also has a high concentration of xenobiotic-metabolizing enzymes (mainly cytochrome P-450), which render most toxicants less toxic and more water-soluble, and thus more readily excretable. But in some cases the toxicants are activated to be capable of inducing lesions (see also Chapter 3). The fact that hepatic lesions are often centrilobular has been attributed to the higher concentration of cytochrome P-450 there. In addition, the relatively lower concentration of glutathione there, compared to that in other parts of the liver, may also play a role (Smith *et al.*, 1979).

Types of liver injury

Toxicants can induce a variety of toxic effects on different organelles in the cells in liver (as shown in Table 13.1), exhibiting different types of liver injury as described below. These liver injuries are mediated through a number of biochemical reactions, such as lipid peroxidation, covalent binding, inhibition of protein synthesis, disturbance of biliary production and/or flow, immunologic reaction, and perturbation of calcium homeostasis.

Fatty liver (steatosis)

A fatty liver is one that contains more than 5% lipid by weight. The presence of an excess stainable fat in such liver is demonstrable histochemically. The lesion can be acute, such as that induced by ethionine, phosphorus, or tetracycline. Ethanol and methotrexate can cause either

Table 13.1 Effects of toxicants on subcellular organelles in liver cells

Organelle	Effect	Examples of toxicants
Plasma membrane	Enzyme leakage	Acetaminophen, carbon tetrachloride, phalloidin
Nucleus	Neoplasia	Aflatoxin, beryllium, cycasin, dimethyl-nitrosamine, tannic acid
Mitochondria	Swelling	Carbon tetrachloride, cycasin, dimethyl-nitrosamine, diquat, ethionine, phosphorus
Lysosomes	Accumulation	Beryllium, carbon tetrachloride, ethionine, phosphorus
Peroxisomes	Proliferation	Clofibrate, trichloroethylene, high-fat diet
Endoplasmic reticulum	Degranulation; proliferation	Carbon tetrachloride, dimethyl-nitrosamine, ethionine, phosphorus
Cytoskeleton	Derangement	Cytochalasin B, phalloidin
Bile canaliculi	Dilatation	Lithocholate, taurocholate

Source: Adapted from de la Iglesia *et al.*, 1982; Stott, 1988; and Plaa, 1993.

acute or chronic lesions. Some toxicants, such as tetracycline, produce many small fat droplets in a cell, whereas others, such as ethanol, induce large fat droplets, which displace the nucleus.

Although lipid accumulation in the liver is the common end point of these toxicants, the underlying mechanisms are varied. One of the mechanisms is an increased synthesis of triglyceride and the other lipid moieties. However, the most common mechanism is impairment of the release of hepatic triglyceride to the plasma. Since hepatic triglyceride is secreted only when it is combined with lipoprotein (forming *very low density lipoprotein* (VLDL)), accumulation of hepatic lipid can occur as a result of a number of mechanisms:

1   Inhibition of the synthesis of the protein moiety of lipoprotein;
2   depressed conjugation of triglyceride with lipoproteins; and
3   loss of potassium from hepatocytes, resulting in an interference of transfer of the VLDL across the cell membrane (Plaa, 1993).

Liver necrosis

Liver necrosis involves the death of hepatocytes. The necrosis can be focal (central, mid-zonal, peripheral) or massive. It is usually an acute injury. A number of chemicals have been demonstrated or reported to cause liver necrosis. It is a serious toxic manifestation but is not necessarily critical because of the remarkable regenerating capacity of the liver.

Cell death occurs along with rupture of the plasma membrane. No ultrastructural changes of the membrane per se have been detected prior to its rupture. There are, however, a number of changes that precede cell death. Early morphologic changes include cytoplasmic edema, dilatation of endoplasmic reticulum, and disaggregation of polysomes. There is an accumulation of triglycerides as fat droplets in the cells. Late changes are progressive swelling of mitochondria with cristae disruption, cytoplasmic swelling, dissolution of organelles and nucleus, and rupture of plasma membrane (see Bridges *et al.*, 1983).

The biochemical changes are complex, and various hepatotoxicants apparently act through different mechanisms. Carbon tetrachloride (CCl_4) has been shown to act primarily through its reactive metabolite, the trichloromethyl radical $^{\bullet}CCl_3$ (Recknagel and Glende, 1973), which covalently binds with proteins and unsaturated lipids and induces lipid peroxidation. Subcellular membranes are rich in such lipids and are therefore susceptible (see Table 13.1). Recknagel *et al.* (1982), however, suggested that microsomal lipid peroxidation might lead to a depression of microsomal Ca^{2+} pump resulting in an early disturbance of liver cell Ca^{2+} homeostasis, which might then induce cell death. In addition, Shah *et al.* (1979)

suggested that the toxicity of CCl_4 might be mediated through another metabolite, namely phosgene.

A number of chemically related compounds, such as chloroform, tetra-chloroethane, and carbon tetrabromide, as well as phosphorus, appear to act in similar ways. Acetaminophen also induces liver necrosis but apparently not through lipid peroxidation (Kamiyama *et al.*, 1993). At low doses, its reactive metabolite conjugates with sulfate and glutathione. With increasing doses, the level of glutathione reduces, and the covalent binding of the chemical to the proteins rises, as is dramatically shown in Figure 3.2. Bromobenzene is also bioactivated in the liver. Its 3,4-epoxide covalently binds to proteins and lipids and causes necrosis (see also Chapter 3). Other examples include isoniazid and iproniazid, both of which undergo bioactivation and form metabolites that bind with macromolecules and cause necrosis (Mitchell *et al.*, 1976).

Disturbance of Ca^{2+} homeostasis may also play an important role through an activation of molecular oxygen resulting in an oxidative stress, as discussed in Chapter 4 (Thomas and Reed, 1989).

Other biochemical changes include depletion of adenosine triphosphate (ATP), shifts of the Na^+ and K^+ balance between hepatocytes and blood, depletion of glutathione, damage to cytochrome P-450, and loss of NAD and NADP (Kulkarni and Hodgson, 1980).

Cholestasis

This type of liver damage, usually acute, is less common than fatty liver and necrosis, and it is more difficult to induce in animals with the possible exception of the steroids. The cholestatic agents appear to act through several mechanisms. For example, ANIT (α-naphthylisocyanate) can induce cholestasis, hyperbilirubinemia, and inhibition of microsomal mixed-function oxygenases. Reduction of biliary excretory activity of the canalicular membrane appears to be the predominant mechanism for cholestasis. Furthermore, ANIT seems to alter ductular cell permeability. More recently, it has been shown that platelets seem to contribute to ANIT-induced liver injury (Bailie *et al.*, 1994).

A number of anabolic and contraceptive steroids as well as taurocholate, chlorpromazine, and erythromycin lactobionate have been found to cause cholestasis and hyperbilirubinemia associated with canalicular bile plugs. Ethinyl estradiol and chlorpromazine seem to impair the permeability of the biliary tract, thus reducing bile salt-independent bile flow (Plaa and Priestly, 1976; Plaa, 1993).

Cirrhosis

Cirrhosis is characterized by the presence of septae of collagen distributed throughout most of the liver. Separated by these fibrous sheaths, clusters of hepatocytes appear as nodules.

The pathogenesis is not fully understood, but in a majority of cases, cirrhosis seems to originate from single-cell necrosis associated with a deficiency in the repair mechanism. This condition then leads to fibroblastic activity and scar formation. Inadequate blood flow in the liver may be a contributing factor.

Several chemical carcinogens and long-term administration of CCl_4 can induce cirrhosis in animals. The most important cause of human cirrhosis is chronic ingestion of alcoholic beverages. The mechanism is not fully understood, but ethanol may damage mitochondria and increase local production of reactive oxygen species. These may lead to steatosis, necrosis and cirrhosis. This pathologic condition can be induced in animals only with ethanol in combination with diets deficient in choline, proteins, methionine, vitamin B_{12}, and folic acid. Since this type of nutritional deficiency is common in alcoholism, Hartroft (1975) suggested the nutritional deficiency as the primary cause. Lieber and DiCarli (1976) were able to induce cirrhosis in baboons with ethanol alone and claimed, therefore, that alcohol has direct hepatotoxicity.

Viral-like hepatitis

A clinical syndrome indistinguishable from viral hepatitis has been known to be associated with various drugs. In general, they have the following characteristics (Plaa, 1993):

1   Such liver injuries are not demonstrable in animals,
2   the effects in humans do not seem to be related to the dose,
3   the latent period varies greatly,
4   the toxicity is manifest in only a few susceptible individuals,
5   the histologic picture is more variable,
6   the patients usually show other signs of hypersensitivity and sometimes respond to a challenge dose, and
7   fever, rash, and eosinophilia are present in many cases.

The clinical picture may vary from patient to patient. For example, among those with halothane-induced hepatotoxicity, 50% of the patients had signs of typical immunologic reaction: fever, eosinophilia, prior exposure to this anesthetic. Others did not exhibit these signs and the livers of fatal cases showed lesions similar to those induced by CCl_4 (Lewis and Zimmerman, 1989).

Halothane may induce a mild hepatotoxicity which is reproducible in animals. In addition, it may act through an immune-mediated mechanism to produce the viral-like liver toxicity, which is more severe and delayed in onset (Hubbard *et al.*, 1988).

Carcinogenesis

Hepatocellular carcinoma and cholangiocarcinoma are the most common types of primary malignant neoplasms of the liver. Others include angiosarcoma, glandular carcinoma, trabecular carcinoma, and undifferentiated liver cell carcinoma. The significance of adenoma, focal basophilic hyperplasia, and hyperplastic nodule is as yet uncertain, whereas bile duct hyperplasia is likely to be a physiologic response to toxic exposure (Newberne, 1982).

As discussed in Chapter 7, a large number of toxicants are known to induce liver cancers in animals. However, the carcinogenicity of these chemicals in humans with respect to liver has not been well established (Wogan, 1976). On the other hand, the role of vinyl chloride in causing angiosarcoma in humans is beyond doubt.

Hepatotoxicants

Some of the liver injuries described above, namely, steatosis, necrosis, cirrhosis, and neoplasia, have a number of common features. (1) These injuries are relatively easily produced in experimental animals. (2) Many toxicants can induce several types of such injuries. For example, steatosis, necrosis, and cirrhosis can result from exposure to CCl_4 (and related chemicals such as chloroform), aflatoxins, and phosphorus. Aflatoxins and dioxins can induce necrosis, cirrhosis, and neoplasm. Steatosis and cirrhosis are seen after exposure to ethanol, and bromobenzene is known to induce necrosis and cirrhosis.

Cholestasis is induced mainly by certain bile salts, α-naphthylisocyanate, certain anabolic and contraceptive steroids, manganese, and a number of drugs. Some of these drugs and other substances are also known to induce viral-like hepatitis. For example, *p*-aminosalicylic acid, chlorpromazine, erythromycin, and phenytoin (diphenylhydantoin) appear to produce viral-like hepatitis through a type of hypersensitivity reaction. On the other hand, iproniazid, isoniazid, and hydrazine derivatives induce this effect perhaps through a metabolic abnormality.

Examples of the various types of hepatotoxicants are listed in Appendix 13.1.

Testing procedures

Animals and doses

The animals most commonly used are rats and mice. This is because of their ready availability, small size, low cost, ease in handling, and the relative abundance of toxicologic data. Furthermore, determinations of toxicities on the liver are often a part of short-term and long-term studies, which are usually carried out in rats and mice. Sometimes dogs are used because of their greater susceptibility to a number of toxicants. Rhesus monkeys do not appear to be preferable to dogs because they are less susceptible and are more variable in their response (Gray, 1976). The chemical to be tested should be administered to the animals by the same route as the expected human exposure.

Examinations

Gross pathology

The color and appearance can often indicate the nature of toxicity, such as fatty liver, or cirrhosis. The organ weight is usually a very sensitive indicator of effect on the liver. Whereas an effect does not necessarily indicate toxicity, an increase in liver weight has been shown in certain cases to be the most sensitive criterion of toxicity. For instance, DA 1627 [α-methyl-(α-morpholinoethyl)-1-naphthyl acetic acid] was found to significantly increase the absolute and relative liver weight at a dose level of 250 mg/kg/day without histologic changes. Fatty degeneration was observed in the animals dosed at a higher level, 1,000 mg/kg (Bianchi et al., 1968).

Microscopic examinations

Light microscopy can detect a variety of histologic abnormalities, such as fatty change, necrosis, cirrhosis, hyperplastic nodules, and neoplasia. Korsrud et al. (1972) found that CCl_4 produced histopathologic changes in the liver of rats at doses lower than those that induced changes in serum enzymes. Grice (1972) confirmed this finding with CCl_4 as well as with mercuric chloride, thioacetamide, and diethanolamine.

Electron microscopy can detect changes in various subcellular structures. Observations of subcellular changes, along with biochemical findings, are often useful in delineating the mechanism of action of toxicants.

Biochemical tests

Serum enzymes

A number of serum enzymes have been used as indicators of hepatic injuries. These enzymes are released to the blood from the cytosol and subcellular organelles. The serum level of alanine aminotransferase (ALT) is increased in good correlation with the severity of hepatic necrosis as determined histologically. It is therefore the choice test in liver necrosis. In addition, ornithine carbamoyl transferase (OCT) and sorbitol dehydrogenase (SDH) are more sensitive, but less specific, than ALT. They are therefore often used in conjunction with ALT when testing new toxicants. The enzyme levels in blood are often used as biomarkers among humans exposed to hepatoxicants.

In cholestatic lesions, both ALT and alkaline phosphatase (AP) are greatly elevated. On the other hand, serum cholinesterase may be reduced in certain cases of liver diseases. For additional details, see Plaa and Charbonneau (1994).

Other tests

The liver is involved in the metabolism of carbohydrate, fat, and protein as well as in the formation of prothrombin and the excretion of bilirubin and certain foreign chemicals. It is also the major site of biotransformation of toxicants. Tests have thus been devised to determine these hepatic functions.

For example, bilirubin is excreted by the liver, hence its level in the blood is an index of liver function, but it is relatively insensitive. The rate of excretion of BSP is a more sensitive indicator of liver damage. Clinically, the prolongation of prothrombin time, after excluding vitamin K deficiency, has been used in detecting acute hepatic lesions. A chemical may either potentiate or inhibit the pharmacologic and toxicologic actions of another by stimulating the hepatic microsomal enzymes (see Chapter 5). Measurements of barbiturate-induced sleeping time and the duration of zoxazolamine-induced paralysis have been used as indications of hepatic effects.

In addition, a number of biochemical tests can be performed on the liver tissue itself:

1   level of triglycerides,
2   activity of glucose 6-phosphatase,
3   level of microsomal conjugated dienes, resulting from peroxidation of microsomal lipids,
4   covalent binding of reactive metabolites to tissue macromolecules,

5   arylation or alkylation of purine and pyrimidine components of DNA and RNA (carcinogenicity), and
6   arylation or alkylation of other macromolecules (necrosis?).

Because of the importance of lipid peroxidation in liver lesions, the extent of this reaction is often determined, using thiobarbituric acid (TBA). It combines with malonaldehyde, a degradation product of the lipid, to form a colored complex, which can be measured quantitatively.

In vitro tests

The rat liver can be isolated and perfused in the study of a wide range of effects on a variety of hepatotoxicants. For example, the effects of CCl_4 on the transport and metabolism of triglycerides and fatty acids have been studied by Heimberg et al. (1962). Frazier and Kingsley (1976) reported on the transport of cadmium by the isolated liver to the bile. Isolated rat and human hepatocytes, in suspension or in culture, have been used in a variety of biochemical studies. Freshly isolated hepatocytes are often used, but they can be maintained for only 26 hours. However, they can survive 15 days if kept in culture media. Normal hepatocytes have little or no mitotic activity. To study the effects on dividing liver cells, hepatocytes from very young animals or from liver tumors are used. The techniques involved in isolating and incubating these cells and in testing their viability are given by Greim (1980).

The isolated hepatocytes can be used to determine the nature of various toxic effects:

1   Membrane damages can be detected microscopically or biochemically. Biochemical procedures include measuring the ability of the cells to take up cofactors (e.g., NADPH), polar dyes (e.g., trypan blue), and substrates (e.g., succinate) and leakage of cytoplasmic enzymes.
2   There may be changes in cellular macromolecules such as inhibition of protein and RNA synthesis, and increased synthesis of DNA.
3   Other effects include alterations of intermediary metabolism and changes in the activity and growth of the hepatocytes.

Evaluation

Nature of toxicity

The seriousness of various types of liver lesion differs markedly. Thus, certain effects on the liver, such as malignant neoplasm, are irreversible and serious. Necrosis may or may not be serious, depending on the extent of the effect. Local necrotic cells may be replaced by new cells through mitosis of adjacent hepatocytes. An accumulation of triglycerides per se is not necessarily indicative of damage. Under certain conditions the hepatocytes, with accumulated fat, function normally (Ingelfinger, 1971). The mortality rate in drug-induced cholestatic jaundice is less than 1%, whereas that in hepatocellular jaundice (viral-like hepatitis) ranges from 10% to 50%.

As noted above, changes in organ weight are often a very sensitive indicator of toxicity. However, it is important to bear in mind that some enzyme inducers such as phenobarbital may increase the liver weight associated with biological effects that are generally considered as adaptive rather than toxic. These effects generally include proliferation of the smooth endoplasmic reticulum, increased cytochrome P-450 content, increased drug-metabolizing activity, and increased amount of polyunsaturated acyl side chains. On the other hand, hepatotoxicants generally disturb the structure of the endoplasmic reticulum membranes, decrease the cytochrome P-450 content, decrease drug-metabolizing activity, and increase the amount of saturated acyl side chains (de la Iglesia et al., 1982).

Quantitative assessment

In general, microscopic changes are difficult to quantify. However, pathologic lesions can be graded according to their nature and extent (Grice, 1972). Quantitative stereology can be applied to light and electron microscopy. The tissue composition can be characterized in terms of volume, surface, and population density (de la Iglesia et al., 1982).

Biochemical findings can be readily analyzed statistically. The biochemical effects, when plotted against log dose, usually show linear dose–response relationship. This has been demonstrated, for example, in CCl_4-treated mice, with the following parameters: BSP retention, SGPT, bilirubinemia and triglycerides, glucose 6-phosphatase, and peroxidation (Plaa and Priestly, 1976).

These dose–response relations can be used in comparing the relative toxicity of different chemicals. They can also be used in the assessment of the relative sensitivity of different parameters. For example, with a 10-fold increase in the dose of CCl_4, there was a four- to five-fold increase in ALT, but only a 50% decrease in liver glucose 6-phosphatase (Plaa and Priestly, 1976).

References

Bailie, M. B., Pearson, J. M., Lappin, P. B., Killam, A. L., and Roth, R. A. (1994) Platelets and α-naphthylisothiocyanate-induced liver injury. *Toxicol. Appl. Pharmacol.* 129:207–213.

Bass, N. M. (1996) Toxic and drug induced liver disease, in *Cecil's Textbook of Medicine*, J. C. Bennett and F. Plumm (eds), Philadelphia, PA: W.B. Saunders, pp. 772–776.

Bianchi, C., Bonardo, G., and Marazzi-Uberti, E. (1968) Toxicology of α-methyl-α-(2-morpholinoethyl)-1-naphthyl-acetic acid hydrochloride. *Toxicol. Appl. Pharmacol.* 12:331–336.

Bridges, J. W., Benford, D. J., and Hubbard, S. A. (1983) Mechanisms of toxic injury. *Ann. NY Acad. Sci.* 407:42–63.

de la Iglesia, F., Sturgess, J. M., and Feuer, G. (1982) New approaches for assessment of hepatotoxicity by means of quantitative functional–morphological interrelationship, in *Toxicology of the Liver*, G. L. Plaa and W. R. Hewitt (eds), New York, NY: Raven Press.

Deng, D. J., Yang, S. M., Li, T., and Xin, H. J. (1999) Confirmation of N-(Nitrosomethyl)urea as a nitrosourea derived by nitrosation of fish sauce. *Biomed. Envir. Sci.* 12:54–61.

Frazier, J. M. and Kingsley, B. S. (1976) Kinetics of cadmium transport in the isolated perfused rat liver. *Toxicol. Appl. Pharmacol.* 38:583–593.

Gray, J. E. (1976) Assessment of hepatotoxic potential. *Environ. Health Perspect.* 15:47–54.

Greim, H. (1980) Isolated cell systems as a tool in toxicological research. *Arch. Toxicol.* 44:209–210.

Grice, H. C. (1972) The changing role of pathology in modern safety evaluation. *CRC Crit. Rev. Toxicol.* 1:119–152.

Hartroft, W. S. (1975) On the etiology of alcoholic liver cirrhosis, in *Alcoholic Liver Pathology*, J. M. Khanna, Y. Israel, and H. Kalant (eds), Toronto: Addiction Research Foundation.

Heimberg, M., Weinstein, I., Dishmon, G., and Dunkerly, A. (1962) The action of carbon tetrachloride on the transport and metabolism of triglycerides and fatty acids by the isolated perfused rat liver and its relationship to the etiology of fatty liver. *J. Biol. Chem.* 237:3623–3627.

Hubbard, A. K., Gandolfi, A. J., and Brown, R. R. (1988) Immunological basis of anesthetic-induced hepatotoxicity. *Anesthesiol.* 69:814–817.

Ingelfinger, F. J. (1971) Forward, in *Regeneration of Liver and Kidney*, N. L. R. Butcher and R. A. Malt (eds), Boston, MA: Little, Brown.

Kamiyama, T., Sato, C., Liu, J., Tajiri, K., Miyakawa, H., and Marumo, F. (1993) Role of peroxidation in acetaminophen-induced hepatotoxicity: comparison with carbon tetrachloride. *Toxicol. Lett.* 66:7–12.

Klaassen, C. D. and Watkins, J. B. (1984) Mechanisms of bile formation, hepatic uptake and biliary excretion. *Pharmacol. Rev.* 36:1–67.

Korsrud, G. O., Grice, H. C., and McLaughlan, J. M. (1972) Sensitivity of several serum enzymes in detecting carbon tetrachloride-induced liver damage in rats. *Toxicol. Appl. Pharmacol.* 22:474–483.

Kulkarni, A. P. and Hodgson, E. (1980) Hepatoxicity, in *Introduction to Biochemical Toxicology*, E. Hodgson and F. E. Guthrie (eds), New York, NY: Elsevier.

Leonard, T. B., Hewitt, W. R., Dent, J. G., and Morgan, D. G. (1986) Serum alanine aminotransferase (ALT) as a quantitative indicator to hepatic necrosis. *Toxicologist* 6:184.

Levi, P. E. (1987) Types of liver injury, in *A Textbook of Modern Toxicology*, E. Hodgson and P. E. Levi (eds), New York, NY: Elsevier.

Lewis, J. H. and Zimmerman, H. J. (1989) Drug-induced liver disease. *Med. Clin. North Am.* 73:775–792.

Lieber, C. S. and DiCarli, L. M. (1976) Animal models of ethanol dependence of liver injury in rats and baboons. *Fed. Proc.* 35:1232–1236.

Mitchell, J. R., Snodgrass, W. R., and Gillette, J. R. (1976) The role of biotransformation in chemical-induced liver injury. *Environ. Health Perspect.* 15:27–38.

Newberne, P. M. (1982) Assessment of the hepatocarcinogenic potential of chemicals: Response of the liver, in *Toxicology of the Liver*, G. L. Plaa and W. R. Hewitt (eds), New York, NY: Raven Press.

Plaa, G. L. (1976) Quantitative aspects in the assessment of liver injury. *Environ. Health Perspect.* 15:39–46.

Plaa, G. L. (1993) Toxic responses of the liver, in *Casarett and Doull's Toxicology*, 4th edn, M. O. Amdur, J. Doull, and C. D. Klaassen (eds), New York, NY: McGraw-Hill, pp. 334–353.

Plaa, G. L. and Charbonneau, M. (1994) Detection and evaluation of chemically induced liver injury, in *Principles and Methods of Toxicology*, A. W. Hayes (ed.), New York, NY: Raven Press, pp. 839–870.

Plaa, G. L. and Priestly, B. G. (1976) Intrahepatic cholestasis induced by drugs and chemicals. *Pharmacol. Rev.* 28:207–273.

Recknagel, R. O. and Glende, E. A., Jr. (1973) Carbon tetrachloride hepatotoxicity: An example of lethal cleavage. *CRC Crit. Rev. Toxicol.* 2:263–297.

Recknagel, R. O., Glende, E. A., Waller, R. L., and Lowrey, K. (1982) Lipid peroxidation: Biochemistry, measurement, and significance in liver cell injury, in *Toxicology of the Liver*, G. L. Plaa and W. R. Hewitt (eds), New York, NY: Raven Press.

Shah, H., Martman, S. P., and Weinhouse, S. (1979) Formation of carbonyl chloride in carbon tetrachloride metabolism by rat liver *in vitro*. *Cancer Res.* 39:3942–3947.

Smith, M. L., Loveridge, N., Wills, E. D., and Chayen, J. (1979) The distribution of glutathione in rat liver lobule. *Biochem. J.* 182:103–108.

Stott, W. T. (1988) Chemically induced proliferation of peroxisomes: Implications for risk assessment. *Regul. Toxicol. Pharmacol.* 8:125–159.

Thomas, C. E. and Reed, D. J. (1989) Current status of calcium in hepatocellular injury. *Hepatology* 10:375–384.

Wogan, C. N. (1976) The induction of liver cell cancer by chemicals, in *Liver Cell Cancer*, H. M. Cameron, D. A. Linsell, and G. P. Warwick (eds), Amsterdam: Elsevier.

Appendix 13.1 Examples of hepatotoxic agents and associated liver injury

Necrosis and fatty liver

Acetaminophen*
Aflatoxin
Allyl alcohol*
Azaserine
Beryllium*
Bromobenzene*
Carbon disulfide
Carbon tetrachloride
Chloroform
Corticosteroid
Cycloheximide[†]
Dichloriobenzene
Dimethylnitrosamine
Diquat

Ethanol[†]
Ethionine[†]
Furosemide*
Galactosamine
Phosphorus
Puromycin[†]
Pyrrolizidine alkaloids
Tannic acid*
Tetrachloroethane
Tetracycline[†]
Thioacetamide*
Trichloroethylene
Valproic acid[†]

Cholestasis (drug-induced)

p-Aminosalicylic acid[‡]
Amitriptyline
Carbamazepine[‡]
Carbarsone
Chlorpromazine[‡]
Chlorthiazide
Diazepam
Erythromycin estolate[‡]
Estradiol
Ethacrynic acid[‡]
Imipramine[‡]
Mepazine

Mestranol
Methandrolone
Methimazole
Oxyphenisatin[‡]
Perphenazine
Phenindione[‡]
Promazine
Steroids, androgenic and anabolic
Sulfanilamide
Thiabendazole
Thioridazine

Viral-like hepatitis (drug-induced)

Colchicine
Halothane
Imipramine
Indomethacin
Iproniazid
Isoniazid
6-Mercaptopurine

Methoxyflurane
α-Methyldopa
Papaverine
Phenylbutazone
Phenytoin
Sulfonamides
Zoxazolamine

Carcinogenesis (in experimental animals)

Acetylaminofluorene
Aflatoxin B₁**
Cycasin
Dialkyl nitrosamines
N(Nitrosomethyl)urea**

Polychlorinated biphenyls
Pyrrolizidine alkaloids
Safrole
Urethane
Vinyl chloride**

Source: Adapted from Levi, 1987; Plaa, 1993; Bass, 1996; Deng, 1999.

Notes
*Primary effect is necrosis.
[†]Primary effect is fatty liver.
[‡]Also induces viral-like hepatitis.
**In humans also.

Chpater 14

Toxicology of the kidney

CONTENTS

Introduction

As noted in Chapter 2, urine is the principal route by which most toxicants are excreted. As a result, the kidney has a high volume of blood flow, concentrates toxicants in the filtrate, transports toxicants across the tubular cells, and bioactivates or detoxifies certain toxicants. It is therefore a major target organ of toxic effects. To facilitate discussions on these effects, the renal structure and functions are briefly reviewed.

The structure

The predominant structures in the kidney are the nephrons, numbering approximately 1.3×10^6. Each nephron consists of a glomerulus and a series of tubules (see Figure 14.1). The glomerulus is supplied with a high-pressure capillary system that produces an ultrafiltrate from the plasma. The filtrate collected in the Bowman's capsule flows through the proximal convoluted tubule, the loop of Henle, and the distal convoluted tubule, and then drains through a collecting tubule into the renal pelvis for excretion as urine.

The proximal tubule is divided into three sections (S_1, S_2, and S_3). S_1 and S_3 consist of major portions of the convoluted tubule and the straight portion, respectively. S_2 consists of the end of the convoluted portion and the beginning of the straight portion.

The major function of the kidney is to eliminate wastes resulting from normal metabolism and to excrete xenobiotics and their metabolites. These are effected through the production of urine, a process that also contributes to the maintenance of the homeostatic status of the body. In addition, it has several nonexcretory functions.

The production of urine

The production of urine is a complex process. It begins with filtration in the glomeruli. In humans, approximately 180 liters of filtrate is formed per day. Since only 500–2,500 ml of urine is excreted, some 99% of the filtered water is reabsorbed.

The reabsorption of water, through diffusion, takes place first at the

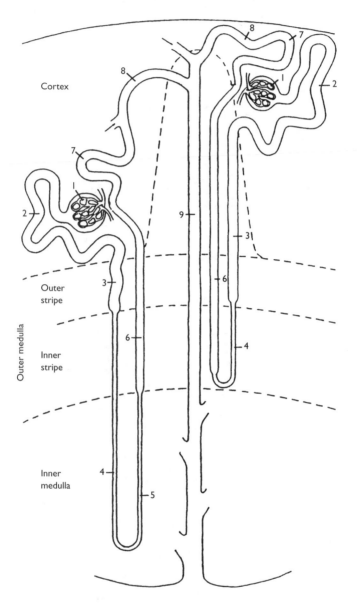

Figure 14.1 Schematic presentation of a cortical (short-looped) and a juxtamedallary (long-looped) nephron together with the collecting system. (1) glomerulus with Bowman's capsule, (2) proximal tubule, convoluted portion, (3) proximal tubule, straight portion, (4) descending thin limb (loop of Henle), (5) ascending limb (loop of Henle), (6) thick ascending limb, (7) distal convoluted tubule, (8) connecting tubule, (9) collecting tubule.

Source: Adapted from Kriz and Bankir, 1988.

proximal tubules, where Na^+ is actively reabsorbed. Further diffusion of water takes place at the descending limb of the loop of Henle to the hyperosmolar interstitium. The hyperosmolarity is produced by the active reabsorption of Cl^- (along with Na^+) at the ascending limb of the loop (Berndt, 1976). The spatial arrangement of the loops and the vasa recta provides an effective countercurrent multiplier mechanism.

Additional water is removed from the filtrate in the distal and the collecting tubules as Na^+ is actively reabsorbed. The extent of the removal of water from these tubules depends on the activity of antidiuretic hormone (ADH). ADH reduces the urine volume by increasing the permeability of these structures to water.

Tubular resorption and secretion

As the glomerular capillaries have large pores (70 nm), substances with molecular weights under 60,000 are filtered into Bowman's capsules. Some of the filtered substances such as glucose and amino acids, which are vital to the body, are reabsorbed by the tubules. On the other hand, ammonia (NH_3), a metabolic waste of amino acids, diffuses through the cells to the filtrate, where it reacts with H^+ to form NH_4^+, which is nondiffusible, hence excreted.

To facilitate the passive reabsorption of water and to maintain homeostasis, various electrolytes in the glomerular filtrate are reabsorbed nearly completely or to a great extent. The reabsorption of Na^+ at the distal and collecting tubules is regulated by mineralocorticoids, that of phosphorus by parathyroid hormone, and that of bicarbonate (HCO_3^-) by the acid-base balance. In addition, K^+ and H^+ are secreted by the tubules.

Nonexcretory functions

The kidney possesses other functions, such as the regulation of blood pressure and volume. This is mediated through the renin-angiotensin-aldosterone system. Renin, a proteolytic enzyme, is formed in the cells of the juxtaglomerular apparatus and catalyzes the conversion of a plasma angiotensin prohormone to angiotensin I. The latter, a decapeptide, is converted in the lung to angiotensin II by an enzyme that removes a dipeptide from the C-terminal end.

A renal erythropoietic factor (REF) also acts on a plasma protein to form erythropoietin, which increases the production of normoblasts and the synthesis of hemoglobin. Renal prostaglandins are produced in the interstitial cells in the medulla and appear to have the capability of regulating renal blood flow and the excretion of Na^+ and urine. The kidney is also involved in the conversion of the relatively inactive 25-hydroxy-vitamin D_3 to the active 1,25-dihydroxy-vitamin D_3.

Nephrotoxicants: mechanism and site of action

The major groups of nephrotoxicants are heavy metals, antibiotics, analgesics, and certain halogenated hydrocarbons (Table 14.1). All parts of the nephron are potentially subject to the detrimental effects of toxicants. However, most toxicants preferentially affect specific parts of the kidney. The mechanisms of action of nephrotoxicants include interaction with receptors, inhibition of oxidative phosphorylation, disturbance of Ca^{2+} homeostasis, and adverse effects in plasma and subcellular membranes. Details of these are provided in a review article (Commandeur and

Table 14.1 Nephrotoxicants

Toxicants	Site of action
Heavy metals	
Cadmium	Proximal tubules
Chromium	Proximal tubules
Gold	Glomeruli
Lead	Proximal tubules and blood vessels
Mercury, inorganic	Proximal tubules and glomeruli
Antibiotics	
Aminoglycosides	Glomeruli and proximal tubules
Amphotericin-B	Glomerular blood vessels and distal tubules
Cephaloridine	Proximal tubules
Puromycin	Glomeruli
Tetracycline	Interstitial tissues in medulla
Halogenated hydrocarbons	
Bromobenzene	Proximal tubules
Carbon tetrachloride	Proximal tubules
Chloroform	Proximal tubules
Decalin	Proximal tubules
Hexachlorobutadiene	Pars recta
Hydroquinone	Proximal tubules
Analgesics/anesthetics	
Acetaminophen	Various parts of nephron and blood vessels
Methoxyflurane	Various parts of nephron
Antineoplastics	
Cisplatin	Pars recta and other parts of nephron
Immunosuppressants	
Cyclosporin	Blood vessels and interstitial tissue
Miscellaneous	
Glycol	Tubular blockade
Sulfapyridine	Tubular blockade

Vermeulen, 1990). In general, males are more susceptible to chemical-induced nephrotoxicity. This is especially true among geriatric patients (Kacew *et al.*, 1995).

Glomeruli

The antibiotic puromycin can increase the permeability of the glomerulus to proteins such as albumin. This has been attributed to an alteration in the electrical charge of glomerular basement membrane (Brenner *et al.*, 1977). On the other hand, the aminoglycoside antibiotics, such as gentamicin and kanamycin, decrease the glomerular filtration, in addition to their effects on renal tubules (Humes and O'Connor, 1988). Certain toxicants, e.g., gold, mercury and penicillamine, may induce membranous glomerulonephritis by the deposition of antigen antibody conjugates in the glomerular basement membrane.

Proximal tubules

Because of their active absorptive and secretory activities, the proximal tubules often have higher concentrations of toxicants. Furthermore, they have a higher level of cytochrome P-450 to detoxify or activate toxicants. They are thus often the site of toxic effects. Heavy metals, such as mercury, chromium, cadmium, and lead, can alter the functions of the tubules, characterized by glycosuria, aminoaciduria, and polyuria. After higher doses, they cause tubular cell death, elevated BUN, and anuria. The straight portion (pars recta) of the proximal tubules appears more susceptible than the convoluted portion to the toxicity of mercury (Phillips *et al.*, 1977). The nephrotoxicity may result from a combination of direct cellular toxicity and ischemia secondary to vasoconstriction. Additional information on renal toxicity of metals is given in Chapter 21.

As noted above, certain antibiotics affect the glomerular filtration. In addition, many antibiotics are also secreted by the proximal tubules and can induce alterations in the tubular functions. Various aminoglycoside antibiotics (streptomycin, neomycin, kanamycin, gentomicin, and amphotericin-B) have been reported to affect the proximal tubules. These drugs alter membrane phospholipid compositions, permeability, Na^+- K^+-ATPase activity, adenylate cyclase activity, and transport of K^+, Ca^{2+}, and Mg^{2+} (Kaloyanides, 1984; Mingeot-Leclercq *et al.*, 1995). Cephaloridine, unlike the antibiotics named above, is not secreted from the proximal tubules but is accumulated in these cells, thereby causing damage.

Halogenated hydrocarbons such as carbon tetrachloride and chloroform are mainly hepatotoxic, but in certain animal species they may also exert toxic effects on the kidney, especially on the proximal tubules, as reflected in functional changes. At higher doses, however, morphologic changes may be produced in other parts of the nephron. Hexachlorobutadiene damages mainly the pars recta of the proximal tubules, resulting in decreased urinary concentrating ability. Bromobenzene as hexachlorobutadiene, is also nephrotoxic, acting on the proximal tubules, while the former is bioactivated in the liver, the latter is bioactivated in the kidney, via a renal enzyme (C-S lyase) after biotransformation in the liver (Hook *et al.*, 1982).

Other sites

Tetracycline, especially outdated products, may affect the renal medulla and induce interstitial nephritis. Amphotericin-B induces renal toxicity in a majority of the patients, affecting various renal structures.

Methoxyflurane, an anesthetic, is known to be nephrotoxic in humans and certain animals, causing *high-output* renal failure. This chemical has been shown to be biotransformed to inorganic fluoride and oxalate. Experimental data suggest that the F^- acts on several parts of the nephron to reduce the reabsorption of water. First, it interferes with the capability of the proximal tubules to reabsorb water. Second, it inhibits the enzymes involved in the transport of ions at the ascending limb of the loop of Henle, thus reducing the interstitial osmolarity, thereby decreasing water reabsorption. It also damages the collecting tubules, rendering them insensitive to antidiuretic hormone (ADH) (Mazze, 1976).

Analgesic mixtures containing aspirin and phenacetin, a derivative of acetaminophen, can cause chronic renal failure, with the toxic effects located predominantly in the medulla, i.e., loop of Henle, vasa recta, interstitial cells, and collecting tubules. The effects might be a result of vasoconstriction of the vasa recta (the blood vessels surrounding the loop of Henle) due to an inhibition of the synthesis of vasodilator prostaglandin (Nanra, 1974). Cisplatin affects many parts of the tubules in patients taking this chemotherapeutic agent (Tanaka *et al.*, 1986). Cyclosporin causes acute thrombotic microangiopathy and chronic nephropathy with interstitial fibrosis (Racusen and Solez, 1988).

Other types of toxicity include renal carcinogenicity of DMN (dimethylnitrosamine), and tubular blockade induced by the metabolites of sulfapyridine (acetylsulfapyridine) and glycols (oxalic acid). Penicillins and sulfonamides have been reported to cause inflammatory interstitial nephritis in humans. An immunologic mechanism has been suggested as responsible for this toxicity (Appel and Neu, 1977).

Testing procedure

Functional and morphologic examinations of the kidney are routinely carried out as an integral part of short-term and long-term toxicity studies.

The types of examinations involved are described in Chapter 6 and are further elaborated here.

In studies designed specifically for nephrotoxicity, dogs, rabbits, and rats are the commonly used animals. Examinations of kidney functions may be done in a number of ways.

Urinalysis

Proteinuria

Because of the size of their molecules, only a very small amount of proteins of low molecular weight pass through the glomerular filter. The low-molecular-weight proteins are readily reabsorbed by the proximal tubules. The occurrence of large amounts of such protein in the urine is thus an indication of a loss of tubular reabsorptive function, as in cadmium poisoning. On the other hand, excretion of high-molecular weight protein indicates a loss of integrity of glomeruli. It is to be noted that normal rat urine may contain some protein. A critical comparison of the treated animals with the controls is therefore important.

Glycosuria

Glucose in the glomerular filtrate is completely reabsorbed in the tubules, provided the amount of glucose to be reabsorbed does not exceed the *transport maximum* (Tm). Glycosuria in the absence of hyperglycemia thus indicates tubular dysfunction.

Urine volume and osmolarity

These two values are usually inversely related and are useful indicators of renal function in a *concentration test*, wherein water is withheld from the animal, and also in a *dilution test*, wherein a large amount of water is given to the animal. The osmolarity can be estimated from the specific gravity, but the freezing point of urine provides a more accurate measurement. A toxicant may cause high-output renal failure as noted above. On the other hand, it may cause oliguria or even anuria, resulting from tubular injury, with concomitant interstitial edema and intraluminal sediment or debris, which blocks urine flow.

Acidifying capacity

This can be assessed from urine pH, titratable acids, and NH_4^+. This capacity is reduced when there is distal tubular dysfunction.

Enzymes

Enzymes such as maltase and acid phosphatase in urine may indicate destruction of proximal tubules. Urine alkaline phosphatase, on the other hand, may be renal or hepatic in origin. Plummer (1981) suggests that the urinary enzymes not only are useful indicators of renal damage but also indicate the subcellular site of origin. For example, alkaline phosphatase is located in endoplasmic reticulum, glutamate dehydrogenase in mitochondria, and lactate dehydrogenase in cytoplasm. In general, urinary enzymes are more useful measures in acute nephrotoxic conditions.

Blood analysis

Blood urea nitrogen (BUN)

Blood urea nitrogen is derived from normal metabolism of protein and is excreted in the urine. Elevated BUN usually indicates glomerular damage. However, its level can also be affected by poor nutrition and hepatotoxicity, which are common effects of many toxicants.

Creatinine

Creatinine is a metabolite of creatine and is excreted completely in the urine via glomerular filtration. An elevation of its level in the blood is thus an indication of impaired kidney function. Furthermore, data on its level in blood and its amounts in urine can be used to estimate the glomerular filtration rate. One drawback with this procedure is the fact that some creatinine is secreted by the tubules.

Special tests

Glomerular filtration rate (GFR)

The glomerular filtration rate can be more accurately determined by the clearance of inulin, a polysaccharide. It is diffused into the glomerular filtrate and is neither reabsorbed nor secreted by the tubules. Reduced GFR indicates impairment of glomerular filtration.

Renal clearance

This is the volume of plasma that is completely cleared of a substance in a unit of time. The renal clearance of p-aminohippuric acid (PAH) exceeds that of inulin because it is not only filtered through the glomeruli but also secreted by the tubules. A reduction of PAH elimination without a concomitant decrease of GFR indicates tubular dysfunction. PAH is nearly completely (up to 90%) removed from the blood in one passage. The rate of its clearance is therefore useful in determining the effective renal plasma flow (ERPF). The renal blood flow can also be determined by the use of radiolabeled microspheres or an electromagnetic flowmeter.

PSP excretion test

The rate of excretion of phenolsulfonphthalein is related to renal blood flow. It is, therefore, often used in the assessment of renal function. However, a reduced secretion rate can also result from cardiovascular diseases.

Morphologic examinations

Gross examination

The organ weight of the kidney per se, or in terms of body weight of the animal, as a rule, is routinely determined at the end of short-term and long-term toxicity studies. Alterations in the organ weight, when compared to the controls, often suggest kidney lesions. A number of other pathologic lesions can also be detected on gross examination.

Microscopic examination

Light microscopy can reveal the site, extent, and morphologic nature of renal lesions. Electron microscopy is useful in assessing ultrastructural changes in the cells. For example, prolonged exposure to methyl mercury increased the volume density of mitochondria and lysosomes. Concomitantly, there were changes in various enzyme activities, the most notable of which was the marked increase in the specific activity of δ-aminolevulinic acid synthetase (Fowler, 1980).

In vitro studies

Kidney slices

Tissue slices provide a useful tool for the study of renal tubular function. In spite of the relatively artificial conditions imposed by *in vitro* studies, Berndt (1976) compiled data demonstrating that the *in vitro* uptakes of various organic acids, bases, sugars, amino acids, and inorganic electrolytes were essentially identical to those under *in vivo* conditions.

A toxicant to be studied can be added to the medium in which the slices are immersed, or it can be administered to the animal prior to the removal of the kidney for the preparation of the slices. For example, Koschier and Berndt (1976) reported that renal slices from animals pretreated with 2,4,5-trichlorophenoxyacetic acid (2,4,5-T) showed impaired renal transport of 2,4,5-T, 2,4-dichlorophenoxyacetic acid (2,4-D), and TEA in the absence of morphologic changes. A description of the method used in studying nephrotoxicants on kidney slices and the results obtained thereof, as well as extensive literature citations, are provided by Kacew and Hirsch (1982).

Perfused renal tubules

Various sections of the renal tubules of the rabbit have been isolated and their transport functions studied. In addition, other species of animals have been used; these include the mouse, rat, hamster, snake, flounder, frog, salamander, and humans. Schafer (1981) described the technique and outlined the pros and cons of this procedure.

Isolated nephrons

Endou *et al.* (1983) isolated nephrons from rat kidney after perfusing it with 0.1% collagenase to facilitate the dissection. They found cytochrome P-450 existent only in the proximal tubules, the straight portion containing more than the convoluted portion.

Evaluation

Nature of toxicity

The kidney has a remarkable compensatory capability. Even after appreciable changes in renal functions and morphology, the kidney may compensate and regain normal functions. Therefore, it is important to perform tests at repeated and appropriate time intervals.

Nephrotoxicants can exert adverse effects on various parts of the kidney, resulting in alterations of different functions. A variety of tests should therefore be performed. The most sensitive and reliable tests appear to vary depending on the nature of the nephrotoxicants as well as the experimental conditions (e.g., animal species, duration of exposure). Kluwe (1981) concluded from his studies that *in vitro* accumulation of organic ions (e.g., PAH, TEA), urinary concentrating ability, and kidney weight were the most sensitive and consistent indicators of nephrotoxicity. Standard urinalysis, serum analyses, qualitative enzymuria, and histopathologic changes were less sensitive and less consistent. Goldstein *et al.* (1981) observed that urine osmolarity was the most sensitive indicator of the nephrotoxicity of a platinum complex, whereas GFR and ERPF were affected only later and at higher doses.

In assessing the renal effects of a toxicant, extrarenal factors that might affect the blood volume or blood pressure should be taken into account, since they may indirectly impair renal functions. Furthermore, kidney diseases, such as those associated with aging, may be prevalent and should also be considered.

Quantitative assessment

In general, morphologic changes are difficult to quantify. However, criteria for grading the microscopic changes have been suggested by Zbinden (1976). On the other hand, biochemical and functional tests usually yield data that can be readily analyzed statistically. Since nephrotoxicants may affect several renal functions differently, quantitative comparison of relative toxicity should be done with caution.

References

Appel, G. B. and Neu, H. C. (1977) The nephrotoxicity of antimicrobial agents (parts 1 and 2). *N. Engl. J. Med.* 296:663–670, 722–728.

Berndt, W. O. (1976) Use of tissue slice technique for evaluation of renal transport processes. *Environ. Health Perspect.* 15:73–88.

Brenner, B. M., Bohrer, M. P., Baglis, C., and Deen, W. M. (1977) Determinants of glomerular permselectivity: Insights derived from observations *in vivo*. *Kidney Int.* 12:229–257.

Commandeur, J. N. M. and Vermeulen, N. P. E. (1990) Molecular and biochemical mechanisms of chemically induced nephrotoxicity: A review. *Chem. Res. Toxicol.* 3:171–194.

Endou, H., Koseki, C., and Sakai, F. (1983) Effects of 3-methylcholanthrene and starvation on intranephron distribution of cytochrome P-450. *Toxicol. Lett.* 18(Suppl. 1):1–10.

Fowler, B. A. (1980) Ultrastructural morphometric/biochemical assessment of cellular toxicity, in *The Scientific Basis of Toxicity Assessment*, P. R. Witschi (ed.), Amsterdam: Elsevier/North Holland.

Goldstein, R. S., Noordwier, B., Bond, J. T., Hook, J. B., and Mayor, G. H. (1981) cis-Dichlorodiammineplatinum nephrotoxicity: Time course and dose response of renal functional impairment. *Toxicol. Appl. Pharmacol.* 60:163–175.

Hook, J. B., Rose, M. S., and Lock, E. A. (1982) The nephrotoxicity of hexachloro-1:3-butadiene in the rat: Studies of organic anion and cation transport in renal slices and the effects of monoxygenase inducers. *Toxicol. Appl. Pharmacol.* 65:373–382.

Humes, H. D. and O'Connor, R. P. (1988) Aminoglycoside nephrotoxicity, in *Diseases of the Kidney*, 4th edn, vol. 2, R. W. Shrier and C. W. Gottschalk (eds), Boston, MA: Little, Brown.

Kacew, S. and Hirsch, G. H. (1982) Evaluation of nephrotoxicity of various compounds by means of *in vitro* techniques and comparison to *in vivo* methods, in *Toxicology of the Kidney*, J. B. Hook (ed.), New York, NY: Raven Press.

Kacew, S., Ruben, Z., and McConnell, R. F. (1995) Strain as a determinant factor in the differential responsiveness of rats to chemicals. *Toxicol. Path.* 23:701–714.

Kaloyanides, G. J. (1984) Aminoglycoside-induced functional and biochemical defects in the renal cortex. *Fundam. Appl. Toxicol.* 4:930–943.

Kluwe, W. M. (1981) Renal function tests as indicators of kidney injury in subacute toxicity studies. *Toxicol. Appl. Pharmacol.* 57:414–424.

Koschier, E. F. and Berndt, W. O. (1976) *In vitro* uptake of organic ions by renal cortical tissue of rats treated acutely with 2,4,5-trichlorophenoxyacetic acids. *Toxicol. Appl. Pharmacol.* 35:355–364.

Kriz, W. and Bankir, L. (1988) A standard nomenclature for structures of the kidney. *Am. J. Physiol.* 254:F1–F8.

Mazze, R. I. (1976) Methoxyflurane nephropathy. *Environ. Health Perspect.* 15:111–120.

Mingeot-Leclercq, M. P., Brasseur, R., and Schank, A. (1995) Molecular parameters involved in aminoglycoside nephrotoxicity. *J. Toxicol. Envir. Health* 44:263–300.

Nanra, R. S. (1974) Pathology, etiology and pathogenesis of analgesic nephropathy. *Aust. N.Z. J. Med.* 4:602–603.

Phillips, R., Yamaguchi, M., Cote, M. G., and Plaa, G. L. (1977) Assessment of mercuric chloride-induced nephrotoxicity by *p*-aminohippuric acid uptake and the activity of four gluconeogenic enzymes in rat renal cortex. *Toxicol. Appl. Pharmacol.* 41:407–422.

Plummer, D. T. (1981) Urinary enzyme in drug toxicity, in *Testing for Toxicity*, J. W. Gorrod (ed.), London: Taylor & Francis.

Racusen, L. C. and Solez, K. (1988) Cyclosporine nephrotoxicity. *Int. Rev. Expo. Pathol.* 30:107–157.

Schafer, J. A. (1981) Transport studies in isolated perfused renal tubules. *Fed. Proc.* 40:2450–2459.

Tanaka, H., Ishikawa, E., Teshima, S., and Shimizu, E. (1986) Histopathological study of human cisplatin nephrotoxicity. *Toxicol. Pathol.* 14:247–257.

Zbinden, G. (1976) *Progress in Toxicology*, vol. 2. New York, NY: Springer-Verlag.

Additional reading

WHO (1991) Principles and Methods for the Assessment of Nephrotoxicity Associated with Exposure to Chemicals. *Envir. Health Criteria*, 119.

Chapter 15

Toxicology of the skin

General considerations

The body of humans, as well as that of other animals, is almost entirely covered by skin. As a result, it is exposed to a variety of chemicals such as cosmetics, household products, topical medication, and industrial pollutants, especially in certain workplaces. Dermal exposure to chemicals can result in various types of lesions. Furthermore, skin lesions may follow systemic exposure to chemicals.

The skin consists of the epidermis and the dermis, which rests over the subcutaneous tissue (Figure 15.1). The epidermis is relatively thin, averaging 0.1–0.2 mm in thickness, whereas the dermis is about 2 mm thick. These two layers are separated by a basement membrane.

The living layer of epidermis in turn consists of a basal cell layer (stratum germinativum), which provides the other layers with new cells. These new cells become prickle cells (stratum spinosum) and, later, the granular cells (stratum granulosum). The nuclei in these cells disintegrate and dissolve. In addition, these cells produce keratohydrin, which later becomes keratin in the outermost stratum corneum, the horny layer. This layer is gradually shed. This development process takes about four weeks. The epidermis also contains melanocytes, which produce pigments; the Langerhans cells, which act as macrophages; and lymphocytes. The latter two types of cells are involved in immune responses. The epidermis thus forms an important protective cover of the body.

The dermis is mainly composed of collagen and elastin, which are important structures for the support of the skin. In this layer, there are several types of cells, the most abundant being the fibroblasts, which are involved in the biosynthesis of the fibrous proteins and ground substances such as hyaluronic acid, chondroitin sulfates, and mucopolysaccharides.

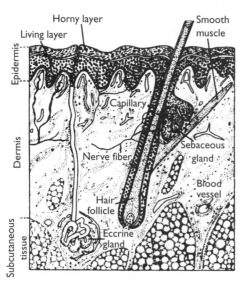

Figure 15.1 Cross section of the skin showing the two major layers of epidermis and dermis, and the various structures in the dermis.

The other types of cells include fat cells, macrophages, histiocytes, and mast cells. Underneath the dermis is the subcutaneous tissue.

There are, in addition, a number of other structures, such as the hair follicles, sweat glands (the exocrine glands), sebaceous glands, small blood vessels, and neural elements.

The possibility of systemic toxicity following dermal exposure to toxicants is discussed in Chapter 2. In addition, dermal reactions may appear following systemic administration of toxicants. The toxicities of pesticides, industrial chemicals, metals, and industrial chemicals from dermal exposure are discussed in Chapters 20, 21 and 24.

Types of toxic effects and dermatotoxicants

A variety of effects can result from dermal exposure to toxicants. Most of the effects involve the skin itself, but some of them affect its appendages – hair, sebaceous glands, and sweat glands.

Primary irritation

Irritation is a reaction of the skin to chemicals such as strong alkalis, acids, solvents, and detergents. It ranges in severity from hyperemia, edema, and vesiculation to ulceration (corrosion). Primary irritations occur at the site of contact and, in general, on the first contact. It is thus different from sensitization.

Sensitization reaction

The skin may show little or no reaction on the first contact with a chemical. However, a reaction or a more severe reaction occurs after a subsequent exposure to the chemical. The induction period ranges from a few days to years. A subsequent exposure to the specific toxicant will elicit a reaction after a delay of 12–48 hours. It is therefore known as "delayed hypersensitivity." A complex immune mechanism is involved in this reaction. Briefly, the toxicant, upon entering the skin, becomes bonded to the surface of certain cells (the APC), which will process it for reaction with T lymphocytes. After such reaction, the sensitized T lymphocytes may release a variety of substances upon reexposure to the same toxicant and result in hyperemia and edema (see also Chapters 4 and 11).

A variety of chemicals, including topical medicaments, can induce sensitization reaction. Table 15.1 lists a number of them. They show positive response in human patch test with a frequency of 5% to 11% (Nethercott et al., 1994).

Toluene diisocyanate (TDI), as noted in Chapter 12, is allergenic causing asthma and other effects in the respiratory tract. In addition, it may cause skin sensitization after inhalation (Ebino et al., 2001)

Table 15.1 Selected dermal sensitizers

Antibiotics	Neomycin
Hair dye ingredient	ρ-Phenylenediamine
Local anesthetics	Benzocaine
Metals	Nickel and nickel salts, beryllium, chromium salts, organomercurials (thimerosol)
Pesticides	Captan, ethylenediamine
Poisonous plants	Poison ivy, poison oak

Phototoxicity and photoallergy

These two types of skin reaction are similar in that both are light-induced and may follow either systemic administration or topical application of the offending chemical. However, photoallergy involves immune reactions, whereas phototoxicity does not. This and other differences have been summarized by Harber and Baer (1972) (Table 15.2).

Phototoxicity is more common than photoallergy. The commonly reported phototoxic chemicals in humans, according to Harber *et al.* (1987), are aminobenzoic acid derivatives, anthraquinone dyes, chlorpromazine, chlorothiazides, phenothiazines, sulfanilamide, and coal tar derivatives (e.g., anthracene, pyridine, acridine, and phenanthrene). The skin reaction consists of a delayed erythema, followed by hyperpigmentation and desquamation.

Table 15.2 Comparison of phototoxic and photoallergic reactions

Reaction	Phototoxic	Photoallergic
Reaction possible on first exposure	Yes	No
Incubation period necessary after first exposure	No	Yes
Chemical alteration of photosensitizer	No	Yes
Covalent binding with carrier	No	Yes
Clinical changes	Usually like sunburn	Varied morphology
Flares at distant previously involved sites possible	No	Yes
Persistent light reaction can develop	No	Yes
Cross-reactions to structurally related agents	Infrequent	Frequent
Concentration of drug necessary for reaction	High	Low
Incidence	Usually relatively high	Usually very low
Passive transfer	No	Possible
Lymphocyte stimulation test	No	Possible
Macrophage migration inhibition test	No	Possible

Source: Adapted from Harber and Baer, 1972.

Table 15.3 Examples of phototoxic photoallergic chemicals

Chemicals	Phototoxicity	Photoallergy
Aminobenzoic acid derivatives	+	+
Chlorpromazine	+	+
Chlorothiazide	+	+
Methoxypsoralens	+	−
Psoralens	+	−
Sulfonamides	+	+
Tetracyclines	+	−
Coal tar derivatives	+	−
Nonsteroidal anti inflammatory drugs	+	−

The commonly reported photoallergic chemicals include aminobenzoic acids, chlorpromazine, chlorpropamide, 2,2-thiobis(4-chlorophenol) (Fentichlor), halogenated salicylanilides, promethazine, sulfanilamide, and thiazides (Harber *et al.*, 1987). Many compounds are therefore both phototoxic and photoallergic. Clinically, photoallergy usually manifests as delayed papules and eczema, but it may also appear as immediate urticarial reaction. Histologically it is characterized by a dense perivascular round cell infiltrate in the dermis. The delayed reactions are Type IV T-cell-mediated immune response, whereas the immediate reaction is probably antibody-mediated (Chapter 11).

The most biologically active rays that cause erythema and pigmentation are in the shorter ultraviolet range, that is, wavelengths below 320 nm. The sunlight ranges from 290 nm upward, but the UV rays emitted by artificial light sources may be shorter. However, the longer UV rays (320–400 nm) per se are less erythrogenic, but are responsible for both phototoxic and photoallergic reactions to chemicals (see "Testing procedures," see p. 216).

Contact urticaria/urticarial reactions

These skin reactions, in the form of urticaria or eczema, appear within minutes to an hour after contact with the offending substance. Hence they are different from the sensitization reaction described above. The mechanism may be non-immunologic, such as the case with aspirin and methyl nicotinate. In other cases, e.g., latex rubber and penicillin, an immunologic mechanism is involved. However, unlike the sensitization reaction described above, an antibody (IgE), rather than T cell, is involved. In both immunologic and non-immunologic cases, the dermal reactions are elicited by vasoactive substances, e.g., histamine along with prostaglandins, leukotrienes, and kinins. A great variety of substances have been reported to induce these reactions, including metals (copper, platinum), medicaments (antibiotics, local anesthetics) and biogenic polymers released from arthropods (jellyfish). Amin *et al.* (1995) have provided extensive lists of agents that induce immunologic and non-immunologic immediate contact reactions. Urticarial actions may also follow ingested or parenterally administered agents.

Cutaneous cancer

It has been known for over two centuries that soots can cause skin cancer (Chapter 7). More recent studies confirm that soots and related substances, such as coal tars, creosote oils, shale oils, and cutting oil, cause cancers of the skin and other sites in animals and humans. In addition, arsenic and certain arsenic compounds have been reported to be associated with skin cancer in humans (Chapter 21).

A number of polycyclic aromatic hydrocarbons (e.g., benzo[a]pyrene) and heterocyclic compounds (e.g., benz[c]acridine) are known to induce skin cancer after topical applications on animals (IARC, 1973). UV radiation is an important cause of skin cancer in humans, and a number of chemicals can influence the effect of UV light and vice versa (Forbes, 1995).

Effects on epidermal adnexa

Hair

Loss of hair may result from various antimitotic agents used in cancer chemotherapy. These agents affect the anagen phase of hair growth. The affected hair starts to shed after about two weeks of therapy, but hair growth resumes about two months after the suspension of therapy.

A number of other medications are known to cause hair loss by converting hair follicles in anagen phase to telogen phase. In such cases, hair shedding generally starts 24 months after therapy. The medications involved in this type of hair loss include oral contraceptives, anticoagulants, propranolol, and triparanol.

Sebaceous glands

These glands secrete lipid through expulsion of their lipid-laden cells and are therefore known as *holocrine*. Their activity is hormone-dependent. For example, androgens stimulate and estrogens inhibit the excretion. Adrenocortical steroids and thyroid hormones also have some stimulatory activity. Acne may be formed as a result of proliferation of the follicular epithelium of the sebaceous gland. Topically applied substances such as greases and oils, and systemically administered substances such as iodides and bromides, may increase the formation of acnes.

A number of chlorinated aromatic hydrocarbons can cause various skin lesions, including *chloracne*, which is characterized by small straw-colored cysts and comedones, and in which the sebaceous gland is replaced by a keratinous cyst. The severity of chloracne varies, but it has been noted among occupational workers. However, it was more notable in the outbreaks in Japan among individuals after their consumption of a batch of rice oil contaminated with polychlorinated biphenyls (PCB) (WHO, 1976), and in Seveso, Italy, among residents near a factory that accidentally released a large amount of TCDD (2,3,7,8-tetrachlorodibenzo-*p*-dioxin) (Pocchiari, 1980).

Sweat glands

Sweating serves useful physiologic functions such as regulation of body temperature. Blockage of the sweat ducts, a disorder known as miliaria, may occur after topical application of 95% phenol and chloroform (Shelley and Horvath, 1950).

Testing procedures

For most effects on skin, the test animal of choice is the albino rabbit, although albino guinea pigs, white mice, and others are also used.

Primary irritation

This effect is in general measured by a patch test on the skin of rabbits (Draize, 1959). A small amount (0.5 g or 0.5 ml) of the chemical to be tested is introduced under a 1-square-inch gauze pad that is placed over a shaved part of the skin. The pad is suitably fastened over the animal for 24 hours. At the end of this period, the pad is removed and the skin reaction is graded according to the extent of (1) erythema and eschar formation, and (2) edema formation. The skin reaction is read again at the end of 72 hours. The same test is done on other rabbits, except that the skin has been abraded. The 24- and 72-hour readings from both groups are added to obtain the *primary irritation index*. The test procedure, grading of skin reaction, and interpretation of the grading are given in Appendix 14.1.

There are a number of modified skin irritation tests based on the Draize procedure. The modifications involve the animal species and the number of animals used, amount of test material applied, repetitive applications, and types of examinations. For details, see Henry (1992).

Sensitization reaction

The procedure described by Draize (1959) calls for the use of guinea pigs that are given the chemical by 10 repeated intradermal injections on one flank and a challenging dose on the other flank after a 10- to 14-day resting period. A greater reaction after the challenging dose, in comparison with that after the sensitizing doses, indicates sensitization.

The *Draize test* is generally considered insufficiently sensitive to identify allergic potential. Magnusson and Kligman (1969) therefore recommended the use of the *maximization test*, in which the guinea pigs are given intradermally on day 0 the test substance with and without Freund's complete adjuvant. On day 7 the substance is applied at the same site occlusively. Two weeks later, the test substance is applied topically over the pretreated areas in these animals. Different concentrations of the agent are used in the challenge. Recently, OECD (1992) has adopted this and the Buehler test which requires the application of the chemical under closed patches.

Human experience is obtained either in patch tests or in a controlled population. In the latter case, the substance is widely distributed to the target population for use as directed. Their skin reactions are examined and evaluated. A patch test usually involves 100 males and 100 females, covering a wide age range. The test material (0.5 ml or 0.5 g) is applied by patch to an area on the arm or back. The skin reaction is examined on the following day after the removal of the patch.

Phototoxicity and photoallergy

Phototoxicity appears to be more readily demonstrable in the hairless mouse, the rabbit, and the guinea pig. The substance to be tested may be administered topically or by a systemic route. The reaction of the skin to nonerythrogenic light (wavelength greater than 320 nm) is then determined. Significant erythema, compared to controls, indicates phototoxicity.

For the detection of photoallergy, albino guinea pigs are especially useful. The procedure involves, in principle, an induction of photosensitization by repeatedly applying a small amount of the chemical on a shaved and depilated area of the skin and exposing that area to appropriate UV rays. After a three-week interval, the guinea pigs are exposed to the chemical and the UV rays to elicit photoallergy.

Contact urticaria

A number of animal models have been proposed based on the procedure devised by Jacobs (1940). These generally involve a patch test on the flank and nipples of guinea pigs. Recently, a test using guinea pig ears has been found satisfactory in screening human contact urticarigenic substances (Lahti and Maibach, 1984).

The open patch test can be applied to human volunteers or to patients suspected of being susceptible to the chemical. In the latter case, all necessary resuscitation equipment and qualified personnel should be available to respond to anaphylactoid reaction.

Any immunologic involvement can be demonstrated by the passive transfer test, in which 0.1 ml fresh serum from the patient is injected intra-dermally into the forearm of a volunteer and challenged 24 hours later by applying the suspect chemical to the injection site.

Cutaneous cancer

The procedure involves topical application of the substance on a shaved area of the skin. The substance per se, if a liquid, is applied directly. Otherwise, it is dissolved or suspended in a suitable vehicle. The skin painting is usually done once a week or more frequently. The commonly used animal is the mouse. It is advisable to include a vehicle control group as well as a positive control group, which is treated with a known skin car-cinogen such as benzo[a]pyrene.

Evaluation

Although various tests for primary irritation and sensitization reaction have been in use for many years, their reliability and reproducibility have been questioned. For example, Nixon et al. (1975) and Griffith and Buehler (1977) found the rabbit to be generally more susceptible than the guinea pig and humans, and the use of these two species is more reliable in predicting human reactions. Furthermore, the use of abraded skin did not enhance the value of the animal tests.

The various sensitization tests in guinea pigs and the human patch test yielded comparable results to a variety of chemicals. However, these tests appear to be more likely to yield false-positive results than false-negatives, compared to use experience in humans. There is less information compar-ing results from the various tests in animals and human experience with respect to the other types of dermal effects. However, the available information indicates that they are useful as screening procedures.

In vitro tests

In order to reduce the use of intact animals in dermal irritancy tests, several in vitro procedures have been developed. One of them involves the determination of the uptake of neutral red by normal human ker-atinocytes. Chemicals that damage these isolated cells will reduce the uptake of the dye (Borenfreund and Puerner, 1984; Shopsis et al., 1987). A method using cultured rat epidermal keratinocytes to measure toxic effects in terms of plasma membrane integrity and lysosomal and mitochondrial functions has been described (Hsieh and Acosta, 1991).

References

Amin, S., Lahti, A., and Maibach, H. I. (1995) Immediate contact reactions: Contact urticaria and the contact urticaria syndrome, in *Dermatotoxicology*, 5th edn, F. N. Marzulli and H. I. Maibach (eds), Washington, DC: Taylor & Francis.

Borenfreund, E. and Puerner, J. (1984) A simple quantitative procedure using monolayer cultures for cytotoxicity assays. *J. Tissue Culture Methods* 9:7–9.

Draize, J. H. (1959) Dermal toxicity, in *Appraisal of the Safety of Chemicals in Foods, Drugs and Cosmetics*, Editorial Committee of the Association of Food and Drug Officials of the United States (eds), P.O. Box 3425, York, PN. 17402.

Ebino, K., Ueda, H., Kawakatsu, H. *et al.* (2001) Isolated airway exposure to toluene diisocyate results skin sensitization. *Toxicol. Letters* 121:79–85.

Forbes, P. D. (1995) Carcinogenesis and photocarcinogenesis test methods, in *Dermatotoxicology*, F. N. Marzull and H. I. Maibach (eds), Washington, DC: Taylor & Francis.

Griffith, J. F. and Buehler, E. V. (1977) Prediction of skin irritancy and sensitizing potential by testing with animals and man, in *Cutaneous Toxicity*, V. A. Drill and P. Lazar (eds), New York, NY: Academic Press, pp. 155–174.

Harber, L. C. and Baer, R. L. (1972) Pathogenic mechanisms of drug-induced photosensitivity. *J. Invest. Dermatol.* 58:327–342.

Harber, L. S., Shalita, A. R., and Armstrong, R. B. (1987) Immunologically mediated contact photosensitivity in guinea pigs, in *Dermatotoxicology*, F. N. Marzulli and H. I. Maibach (eds), Washington, DC: Hemisphere, pp. 413–430.

Henry, M. C. (1992) USEPA efforts in harmonization of acute toxicity test guidelines with OECD. *J. Am. College Toxicol.* 11:285–291.

Hsieh, G. C. and Acosta, D. (1991) Dithral-induced cytotoxicity in primary cultures of rat epidermal keratinocytes. *Toxicol. Appl. Pharmacol.* 107:16–26.

IARC (1973) *Certain Polycyclic Aromatic Hydrocarbons and Heterocyclic Compounds*. IARC Monographs on the Evaluation of Carcinogenic Risk of the Chemical to Man, vol. 3. Lyon, France: International Agency for Research on Cancer.

Jacobs, J. L. (1940) Immediate generalized skin reactions in hypersensitive guinea pigs. *Proc. Soc. Exp. Biol. Med.* 43:641–643.

Kligman, A. M. and Katz, A. G. (1968) Pathogenesis of acne vulgaris. I. Comedogenic properties of human sebum in external ear canal of the rabbit. *Arch. Dermatol.* 98:53–57.

Lahti, A. and Maibach, H. I. (1984) An animal model for nonimmunologic contact urticaria. *Toxicol. Appl. Pharmacol.* 76:219–224.

Magnusson, B. and Kligman, A. M. (1969) The identification of contact allergens by animal assay. The guinea pig maximization test. *J. Invest. Dermatol.* 52:268–276.

Montagna, W. (1965) The skin. *Sci. Am.* (Feb.):60.

Nethercott, J. R., Holness, D. L., Adams, R. M. *et al.* (1994) Multivariate analysis of the effect of selected factors on the elicitation of patch test response to 28 common environmental contactants in North America. *Am. J. Contact Dermatitis* 5:13–18.

Nixon, G. A., Tyson, C. A., and Werz, W. C. (1975) Interspecies comparisons of skin irritancy. *Toxicol. Appl. Pharmacol.* 31:481–490.

OECD (1992) *OECD Guidelines for Testing Chemicals.* Paris: Organization for Economic Cooperation and Development.

Pocchiari, F. (1980) Accidental release of 2,3,7,8-tetrachlorodibenzo-*p*-dioxin (TCDD) at Seveso, Italy. *Ecotoxicol. Environ. Safety* 4:282.

Shelley, W. B. and Horvath, P. N. (1950) Experimental miliaria in man. II. Production of sweat retention anhidrosis and miliaria crystallina by various kinds of injury. *J. Invest. Dermatol.* 1:9–20.

Shopsis, C., Borenfreund, E., and Stark, D. M. (1987) Validation studies on a battery of potential *in vitro* alternatives to the Draize test, in *Alternative Methods in Toxicology*, vol. 5, A. M. Goldberg (ed.), New York, NY: Mary Ann Liebert, pp. 31–44.

von Krogh, G. and Maibach, H. I. (1987) The contact urticaria syndrome, in *Dermatotoxicology*, F. N. Marzulli and H. I. Maibach (eds), Washington, DC: Hemisphere.

WHO (1976) *Polychlorinated Biphenyls and Terphenyls.* Environmental Health Criteria 2. Geneva: World Health Organization.

Appendix 15.1 Primary irritation

Primary irritation of the skin is measured by a patch-test technique on the abraded and intact skin of the albino rabbit clipped free of hair. A minimum of six subjects is used per preparation tested. The method consists in introducing under a one-inch patch 0.5 ml (in case of liquids) or 0.5 g (in cases of solids and semisolids) of the test substance. It is also desirable in the case of solids to attempt solubilizing in an appropriate solvent and to apply the solution as for liquids. The animals are immobilized in an animal holder with patches secured in place by adhesive tape. The entire trunk of the animal is then wrapped with rubberized cloth for the entire 24 hour period of exposure. This latter procedure aids in maintaining the test patches in position, and, in addition, retards the evaporation of volatile substances. After the 24 hours of exposure, the patches are removed and the resulting reactions are evaluated on the basis of scores in Table A15.1. Readings are made also after 72 hours, and the final score represents an average of 24- and 72-hour readings. An equal number of exposures are made on areas of skin which have been previously abraded. The abrasions are minor incisions through the stratum corneum, but not sufficiently deep to disturb the derma (that is, not sufficiently deep to produce bleeding).

The total erythema and edema scores are added in both the 24- and 72-hour readings, and the averages of the scores for intact and abraded skin are combined; this combined average is referred to as the primary irritation index. It is useful for placing compounds in general groups with reference to irritant properties.

Table A15.1 Evaluation of skin reactions

1 *Erythema and eschar formation*	
No erythema	0
Very slight erythema (barely perceptible)	1
Well-defined erythema	2
Moderate to severe erythema	3
Severe erythema (beet redness) to slight eschar formation (injuries in depth)	4
Total possible erythema score	4
2 *Edema formation*	
No edema	0
Very slight edema (barely perceptible)	1
Slight edema (edges of area well defined by definite raising)	2
Moderate edema (raised approximately 1 mm)	3
Severe edema (raised more than 1 mm and extending beyond area of exposure)	4
Total possible edema score	4

Source: Draize, 1959.

Compounds producing combined averages (primary irritation indexes) of 2 or less are only mildly irritating; whereas those with indexes from 2 to 5 are moderate irritants, and those with scores above 6 are considered severe irritants.

Chapter 16

Toxicology of the eye

General considerations

Although the eyes are relatively small, they are important to one's well-being and they are complex in structure.

The eye is a spherical body that is covered mainly by three coats of tissues: the sclera, choroids, and retina. These coats mainly consist of, respectively, fibrous tissues, pigments and blood vessels, and nerve fibers, cells, and special receptors. They are nontransparent. However, light is admitted through the front of the eye, where the three coats are replaced by a number of tissues, notably the cornea and the lens (Figure 16.1a).

The cornea is a continuum of the sclera. It consists of a relatively thick stroma and is covered, in front, by an epithelium, consisting of several layers of cells and Bowman's membranes, and, behind, by Descemet's membrane and an endothelium. The cornea and the front portion of the sclera as well as the inside of the eyelids are covered by a thin layer of conjunctiva.

The lens consists of transparent fibers enclosed in the lens capsule. It is suspended by the ciliary zonule to the ciliary body and its curvature is adjustable by the contraction and relaxation of the ciliary muscle.

The space between the lens and the cornea is filled with the aqueous humor. Also in this space and immediately in front of the lens is the iris. It is rich in blood vessels and heavily pigmented. The iris has a central opening, the pupil. Filling the space between the lens and retina is the vitreous humor.

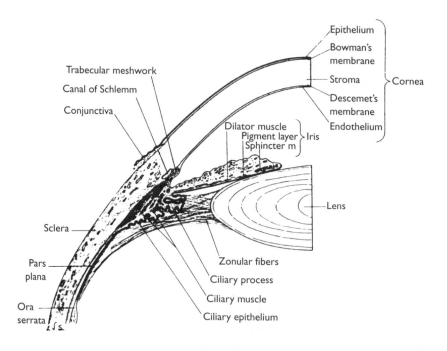

Figure 16.1a Cross section of the anterior chamber angle and surrounding structures.

Source: Reproduced, with permission, from Vaughan, D., Asbury, T., General Ophthalmology, 10th edn. © 1983 by Lange Medical Publications, Los Altos, CA.

The retina is the ocular structure that responds to light stimuli. It consists of several layers (Figure 16.1b). The outermost is a pigmented epithelium. Next to it are the retinal rods and cones, which are the light-responsive neural structures. They are connected via the bipolar cells to the ganglion cells. The axons from the latter cells converge and exit from the eye at the optic papilla as the optic nerve.

Because of their diverse physiologic nature and spatial relations, these various ocular structures may exhibit a variety of effects as a result of exposure to toxicants.

Toxicants and site of their effects

Cornea

The cornea is a delicate structure and is subject to toxic effects of chemicals, mainly from external exposure. Chemicals that affect the cornea include acids and alkalies, detergents, organic solvents, and smog. Acids and alkalies can readily damage the cornea. The extent of damage ranges from minor, superficial destruction of the tissue, which heals completely, to opacity of the cornea or even perforation. Acid burns are related to the low pH as well as the affinity of the anion for the corneal tissue. The effects of alkalies usually have slower onset than those caused by acids and

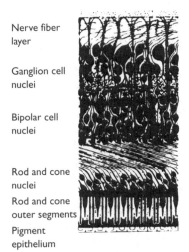

Nerve fiber layer

Ganglion cell nuclei

Bipolar cell nuclei

Rod and cone nuclei

Rod and cone outer segments

Pigment epithelium

Figure 16.1b Cross section of the retina.

Source: Reproduced, with permission of the author, from Polyak, S. *The Retina*. © 1940 by University of Chicago Press, Chicago, IL.

are essentially pH-dependent. However, ammonium ion, which is present in many household products, penetrates the cornea more readily and can thereby affect the iris (Potts, 1996).

Detergents are useful household and industrial products. In general, the nonionic detergents are less damaging than the ionic agents, and the cationics are more damaging than the anionics (Draize and Kelley, 1952). Organic solvents, such as acetone, hexane, and toluene, may enter the eye as a result of industrial or laboratory accidents. These substances can dissolve fat and damage the corneal epithelial cells.

Smog is a mixture of industrial smoke and fog. However, it now refers more often to the photochemical reaction products of automobile exhaust (see Chapter 23). These products accumulate under certain meteorologic conditions. They affect mainly the respiratory tract, but even at low concentrations they irritate the corneal sensory nerve endings and cause reflex lacrimation.

Other chemicals can affect the cornea following *systemic administration*. These include quinacrine, chloroquine, and chlorpromazine. Potts (1996) reviewed the corneal effects of these drugs and other chemicals. They affect the cornea via tears and/or after passing through the blood–aqueous barrier. However, they affect humans only rarely and only after large doses.

Iris, aqueous humor, and ciliary body

Because of its proximity to the cornea, the iris is susceptible to physical trauma and chemical irritation. The effects of such irritation consists of leakage of serum proteins and fibrin as well as leukocytes from the blood vessels. These may be followed by fibroblast metaplasia. Severe damages to the iris cause liberation of melanin granules from the posterior epithelium of the iris.

The iris is innervated by sympathetic nerves (for the dilator muscles) and parasympathetic nerves (for the constrictor muscles). Therefore, the pupil can be dilated by chemicals that are sympathomimetic or parasympatholytic, and it can be constricted by parasympathomimetic and sympatholytic chemicals. Furthermore, the size of the pupil can be altered via the central nervous system by chemicals such as morphine and general anesthetics.

The aqueous humor is secreted by the epithelium of the ciliary body into the posterior chamber. It flows through the pupil into the anterior chamber and drains through the canal of Schlemm at the angle of the anterior chamber. Inflammatory changes of the iris can block the drainage of the fluid through the canal of Schlemm and raise the intraocular pressure, thereby inducing glaucoma. Atropine and other mydriatics may also precipitate glaucoma by dilating the pupil, thus blocking the drainage. Corticosteroids, applied topically or systemically, can also increase the intraocular pressure and cause glaucoma.

In the ciliary body is the ciliary muscle, the contraction of which allows relaxation of the ciliary zonule, which in turn allows the lens capsule to assume a more spherical form. This muscle is parasympathetically innervated; therefore, acetylcholinesterase inhibitors and parasympatholytic agents such as atropine can cause the lens to be fixed in different states of visual accommodation.

Lens

A number of chemicals are known to alter the lenticular transparency, resulting in the formation of cataract. Examples are 2,4-dinitrophenol, corticosteroids, busulfan, triparanol, and thallium. Their cataractogenic property has been noted in humans as well as animals, such as the rabbit, rat, and young fowl. The effects generally follow systemic exposure, but with certain chemicals (e.g., corticosteroids, anticholinesterases), they may occur after topical application (Woods *et al.*, 1967; Axelsson, 1968).

Diabetic patients are more likely to have cataracts, which can also be produced in rats and rabbits rendered diabetic with alloxan or streptozotocin (Heywood, 1982).

In addition, rats fed large amounts of galactose develop cataract (Sippel, 1966). This condition may be comparable to the cataract observed in infants with galactosemia. Such galactosemia results from a metabolic inability, inherited as an autosomal recessive trait, to convert galactose to glucose because of an absence of the enzyme galactose-1-phosphate uridylyl transferase (Kinosita, 1965).

On the other hand, deficiencies of certain nutrients may also induce cataract. These nutrients include tryptophan, proteins, vitamin E, riboflavin, and folic acid (Gehring, 1971).

The mechanism underlying the formation of cataract is not fully understood. It is likely that it varies with the nature of the toxicant. For example, corticosteroid cataract may be mediated through an inhibition of protein synthesis in the lens (Ono, 1972). Busulfan may act through an interference of mitosis of the lenticular epithelial cells (Grimes and von Sallmann, 1966). Triparanol may interfere with the Na^+ pump, resulting in an increase of Na^+ and water in the lens (Harris and Gruber, 1972). The effect of dinitrophenol is likely to be mediated through the uncoupling of oxidative phosphorylation (see also Chapter 4).

An extensive review of cataractogenic chemicals has been prepared by Gehring (1971). The cataratogenic chemicals are listed in Appendix 16.1.

Apart from cataractogenic effects, which are permanent, transient lens opacity has been noted in young beagle dogs following administration of some tranquilizers, some diuretics, and diisophenol. In addition, the transparency and refraction of the lens may also be altered by dimethyl sulfoxide and p-chlorophenylalanine (Heywood, 1982).

Retina

Certain polycyclic compounds, such as chloroquine, hydroxychloroquine, and thioridazine, can induce retinopathy in humans and animals. They affect the visual acuity, dark adaptation, and retinal pigment pattern. Hyperoxia and iodate may also induce retinal changes.

Different mechanisms are involved in these retinal effects. Inhibition of protein metabolism in the pigment epithelium has been suggested as the primary toxic effect of chloroquine and hydroxychloroquine, which have strong affinity for melanin (Meier-Ruge, 1972). Increased oxygen supply to the retina induces vasoconstriction, which is associated with a decrease in the supply of nutrients. The latter effect is probably responsible for the hyperoxia-induced retinal changes. Iodate apparently affects the pigment epithelium, the derangement of which results in degeneration of the rod layer. The various reviewed modes of action has been provided by Heywood (1982). These include the early formation of membranous cytoplasmic bodies (myeloid bodies), degenerative changes in the cell body of the rods and cones, derangement of the intracytoplasmic rods, and the appearance of vacuoles around these rods in the tapetum.

Leong et al. (1987) reported that an important chemical intermediate, 4,4-methylenedianiline, a well known hepatotoxicant, induces degeneration of the inner and outer segments of the photoreceptor cells in albino and pigmented guinea pigs. Other retinal effects include hemorrhage from rupture of blood vessels or disturbance of blood clotting mechanism and exudates, which may cause partial detachment of retina.

Optic nerve

As noted above, the retina contains, among other structures, the ganglion cells, the axons of which form the optic nerve. Toxicants can affect either the ganglion cells or the optic nerve. Damage to one of them often results in the degeneration of the other.

Some toxicants affect mainly the central vision. The most notable example is methanol. Others include carbon disulfide, disulfuram, ethambutol, and thallium. On the other hand, quinine, chloroquine, pentavalent arsenic, and carbon monoxide cause constriction of visual fields by damaging the structures responsible for peripheral vision. Interestingly, nitrobenzol affects both the central and peripheral vision (Harrington, 1976). While methyl mercury also causes constriction of visual field, its toxic effect is on the visual cortex instead of the optic nerve (Chapter 21).

These toxicants can also be classified according to their effects on other peripheral nerves. For example, quinine, ethambutol, and methanol generally do not affect other peripheral nerves, while carbon disulfide, disulfiram, and thallium cause both optic and peripheral neuropathies. It is worthy of note that certain organic solvents can induce peripheral neuropathy but spare the visual system. These include tri-o-cresyl phosphate, acrylamide, n-hexane, and methyl n-butyl ketone (Grant, 1980).

Clioquinol (also known as Vioform and Entero-Vioform) was widely used for the prevention and treatment of "traveler's diarrhea." It has reportedly caused more than 10,000 cases of SMON (subacute myelo-opticoneuropathy), a disease affecting the optic nerves, spinal tracts, and peripheral nerves (Potts, 1996).

Testing procedures

Effects on the eye can be examined after topical application of the toxicants. In addition, systemic administration can also result in ocular alterations. Several types of examinations are available.

Albino rabbits are commonly used to determine the ocular irritancy of ophthalmic medications and other chemicals that might come in contact with the eye. Dogs and nonhuman primates (rhesus monkeys) have also been used. For effects on the lens, retina, and optical nerve, many species of animals are used, such as rat, rabbit, cat, dog, monkey, and pig.

Gross examination

The test described by Draize and Kelley (1952) has been a standard procedure for testing ocular irritancy. It specifies the use of nine rabbits. Into one eye of each rabbit is instilled 0.1 ml of the test material. In three of the nine rabbits, the test material is washed with 20 ml of lukewarm water two seconds after the instillation, and in three others, the washing is done with a four second delay. In the three remaining rabbits, the material is left in the eye. The ocular reactions are read with the unaided eye or with the aid of a slit-lamp at 24, 48, and 72 hours and at four and seven days after treatment. The reactions of the conjunctiva (redness, chemosis, and discharge), cornea (the degree and extent of opacity), and iris (congestion, swelling, and circumcorneal injection) are scored according to a specified scale. A series of colored pictures, originally provided by the U.S. Food and Drug Administration in 1965 as a guide for grading eye irritation, are available from the U.S. Consumer Product Safety Commission, Washington, DC 20207. Samples were reproduced in Hackett and McDonald (1995).

Several modified versions of the Draize and Kelley test have been proposed. Griffith *et al.* (1980) reported on their results of assessing eye irritancy of a large number of substances. The irritancy ranged from nil to corrosive. The authors recommend that the following points be taken into account in conducting eye irritation tests:

1   A 0.01 ml dose, or its weight equivalent for solids and powders, be applied directly to the central corneal surface of at least six eyes without subsequent rinsing or manipulation of the eyelids.
2   Evaluation of the irritancy be based on the median duration for the eyes to return to normal, instead of using a scoring system based on the type and extent of the effects.

The latest U.S. federal agency regulation (CPSC, 1988) requires the use of six albino rabbits for each test substance. For test liquids, 0.1 ml is used, and for solids and pastes, 100 mg. The test material is instilled into one eye of each rabbit without washing. Ocular examinations are done after 24, 48, and 72 hours. A rabbit is considered as having positive reaction if the eye shows, on any examination, ulceration or opacity of the cornea, inflammation of the iris, or swelling of the conjunctiva with partial eversion of the eyelids.

Another variation of the Draize procedure calls for the use of three rabbits whose eyes are examined at 1, 24, 48, and 72 hours. However, only one albino rabbit should be used first, if marked effects are expected. Furthermore, if it is thought that the substance could cause unreasonable pain, a local anesthetic should be used. The grading of the eye irritation is shown in Appendix 16.2 (OECD, 1987).

Instrumental examinations

Ophthalmoscopy

The ophthalmoscope is used in assessing effects of toxicants on various parts of the retina. The examination is generally intended to discover the existence of edema, hyperemia or pallor, atrophy of the optic disk, pigmentation, or the state of the blood vessels. Changes in the vitreous humor, lens, aqueous humor, iris, and cornea can also be revealed.

Visual perimetry

Effect on the visual field can be readily determined in humans, but not in laboratory animals, except the nonhuman primates. Merigan (1979) described a procedure using macaque monkeys to demonstrate the loss of peripheral vision resulting from exposure to methyl mercury.

Other procedures

Visual acuity and color vision are sensitive and useful indicators of effects on the visual system in humans. Procedures involving instrumentation, such as electro-oculography, and visual-evoked responses are also useful and can be incorporated in animal experimentation (Grant, 1980).

Histologic and biochemical examinations

Light microscopy can usually pinpoint the site of action of toxicants, electron microscopy can demonstrate ultrastructural changes, and biochemical studies can reveal the mechanism of toxic effects. For example, with light microscopy, chloroquine has been observed to cause a thickening of the pigment epithelium, followed by migration of the pigment to the outer nuclear layer, and finally total atrophy of the photoreceptors (Meier-Ruge, 1968). Electron microscopy showed mitochondrial swelling and disorganization of the endoplasmic reticulum in the photoreceptor inner segment (Solze and McConnell, 1970). Biochemical studies revealed inhibition of many enzymatic reactions, especially those related to protein metabolism of the pigment epithelium.

In vitro tests

Because of humane concerns about the use of animals in eye irritation tests, a number of *in vitro* tests have been developed. They involve the use of cells from isolated cornea and chorioallantoic membrane and measuring their uptake of dyes, such as neutral red, as an indicator of toxicity. Other proposed procedures include isolated rabbit eye and isolated chicken eye (Green, 1998). However, these tests apparently require much refinement and extensive validation.

Evaluation

Eye irritation tests are widely used to assess the ocular irritancy of chemicals. In general, the albino rabbit is the animal of choice. Some intralaboratory and interlaboratory variations in the scores were noted in a collaborative study (Marzulli and Ruggles, 1973). Nevertheless, periodic collaborative studies tend to improve the reliability of the scores. The various modifications made on the Draize test also tend to reduce the variability of the results.

A large number of animal experimentations and clinical studies indicate that there is a fair correlation between humans and animals in their reactions to toxicants with respect to cataract formation and retinopathy (Grant, 1980; Potts, 1996).

References

Axelsson, U. (1968) Glaucoma, miotic therapy and cataract. III. Visual loss due to lens changes in glaucoma eyes treated with paraoxon (Mintacol), echothiophate or pilocarpine. *Acta Ophthalmol.* 46:831.

CPSC (1988) Consumer Product Safety Commission. Test for eye irritants. Code of Federal Regulations, Title 16. Federal Hazardous Substances Act Regulation, Part 1500.42.

Draize, J. H. and Kelley, E. A. (1952) Toxicity to eye mucosa of certain cosmetic preparations containing surface-active agents. *Proc. Sci. Sect. Toilet Goods Assoc.* 17:1–4.

Gehring, P. J. (1971) The cataractogenic activity of chemical agents. *CRC Crit. Rev. Toxicol.* 1:93–118.

Grant, W. M. (1980) The peripheral visual system as a target, in *Experimental and Clinical Neurotoxicology*, B. S. Spencer and H. H. Schaumburg (eds), Baltimore, MD: Williams & Wilkins.

Green, S. (1998) Update on agency initiatives in alternative methods, in *Dermatology Methods: The Laboratory Worker's Vade McCum*, F. N. Margulli and H. I. Maribach (eds), Philadelphia, PA: Taylor & Francis, pp. 377–382.

Griffith, J. F., Nixon, G. A., Bruce, R. D., Reer, P. J., and Bannan, E. A. (1980) Dose–response studies with chemical irritants in the albino rabbit eye as a basis for selecting optimum testing conditions for predicting hazard to the human eye. *Toxicol. Appl. Pharmacol.* 55:501–513.

Grimes, P. and Von Sallmann, L. (1966) Interference with cell proliferation and induction of polyploidy in rat lens epithelium during prolonged Myleran treatment. *Exp. Cell Res.* 62:265–273.

Hackett, R. B. and McDonald, T. O. (1995) Assessing ocular irritation, in *Dermatotoxicology*, F. N. Marzulli and H. I. Maibach (eds), Washington, DC: Taylor & Francis.

Harrington, D. O. (1976) *The Visual Fields*. St. Louis, MI: Mosby.

Harris, J. E. and Gruber, L. (1972) Reversal of triparanol-induced cataracts in the rat. II. Exchange of ^{22}Na, ^{42}K, ^{86}Rb in cataractous and clearing lenses. *Invest. Ophthalmol. Vis. Sci.* 11:608–616.

Heywood, R. (1982) Histopathological and laboratory assessment of visual dysfunction. *Environ. Health Perspect.* 44:35–45.

Kinosita, J. H. (1965) Cataracts in galactosemia. *Invest. Ophthalmol. Vis. Sci.* 4:786–799.

Leong, B. K. J., Lund, J. E., Groehn, J. A., Coombs, J. K., Sabaitis, C. P., Weaver, R. J., and Griffin, R. L. (1987) Retinopathy from inhaling 4,4′-methylenedianiline aerosols. *Fundam. Appl. Toxicol.* 9:645–658.

Marzulli, F. N. and Ruggles, D. I. (1973) Rabbit eye irritation test: Collaborative study. *J. Am. Assoc. Anal. Chem.* 56:905–914.

Meier-Ruge, M. (1968) The pathophysiological morphology of the pigment epithelium and its importance for retinal structure and function. *Med. Prob. Ophthalmol.* 8:32–48.

Meier-Ruge, W. (1972) Drug-induced retinopathy. *CRC Crit. Rev. Toxicol.* 1:325–360.

Merigan, W. H. (1979) Effects of toxicants on visual systems. *Neurobehav. Toxicol.* 1(Suppl. 1):1522.

OECD (1987) *OECD Guidelines for Testing of Chemicals.* Paris: Organization for Economic Cooperation and Development.

Ono, S. (1972) Presence of corticol-binding protein in the lens. *Ophthalmic Res.* 3:233–240.

Polyak, S. (1940) *The Retina.* Chicago, IL: University of Chicago Press.

Potts, A. M. (1996) Toxic responses of the eye, in *Casarett and Doull's Toxicology*, C. D. Klaassen (ed.), New York, NY: McGraw-Hill.

Sippel, T. O. (1966) Changes in water, protein and glutathione contents of the lens in the course of galactose cataract development in rats. *Invest. Ophthalmol. Vis. Sci.* 5:568–575.

Solze, D. A. and McConnell, D. G. (1970) Ultrastructural changes in the rat photoreceptor inner segment during experimental chloroquine retinopathy. *Ophthal. Res.* 1:140–148.

Vaughan, D. and Ashbury, T. (1983) *General Ophthalmology*, 10th edn. Los Altos, CA: Lange Medical Publications.

Woods, D. C., Contaxis, I., Sweet, D., Smith, J. C. II, and Van Dolah, J. (1967) Response of rabbits to corticosteroids. I. Influence on growth, intraocular pressure and lens transparency. *Am. J. Ophthalmol.* 63:841–849.

Appendix 16.1 Cataractogenic chemicals

Sugars (glucose, galactose, xylose)
Streptozotocin
Corticosteroids
Naphthalene
Mimosine (leucenol)
Methoxsalen
Methionine sulfoximine
Polyriboinosinic acid polyribocytidylic acid
Quietidine (1,4-bis(phenylisopropyl)-piperazine·2HCl)
N-phenyl-β-hydrazinopropionitriles and related compounds
4[3(7-Chloro-5,11-dihydrodibenz[b,e][1,4]-oxyazepin-5-YL)propyl]-1-piperazineethanol dichloride
Tyrosine
2,4-Dinitrophenol (DNP) and related compounds
Alkylating agents
Anticholinesterases
Chlorpromazine
Triparanol
Dimethyl sulfoxide (DMSO)
2,4,6-Trinitrotoluene (TNT)
Sympathomimetic drugs and morphine-like drugs
2,6-Dichloro-4-nitroaniline
Iodoacetic acid
Mephenytoin
Diquat
Oral contraceptives
Sulfaethoxypyridazine
Thallium
Paradichlorobenzene
Heptachlor
Desferal
Thioacetamide

Appendix 16.2 Grading of eye irritation

Cornea	
No ulceration or opacity	0
Scattered or diffuse areas of opacity	1
(other than slight dulling of normal lustre),	
details of iris clearly visible	
Easily discernible translucent area,	2
details of iris slightly obscured	
Nacrous area, no details of iris visible,	3
size of pupil barely discernible	
Opaque cornea, iris not discernible through	4
the opacity	
Iris	
Normal	0
Markedly deepened rugae, congestion, swelling,	1
moderate circumcorneal hyperemia, or injection,	
any of these or combination of any thereof, iris	
still reacting to light (sluggish reaction is positive)	
No reaction to light, hemorrhage, gross destruction	2
(any or all of these)	
Conjunctiva	
Redness (refers to palpebral and bulbar conjunctiva, cornea and iris)	
Blood vessels normal	0
Some blood vessels definitely hyperemic (injected)	1
Diffuse, crimson color, individual vessels not	
easily discernible	2
Diffuse beefy red	
	3
Chemosis: lids and/or nictating membranes	
No swelling	0
Any swelling above normal (includes nictating membranes)	1
Obvious swelling with partial eversion of lids	2
Swelling with lids about half closed	3
Swelling with lids more than half closed	4

Source: OECD, 1987.

Chapter 17

Toxicology of the nervous system

CONTENTS

Introduction

As a vital part of the body, the nervous system is shielded from toxicants in the blood by a unique protective mechanism, namely, the blood–brain and blood–nerve barriers. Nonetheless, it is susceptible to a variety of toxicants. For example, methyl mercury affects mainly the nervous system, although its concentration in the brain is comparable to that in most other tissues, and in fact it is much lower than that in the liver and kidneys.

The greater susceptibility may be attributed partly to the fact that neurons have a high metabolic rate, with little capacity for anaerobic metabolism. Furthermore, being electrically excitable, neurons tend to lose cell membrane integrity more readily. The great length of the axons is another reason why the nervous system is especially susceptible to toxic effects, since the cell body must supply its axon structurally and metabolically.

To facilitate the description of the various types of toxic effects and the procedures for their testing, the various parts of the nervous system are described.

Central and peripheral nervous systems

The system consists of two major parts: the central nervous system (CNS) and the peripheral nervous system (PNS). The CNS is made up of the brain and the spinal cord, and the PNS includes the cranial and spinal nerves, which are either motor or sensory. The neurons of the sensory spinal nerves are located in the ganglia in the dorsal roots. In addition, the PNS also includes the sympathetic nerve system, which arises from neurons in the thoracic and lumbar region of the spinal cord, and the parasympathetic system, which stems from nerve fibers leaving the CNS via the cranial nerves and the sacral spinal roots.

Cells and appendages

The principal cells in the nervous system are neurons, composed of perikarya, along with their dendrites and axons. These structures are responsible for the conduction of nerve impulses. The main supporting structure consists of various types of glial cells. Apart from a lack of conductivity, the glial cells differ from neurons in that the former, as most other types of cells, do reproduce, whereas the latter do not.

In the CNS the glial cells include astrocytes, oligodendrocytes (oligodendroglia), and microglia. Astrocytes help maintain a proper microenvironment around the neurons and support the blood–brain barrier. Oligodendroglia surround the axons in the CNS with a lipid-rich material, the myelin sheath, which provides electrical insulation. Microglia are basically macrophages that are located in the CNS. In the PNS the Schwann cells provide the myelin sheath which wraps around the axon. The myelin sheath is interrupted by the nodes of Ranvier.

Neurotransmitters

Neurons are connected, via their axons, to other neurons at their dendrites or to the receptors in the glands or muscles. At nerve terminals, on excitation by an action potential, chemical neurotransmitters are released. The most common transmitters are acetylcholine and norepinephrine. However, there are several amine neurotransmitters in addition to norepinephrine, i.e., dopamine, serotonin, and histamine. Furthermore, the following amino acids also act as neurotransmitters: γ-aminobutyric acid (GABA), glycine, glutamate and aspartate. These transmitters are small molecules and act rapidly. They are synthesized in the presynaptic terminals. These neurotransmitters are presynthesized, stored in synaptic vesicles, and released upon excitation. Nitric oxide (NO), a recently discovered neurotransmitter, is different from the others in that, as a labile free radical, it is not presynthesized for storage in synaptic vesicles. It is synthesized, on demand, from L-arginine by NO synthase (Zhang and Snyder, 1995).

In addition to these small molecule neurotransmitters, a large number of neuropeptides are slow-acting neurotransmitters/modulators. Some are released by the pituitary gland: ACTH, β-endorphin, growth hormone, thyrotropin, oxytocin, and vasopressin. A number of peptide transmitters act on gut and brain, e.g., leucine enkephalin and methionine enkephalin.

Blood–brain and blood–nerve barriers

These barriers protect the nervous system from certain neurotoxicants. Differences in neurotoxicity sometimes can be explained on the basis of these barriers.

Blood–brain barrier (BBB)

The endothelium in the brain is impermeable to substances of medium molecular weight, such as horseradish peroxidase (mol. wt.: 40,000; diameter: 5–6 nm), because the adjacent cells are tightly joined. Further, these cells have few micropinocytotic vesicles, which in capillaries of other tissues serve as an important transport mechanism across endothelial cells. However, highly lipid-soluble substances and the nonionized fraction of a chemical are more permeable across the BBB. It is, therefore, similar to intact cell membranes in permeability.

The BBB is absent where the cells produce hormones or act as hormonal or chemoreceptors. Glutamate and a number of related compounds, have been shown to affect areas in the brain not protected by the BBB, such as the arcuate nucleus of the hypothalamus and the *area postrema* in various laboratory animals. These effects, while not observed in humans, are of interest because they may be used as tools in the study of such clinical conditions as Huntington's disease, drug-induced Parkinsonism, tardive dyskinesia, and sulfur amino acidopathies.

The BBB is effective in excluding many neurotoxicants, such as diphtheria, staphylococcus, and tetanus toxins. This is also true with doxorubicin, which affects the dorsal root ganglia but not the CNS. Mercury chloride has a small molecule but is hydrophilic and mainly in ionic form. Its concentration in the brain is minimal and so are its CNS effects. On the other hand, methyl mercury is lipophilic and thus readily crosses the BBB, thereby damaging the brain.

Blood–nerve barrier (BNB)

Peripheral nerves are covered by two connective tissue sheaths, the perineurium and epineurium, and interlaced with the endoneurium. The BNB is provided by the blood vessels in the endoneurium and supplemented by the lamellated cells of the perineural sheath. It is not as effective as the BBB; therefore, the dorsal root glanglia are generally more susceptible than the neurons in the CNS to neurotoxicants. For example, doxorubicin affects neurons in the dorsal root ganglia but not those in the brain.

Neurotoxic effects and neurotoxicants

The effects may be classified according to the site of action. These include the neurons, the axons, the glial cells, and the vascular system. A toxicant, however, may affect more than one site. The following is a brief description of certain neurotoxic effects, along with the putative mode of action, grouped according to the site of action.

Figure 17.1 depicts damages to neurons, axons and myelin sheath. *Neu-*

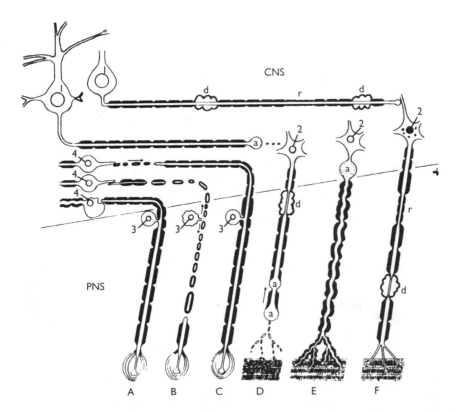

Figure 17.1 Cellular target sites of some neurotoxic chemicals illustrated by upper (1) and lower (2) motor neurons, dorsal root ganglion cells (3), and second-order sensory neurons (4) in the gracile nucleus of the medulla oblongata. The central nervous system (CNS) is represented above the sloping horizontal line, the peripheral nervous system (PNS) below. The peripheral receptors on fibers A–C are pacinian corpuscles. Fibers D–F innervate extrafusal muscle fibers. (a): Axonal degeneration. (d): Demyelination. (r) Remyelination of ventral root, and medulla oblongata.

Source: Adapted from Spencer *et al.*, 1980.

ronopathy is represented by the damage to a second-order sensory neuron (4) which innervates corpuscle A, and a neuron in the dorsal root ganglion (3), which innervates corpuscle B. *Axonopathy* is represented by the damaged central axonal process of a sensory neuron which innervates corpuscle C, and the axons of the lower motor neurons (2) which innervates muscle fibers D and E. *Myelinopathy* is shown along the axons of upper (1) and lower (2) motor neurons which innervates muscle fiber F.

Some neurotoxicants that induce these and other damages are described below.

Neuronopathy

Neurons, being dependent mainly on glucose as an energy source, are susceptible to anoxic and hypoglycemic conditions. A number of chemicals are well known for their anoxigenic effects in the brain. Barbiturates induce anoxia in the brain, especially in hippocampus and cerebellum. Permanent CNS damage even after barbiturate coma, however, is rare, possibly because of the reduced cell metabolism. On the other hand, prolonged exposure to carbon monoxide may induce permanent effects in the brain, arising from the development of a diffuse sclerosis of the white matter (leukoencephalopathy). Cyanide and azide inhibit cytochrome oxidase, thereby producing cytotoxic anoxia.

The cell body of neurons may be affected directly by toxicants. Methyl mercury first causes focal loss of ribosomes and then disintegration and disappearance of the Nissl substances, especially in the small cells. These are followed by nuclear and perinuclear changes and finally by the loss of the entire neuron including its axon (Jacobs et al., 1977). Doxorubicin (Adriamycin) affects neurons by intercalating with DNA, leading to a breakdown of the helical structures (Cho et al., 1980). This derangement inhibits the synthesis of RNA and neuronal protein. Since this drug does not cross the blood–brain barrier, it can affect the neurons in the dorsal root ganglia (Figure 17.1, B) and autonomic ganglia, but not those in the CNS. On the other hand, methyl mercury does penetrate the blood–brain barrier and thus damages the neurons in the CNS as well as those in the dorsal root glanglia.

Organotins are used as pesticides and as plasticizers. Upon entering the nervous system, they accumulate in the Golgi-like structures in the cell body. The cells then undergo swelling and necrosis (Bouldin et al., 1981).

Aluminum also penetrates the BBB and induces encephalopathy with neurofibrillar degeneration in cat and rabbit (DeBoni et al., 1976). Recent reviews conclude that the use of aluminum cooking utensils and the use of various aluminum-containing food additives are safe (Soni et al., 2001).

Glutamate and related chemicals, in very large doses, are known to affect areas of the CNS devoid of BBB (see the "Blood–brain barrier" section, p. 236) and are considered as having neuroexcitatory and neurotoxic effects. The dendrites are the primary site of action. The perikarya are then affected, but the axons are spared (Figure 17.1, A). The toxicity may be mediated through NO (Dawson et al., 1991). Kainic acid is derived from a particular seaweed and it has been used in ascariasis; it is similar to glutamate but much more potent (Olney et al., 1974).

Alcohol in pregnant women may induce in their offspring abnormalities in the nervous system including abnormal neuronal migration and abnormal development of dendritic spines (Abel et al., 1983).

Axonopathy

Some axons are very long (up to 1 m), and the elements in the axons, such as neurofibrils, are synthesized not locally but in the cell body, and are transported along the axon. The axon may therefore be attacked either directly by toxicants or indirectly through damages to the cell body. Lesions may occur either in the proximal or in the distal sections of axons.

Proximal axonopathy

β,β-Iminodiproprionitrile (IDPN) produces typical lesions of this type. It has therefore been used as a model to study motor neuron diseases such as amyotrophic lateral sclerosis. The primary effect of IDPN is the impairment of slow axonal transport of neurofilaments, probably through aberrant phosphorylation of neurofilaments (Gold and Austin, 1991), while their synthesis is continued in the cell body. The accumulation of neurofilaments in the proximal axon causes it to enlarge and the distal axon to atrophy (Figure 17.1, E). The enlarged proximal axon in turn elicits local proliferation of the subpial astrocytic processes and extension of the processes filled with glial filaments along the proximal ventral root. The proximal swelling also stimulates splitting of myelin at the intraperiod line, formation of intramyelinic vacuoles, and ultimate demyelination. The Schwann cells in the demyelinated segment divide and remyelinate, and the repeated demyelination and remyelination give rise to "onion-bulb" formation (Griffin and Price, 1980).

Distal axonopathy

Axons contain three types of neurofibrillary structures, namely, neurotubules, neurofilaments, and microfilaments. In addition, they contain mitochondria and smooth endoplasmic reticulum. These structures are especially susceptible to a variety of neurotoxicants. For example, thallium induces mitochondrial swelling and degeneration, and certain organophosphates and organic solvents cause derangement of the neurofibrillary structures, resulting in distal axonopathy.

An important type of distal axonopathy is produced by certain organophosphorus compounds such as TOCP (tri-o-cresyl phosphate), EPN, and leptophos. These compounds, besides inhibiting acetylcholinesterase, cause *delayed neuropathy*, which manifests mainly as paralysis of muscles. It affects especially long and large nerve fibers, hence the hindlimbs are paralyzed before the forelimbs. TOCP has induced delayed neuropathy in 10,000 humans (see Appendix 1.2). Although a number of other animals may also be affected, especially after repeated exposures, this toxicity can be readily reproduced in hens, usually with a delay of eight to ten days after exposure. Because of the severity of delayed neurotoxicity, new organophosphorus chemicals are routinely tested for this potential hazard. OECD (1984) and EPA (1994) have published guidelines for such tests both after a single dose and after repeated administrations, using domestic hens. The condition is unrelated to acetylcholinesterase inhibition because such potent inhibitors as malathion, parathion, and carbaryl do not possess this toxic property. It is apparently associated with phosphorylation of the enzyme neuropathy target esterase (NTE; formerly known as neurotoxic esterase) (Abou-Donia, 1981; Johnson, 1990).

A different type of distal axonopathy is known to be caused by hexacarbons such as n-hexane and methyl n-butyl ketone. These solvents have caused toxic polyneuropathy among industrial workers, as has acrylamide. Both cause marked neurofilament proliferation in axons, probably as a result of altered phosphorylation of certain proteins (Berti-Mattera et al., 1990). However, giant axonal swellings are common with hexacarbons (Figure 17.1, D), but rare with acrylamide. Furthermore, sensory nerves are involved early with acrylamide but late with hexacarbons, which affect certain motor nerves first. Vincristine may cause accumulation of neurofibrils in the perikarya and axons. It disrupts the axonal neurotubules and neurofilaments and blocks axoplasmic transport of these ultrastructures.

Clioquinol, a popular remedy and preventive for "travelers' diarrhea" in the 1960s and 1970s, induced disorders of the nervous system known as subacute myelo-opticoneuropathy (SMON) in thousands of individuals (Appendix 1.2). In humans and experimental animals, it causes central axonal degeneration of the dorsal root ganglion (Figure 17.1, C), as well as the optic nerves (Worden et al., 1978).

Distal axonopathy has also been hypothesized as resulting from impairment of glycolytic enzyme activities in the axon (Spencer et al., 1979). These enzymes are responsible for the transport of neurofilaments, which are synthesized in the perikaryon and transported along the axon. Impairment of the activities of these enzymes would thus first affect the distal portion of the axon as well as the large, long nerve fibers, which have a greater energy demand on the perikarya. A second hypothesis postulates that the neurofilaments are directly affected by toxicants such as hexacarbons and acrylamide (Savolainen, 1977). Neurofilaments exposed to the toxicant for the longest period, namely those located distally in long fibers, would be affected first.

Interference with impulse conduction

A number of toxicants act mainly on nerve membranes. These membranes normally maintain a negative resting potential. When stimulated, an action potential is generated. The resting and action potentials result from differences in the Na^+ and K^+ concentrations across the membrane, and their concentrations are maintained by the Na^+ channels. Tetrodotoxin, the toxic principle of puffer fish, has been shown to block the action potential by blocking the Na^+ channels. Saxitoxin, the toxic principle produced by the dinoflagellate *Gonyaulax* and taken up by the clam *Saxidomas giganteus*, also acts by blocking the sodium channels. Consumption of improperly cleaned puffer fish or contaminated clam can cause death by respiratory failure. DDT and pyrethroids are markedly different in chemical structure. However, their effects on the nervous systems are similar. They prolong the opening of the sodium channel, thereby initiate repetitive activity at the synapses and neuromuscular junctions (Narahashi, 1992).

Interference with synaptic transmission

Botulinum toxin, the most potent biologic toxin, is produced by *Clostridium botulinum*. It causes paralysis of muscles by impairing the release of acetylcholine from motor nerve endings. Black widow spider venom, on the other hand, causes a massive release of acetylcholine and results in cramps and paralysis.

Tetanoplasmin, from the microbe *Clostridium tetani*, causes tetanus through its effect on the CNS. It blocks release of the inhibitory amino acid transmitters GABA and glycine, thereby causing spastic paralysis. The molecular weight of this proteinaceous dimer is about 150,000, therefore too large to cross the blood–brain barrier. However, it reaches the CNS by retrograde axonal transport (Schield *et al.*, 1977).

Certain neurotoxins (e.g., anatoxin-S) may be produced by cyanobacteria in eutrophied lakes and ponds (Chapter 23). These toxins interfere with transmission of impulses from nerve terminals to muscles, thereby causing muscle paralysis (Carmichael, 1994).

Glial cells and myelin

Myelinating cells

Demyelination can result from injuries to myelinating cells (oligodendrocytes and Schwann cells). Neurotoxins of this type include lead, which affects Schwann cells possibly by interfering with their Ca^{2+} transport. Hypocholesterolemic agents such as triparanol, as expected, disrupt myelin sheath because of the high (70%) lipid content of myelin. However, they produce ultrastructural changes in oligodendrocytes before demyelination occurs. Diphtheria toxin demyelinates possibly by affecting both the myelin and the myelinating cells. Triethyltin, ethidium bromide, and actinomycin are other examples of demyelinating toxins that act on the myelinating cells.

Myelin sheath

Demyelination can also result from effects on the myelin sheath. This type of effect generally involves a disruption of the membrane structure. Other modes of action include (1) inhibition of carbonic anhydrase or other enzymes involved in ion and water transport, (2) inhibition of enzymes involved in oxidative phosphorylation, and (3) chelation of metals. Neurotoxicants that act directly on the myelin sheath include triethyltin, lysolecithin, isoniazid, cyanate, hexachlorophene, and lead. Acetyl ethyl tetramethyl tetralin (AETT) also causes myelinopathy through a complex mechanism (Figure 17.1, F).

Lead has been known for centuries as a neurotoxicant. It affects various parts of the nervous system, including myelin sheath. The PNS is affected before the CNS. In addition, lead affects motor nerves before the sensory, resulting in "wrist-drop" and "foot-drop." Its effects on the blood vessels are discussed below.

Blood vessels and edema

The permeability of the vascular system in the CNS and PNS may be increased by higher blood pressure or lower plasma osmolarity. It may also result from exposure to certain toxins. The greater permeability generally leads to an accumulation of fluids in the extracellular space. In addition, a number of neurotoxicants are known to induce cellular edema.

Extracellular edema

Lead can damage the endothelial cells and cause extravasation of plasma in the brain, especially in the white matter, which has a greater compliance than the gray matter. That suckling rats are more susceptible to lead has been attributed to the immaturity of the vascular system (Press, 1977). Lead has similar effects on the endoneurium, leading to increased endoneural fluid pressure and demyelination. Organic lead, such as tetraethyllead, more readily penetrates the barriers and is therefore more toxic in this respect.

Mercury compounds can damage the endothelial cells and increase their permeability. Organic arsenicals cause edema and focal hemorrhages in the brain. Tellurium causes edema in the endoneurium. Chronic alcoholism is associated with endoneural edema.

Endoneural edema can also result from intramyelinic edema in hexachlorophene intoxication. It may also be associated with Wallerian degeneration due to mechanical injury.

Cellular edema

Various parts of neurons may become edematous following exposure to toxicants. For example, 6-aminonicotinamide affects the perikaryon, cyanide and carbon monoxide affect the axon, and ouabain and methylsulfoxime affect the presynaptic nerve endings.

Edema of astrocytes and oligodendrocytes may be caused by 6-aminonicotinamide. Ouabain can also affect astrocytes. Edema of Schwann cells may be induced by lead, which, as noted above, also may cause extracellular edema.

Triethyltin and isoniazid also cause edema of the myelin sheaths in the CNS. Hexachlorophene induces edema of the myelin sheaths both in the white matter of the brain and in the peripheral nerves.

Testing procedures

Functional Observational Battery (FOB)

A battery of observations has been devised to assess the neurotoxic effects (EPA, 1994; Kallman and Fowler, 1994). These are done in intact animals, usually rats or mice, and can be incorporated in other tests (Chapter 6). These animals are exposed to the toxicant at two or three doses by an appropriate route. The duration of treatment and observation period vary from days to months according to the nature of the toxicant.

The animals are observed for the following abnormalities:

a   Unusual body position, activity level, gait, etc.
b   Unusual behavior such as compulsive biting, self-mutilation, circling, and walking backwards.
c   The presence of convulsions, tremors, lacrimation, red-colored tears, salivation, diarrhea, vocalization, etc.
d   Changes in sensory and motor functions (for details, see the following sections).

Neurologic examinations

These examinations often provide an indication of the site of neurotoxicity. Most of these examinations can be performed in humans as well as in animals. The exceptions relate to the determination of *mental state* and many *sensory functions*, which can be more readily assessed in humans.

Cranial nerves I through XII have different functions, and their tests therefore vary. For example, tests of the acoustic and optic nerves involve the evaluation of responses to sound and light stimuli.

Motor examination includes inspection of muscles for weakness, atrophy, and fasciculation, which indicate dysfunction of the lower motor neuron, that is, the anterior horn cells, motor roots, and peripheral nerves. Spasticity is a sign of dysfunction of the upper motor neurons in the brain and their axons down to the spinal cord. Resting tremor is often associated with lesions in the basal ganglia or cerebellum. Intention tremor occurs during voluntary movement and is a manifestation of cerebellar disease.

Reflex examination includes deep tendon reflexes, the functioning of which involves the intrafusal receptors, dorsal root ganglia, anterior horn cells and their axons, neuromuscular junction, and muscle. Damages to any of these structures will cause these reflexes to be absent or hypoactive. On the other hand, when there is upper motor neuron dysfunction, these reflexes will be exaggerated. The Babinski reflex is the most important superficial cutaneous reflex. Abnormal response is an indication of corticospinal dysfunction.

Gait abnormalities may also aid in locating the site of toxicity. For example, lower motor neuron disease causes high-stepping gait. A scissoring, or stiff, gait indicates upper motor neuron lesion. Cerebellar dysfunction results in an ataxic or reeling gait.

Morphologic examinations

Neurotoxicants may act on the CNS, the PNS, or both. They may induce lesions in the neuronal perikaryon or its axon, either proximally or distally, the myelinating cells or the myelin sheath itself, the astrocytes, or the endothelial cells. Morphologic examinations are therefore important in establishing the precise site of toxic lesions on an anatomic level. Examinations on cellular and ultrastructural levels often facilitate the differential diagnosis of the neuropathy.

Some of the commonly used techniques, along with a list of references, have been provided by Spencer *et al.* (1980). It is worth noting, however, that damages to endothelial cells can be demonstrated not only by signs of edema (fewer cells and nerve fiber per unit area) but also by increases of the pressure of the intracranial and endoneural fluids as well as by the penetration of tracer substances, such as horseradish peroxidase, through the endothelium.

Electrophysiologic examinations

Peripheral nerves

A frequently used examination involves the measurement of *motor nerve* conduction velocity. This can be done on intact animals subjected to short-term or chronic exposure to neurotoxicants or on exposed nerves after local application of the toxicants. *Sensory nerve* conduction velocity and action potentials have also been measured in the study of neurotoxicity.

Electromyography

This procedure calls for the examination of the electrical activities of a muscle, at rest and when contracted, recorded with the aid of a needle electrode inserted into the muscle. Neurotoxicities may manifest as (1) abnormal insertional activity, (2) occurrence of spontaneous electrical activity of a resting muscle, and (3) interference pattern of electrical activity of motor units during voluntary muscle contraction (Goodgold and Eberstein, 1977).

Behavioral studies: testing procedures

There is a large body of information on behavioral toxicology, resulting from a widespread feeling that behavior is a subtle and sensitive indicator of toxicity. However, this view has been questioned, for example, by Norton (1980), who stated: "Scientific data supporting this view are not only scanty but the available evidence often flatly contradicts this assumption." In the hope that improved testing procedures would increase the sensitivity and utility of this approach in neurotoxicology, this branch of neurotoxicology will undoubtedly grow. A few highlights of this subject are presented below.

The tests involve two types of responses: (1) unconditioned responses, which are either emitted (spontaneous) or elicited (reflex), and (2) conditioned responses, which may be considered as either "classic conditioning" (Pavlov) or operant conditioning (Skinner). The extent of training of the experimental animals required and the neurobehavioral function to be assessed are also useful criteria for classification of the tests.

EPA (1994) has provided some guidelines on schedule-controlled operant behavior.

Simple tests

Tilson *et al.* (1980) listed tests that require little or no prior training of the experimental animals (rats and mice) (See Table 17.1).

More involved tests

The tests listed in Table 17.2 require extended or special training, frequent evaluation, and/or manipulation of motivational factors.

Table 17.1 Examples of primary level neurobehavioral tests for rats or mice

Neurobehavioral function	Behavioral test
Sensory	
Visual, olfactory, somatosensory, auditory	Localization
Pain	Tail flick
Orientation in space	Negative geotaxis
Motor	
Spontaneous activity	Activity in Automex
Muscular weakness	Forelimb grip; hindlimb extensor
Fatigability	Swim endurance
Tremor	Frequency of occurrence
Cognitive–associative	
Learning and retention	One-way avoidance; step-through passive avoidance
Affective–emotional	
Responsiveness	Startle to air puff; emergence in a novel environment
Physiologic–consummatory	
Thermoregulation	Body weight; food and water ingestion; core temperature

Source: From Tilson *et al.*, 1980. Reproduced with permission of Peter S. Spencer, Editor.

Table 17.2 Examples of secondary level neurobehavioral tests for rats or mice

Neurobehavioral function	Behavioral test
Sensory	
Visual, auditory, olfactory	Operant psychophysics
Gustatory	Taste discrimination
Somatosensory	T-maze discrimination
Orientation in space	T-maze discrimination
Pain	Operant titration
Motor	
Spontaneous activity	Diurnal cyclicity; patterning
Muscular strength	Operant response force
Tremor	Spectral analysis
Cognitive–associative	
Learning and retention	Autoshaping; temporal discriminating; repeated acquisition
Affective–emotional	
CNS excitability	Brain self-stimulation; aversion thresholds
Physiologic–consummatory	
Thermoregulation	Diurnal patterning; cyclicity; preference

Source: From Tilson *et al.*, 1980. Reproduced with permission of Peter S. Spencer, Editor.

Procedures to enhance sensitivity

Because of the large functional reserve of the brain, focal damages may not result in any overt brain dysfunction. Such damages, however, may be demonstrated clinically with the use of *provocative* tests. These involve administering sodium amobarbital, raising body temperature, or lowering blood pH with the intravenous infusion of ammonium chloride (Lehrer, 1974).

Animals

Apart from rats and mice, other animals such as pigeons, cats, dogs, and monkeys are also commonly used, with testing procedures similar to those listed above.

Evaluation

In view of the wide range of toxic effects on the nervous system, as outlined above, there is clearly a need for a battery of tests for the evaluation of neurotoxicants. It is also worth noting that the choice of animal species is critical in eliciting certain types of toxicity, such as delayed neurotoxicity. Furthermore, the nature of the toxicity on the nervous system, as on other organs, can vary according to the duration of exposure. For example, *n*-hexane and TOCP produce, after acute exposure, narcosis, but they induce axonopathy after repeated exposures.

The significance of a neurotoxic effect depends on its reversibility. In general, irreversible effects are more serious than reversible ones. The site of the effect also plays an important role. There are areas in the nervous system more critical to physiologic function than others. In addition, focal damages in areas with abundant functional reserve are likely to be less serious.

The behavioral effects are especially susceptible to endogenous and environmental variations. For example, Norton (1980) reported data to indicate a large variability of results both between animals of the same species and within the same animal at different times. It is therefore important to adhere to proper experimental procedures, such as sufficiently large number of animals, rigorously controlled experimental environment, and statistical analysis of results.

References

Abel, E. J., Jacobson, S., and Sherwin, B. J. (1983) *In utero* ethanol exposure: functional and structural brain damage. *Neurobehav. Toxicol. Teratol.* 5:139–146.

Abou-Donia, M. B. (1981) Organophosphorus ester-induced delayed neurotoxicity. *Annu. Rev. Pharmacol. Toxicol.* 21:511–548.

Berti-Mattera, L. N., Eichberg, J., Schrama, L., and LoPachin, R. M. (1990) Acrylamide administration alters protein phosphorylation and phospholipid metabolism in rat sciatic nerve. *Toxicol. Appl. Pharmacol.* 103:502–511.

Bouldin, T. W., Gaines, N. D., Bagvell, C. R., and Krigman, M. R. (1981) Pathogenesis of trimethyltin neuronal toxicity. *Am. J. Pathol.* 104:237–249.

Carmicheal, W. W. (1994) The toxins of cyanobacteria. *Scientific American* 270:78–86.

Caroldi, E. J. and Lotti, M. (1982) Neurotoxic esterase in peripheral nerve: assay, inhibition and rate of resynthesis. *Toxicol. Appl. Pharmacol.* 62:498–501.

Cho, E. S., Spencer, P. S., and Jortner, B. S. (1980) Doxorubicin, in *Experimental and Clinical Neurotoxicology*, P. S. Spencer and H. H. Schaumberg (eds), Baltimore, MD: Williams & Wilkins, pp. 440–455.

Dawson, V. L., Dawson, T. M., London, E. D., Bredt, D. S., and Snyder, S. H. (1991) Nitric oxide mediates glutamate neurotoxicity in primary cortical culture. *Proc. Natl. Acad. Sci. USA* 88:6368–6371.

DeBoni, U., Otros, A., Scott, J. W., and Crapper, D. B. (1976) Neurofibrillary degeneration induced by systemic aluminum. *Acta Neuropathol.* 35:285–294.

EPA (1994) Health effects testing guidelines. *Code Federal Retulations, Title 40*, Part 798.

Gold, G. B. and Austin, D. R. (1991) Regulation of aberrant neurofilament phosphorylation in neuronal perikarya. *Brain. Res.* 563:151–162.

Goodgold, J. and Eberstein, A. (1977) *Electrodiagnosis of Neuromuscular Diseases.* Baltimore, MD: Williams & Wilkins.

Griffin, J. W. and Price, D. L. (1980) Proximal axonopathies induced by toxic chemicals, in *Experimental and Clinical Neurotoxicology*, P. S. Spencer and H. H. Schaumberg (eds), Baltimore, MD: Williams & Wilkins, pp. 161–178.

Jacobs, J. M., Carmichael, N., and Cavanagh, J. B. (1977) Ultrastructural studies in the nervous system of rabbits poisoned with methyl mercury. *Toxicol. Appl. Pharmacol.* 39:249–261.

Johnson, M. K. (1990) Contemporary issues in toxicology. Organophosphates and delayed neuropathy – is NTE alive and well? *Toxicol. Appl. Pharmacol.* 103:385–399.

Kallman, M. J. and Fowler, S. C. (1994) Assessment of chemically induced alterations in motor functions, in *Principles of Neurotoxicology*, L. W. Chang (ed.), New York, NY: Marcel Dekker, pp. 373–396.

Lehrer, G. M. (1974) Measurement of minimal brain dysfunction, in *Behavior Toxicology*, C. Xintaras, B. L. Johnson, and I. de Groot (eds), Washington, DC: National Institute for Occupational Safety and Health.

Narahashi, T. (1992) Nerve membrane Na^+ channels as targets of insecticides. *Trends Pharmacol. Sci.* 13:236–241.

Norton, S. (1980) Behavioral toxicology: a critical appraisal, in *The Scientific Basis of Toxicity Assessment*, H. R. Witschi (ed.), Amsterdam: Elsevier/North Holland, pp. 91–107.

OECD (1984) Delayed neurotoxicity of organophosphorus substances, in *Guidelines for Testing Chemicals.* Paris: Organization for Economic Cooperation and Development.

Olney, J. W., Rhee, V., and Ho, O. L. (1974) Kainic acid: a powerful neurotoxic analogue of glutamate. *Brain Res.* 77:507–512.

Press, M. F. (1977) Lead encephalopathy in neonatal Long-Evans rats: morphologic studies. *J. Neuropathol. Exp. Neurol.* 36:169–193.

Savolainen, J. (1977) Some aspects of the mechanism by which industrial solvents produce neurotoxic effects. *Chem. Biol. Interact.* 18:1–10.

Schield, L. K., Griffin, J. W., Drachman, D. B., and Price, D. L. (1977) Retrograde axonal transport: a direct method for measurement of rate. *Neurology* 27:393.

Soni, M. G., White, S. M., Flamm, W. G., and Burdock, G. A. (2001) Safety evaluation of dietary aluminum. *Regul. Toxicol. Pharmacol.* 33:66–79.

Spencer, P. S., Bischoff, M. C., and Schaumberg, H. H. (1980) Neuropathological methods for the detection of neurotoxic disease, in *Experimental and Clinical Neurotoxicology*, P. S. Spencer and H. H. Schaumberg (eds), Baltimore, MD: Williams & Wilkins, pp. 743–757.

Spencer, P. S., Sabri, M. I., Schaumberg, H. H., and Moore, C. (1979) Does a defect in energy metabolism in the nerve fiber cause axonal degeneration in polyneuropathies? *Ann. Neurol.* 5:501–507.

Tilson, H. A. (1989) Screening for neurotoxicity: principles and practices. *J. Am. Coll. Toxicol.* 8:13–17.

Tilson, H. A., Cabe, P. A., and Burne, T. A. (1980) Behavioral procedures for the assessment of neurotoxicity, in *Experimental and Clinical Neurotoxicology*, P. C. Spencer and H. H. Schaumberg (eds), Baltimore, MD: Williams & Wilkins, pp. 758–766.

Worden, A. N., Heywood, R., Prentice, D. E., Chesterman, H., Skerrett, K., and Thomann, P. E. (1978) Clioquinol toxicity in the dog. *Toxicology* 9:227.

Zhang, J. and Snyder, S. H. (1995) Nitric oxide in the nervous system. *Am. Rev. Pharmacol. Toxicol.* 35:213–233.

Appendix 17.1 Select neurotoxicants described in text

Acrylamide-A
Actinomycin-M
AETT-M
Alcohol-N, T
Alanosine-N
Aluminum-N
6-Aminonicotinamide-BV
Anatoxin-C
Arsenic-BV
Azide-N
Barbiturate-N
Botulinum toxin-C
Carbon monoxide-N
Clioquinol-A
Cyanide-N, BV
DDT-C
Diphtheria toxin-M

n-hexane-A
IDPN-A
Kainic acid-N
Lead-MS
Leptophos-A
Lysolecithin-M
Methyl *n*-butyl ketone-A
Methyl mercury-N, BV
Nicotine-C
Organotin-N
Organic solvents-A
Pyrethroids-C
Saxitoxin-C
Tellurium-BV, M
Tetanoplasmin-C
Tetrodotoxin-C
Thallium-A

Doxorubicin-N
EPN-A
Ethidium bromide-M
Glutamate-N
Hexachlorophene-M, BV

Triethyltin-M, BV
Triparanol-M
TOCP-A
Vincristine-A

A: Axonopathy
N: Neuropathy
M: Myelinopathy
C: Conduction and transmission
T: Teratogenicity
BV: Blood vessel and edema
MS: Multiple sites

Chapter 18

Reproductive and cardiovascular systems

REPRODUCTIVE SYSTEM

Introduction

Reproductive process and organs

The reproductive process starts with gametogenesis. In the female animal, oogenesis involves the formation of primary oocytes from the primordial germ cells (oogonia) through mitosis. This development takes place during the fetal period and ceases at birth. Primary oocytes divide by meiosis to form secondary oocytes just before they are ovulated.

On the other hand, spermatogenesis starts with gonocytes during the fetal period, and these cells are transformed to spermatogonia after birth. Spermatogonia remain dormant until puberty, when proliferative activity begins again. Some of the spermatogonia multiply to form additional spermatogonia while others mature to spermatozoa. There are three intermediate stages. Spermatogonia divide by mitosis to form primary spermatocytes, which divide by meiosis to form secondary spermatocytes. These in turn divide to form spermatids. Finally spermatids become spermatozoa by metamorphosis. The entire process is continuous, and the time required for spermatogonia to become spermatozoa is about 60 days (Figure 18.1).

Fertilization requires not only functional ovum and spermatozoa but also effective delivery of the sperm and proper milieu. The conceptus, the fertilized ovum, is then implanted in the uterus and develops through embryonic and fetal stages. At the end of the gestational period, parturition takes place. The pups are suckled until weaning. They then grow and mature to start the reproductive process again, thus completing a reproductive cycle.

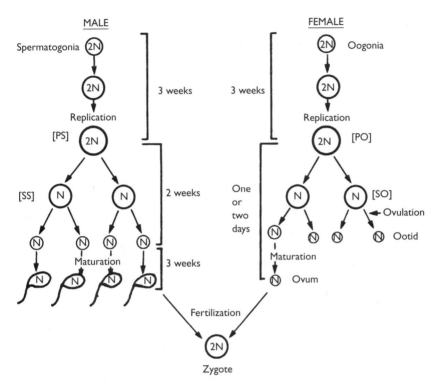

Figure 18.1 Gametogenesis and fertilization. 2N, diploid; N, haploid; PS, primary spermatocyte; SS, secondary spermatocyte; PO, primary oocyte; SO, secondary
oocyte.

Source: From Brusick, 1987, by permission.

Other cells and organs

While gametocytes are the essential elements of the reproductive process,
other cells and organs also play important roles.

In the male reproductive system, spermatogenesis takes place in the
seminiferous tubules in the testis. In these tubules are the Sertoli cells,
which extend from the basement membrane to the lumen of the seminiferous tubules and contain androgen-binding proteins (ABP). The ABP
facilitate the movement of androgen to the spermatocytes for their development.

In addition, there are the Leydig cells, which are located in the interstitial tissue surrounding the seminiferous tubules. These cells are the main
site of synthesis of testosterone, which is essential not only for the development of the reproductive system but also for its proper functioning.

After leaving the testis, spermatozoa are stored in the epididymis to undergo changes in order to gain fertility capacity and for later delivery to the female reproductive system. In addition, the accessory organs prostate and seminal vesicle provide special nutrients and proper milieu for the sperm. These organs respond to the effect of testosterone, and hence their weights are indicators of the blood level of this hormone.

In the female reproductive system the ova can be affected while they are in the ovaries. However, it is more often that the fertilized ova are affected either directly or indirectly through damages to the uterus.

Pharmacokinetics

Throughout the reproductive cycle, toxicants can act directly on the reproductive system or the conceptus, or indirectly via certain endocrine organs. Before chemicals act directly, they must reach the target organs in sufficiently high concentration. This concentration may be higher or lower than that in the blood. For example, with DDT, the concentration is almost 80 times higher in the ovary than in the plasma. A number of other substances have also been shown to penetrate the oocyte, oviduct, uterine fluid, and blastocyst (Fabro, 1978).

Unlike the ovaries, the testis is protected by the blood–testis barrier (BTB) (Lee and Dixon, 1978). The BTB is a complex of a multicellular system composed of capillary endothelial cells, myoid cells and membranes surrounding the seminiferous tubules and the tightly joined Sertoli cells in the tubules. This barrier, however, is less effective than the blood–brain barrier. The penetration rate of chemicals into the testis is governed by their molecular weights, their partition coefficients, and ionic characteristics.

Testis contains both activating and detoxicating enzyme systems. These two enzyme systems, as noted in Chapter 3, are capable of, respectively, increasing and decreasing the toxicities of chemicals. Furthermore, there is an efficient DNA repair mechanism in the premeiotic spermatogenic cells, but there is none in spermatids nor in spermatozoa; mutations can therefore be induced by genotoxic substances on these cells.

Toxicants and their effects

The reproductive functions may be affected by toxicants through their effects on the reproductive system of either sex. In the male, the formation, development, storage and delivery of spermatozoa may be adversely affected. The oocytes, in the females, are also susceptible to certain toxicants. In addition, the implantation of the fertilized ova as well as the growth and development of the conceptus may be affected. In both sexes, some of the toxic effects are mediated through hormonal or nervous system activities.

Male reproductive system

Many chemicals adversely affect spermatogenesis and cause testicular atrophy. These include food colors (e.g., Oil Yellow AB and Oil Yellow OB) (Allmark *et al.*, 1955), pesticides (e.g., DBCP), metals (e.g., lead and cadmium), and organic solvents. A variety of other chemicals affect the testis, such as steroid hormones, alkylating agents, cyclohexylamine, and hexachlorophene.

In addition to reduced sperm count resulting from adverse effects on spermatogenesis, a toxicant may render spermatozoa defective, less mobile, or even dead. For example, methylmethane sulfonate (MMS) and busulfan both cause lethal mutation, but MMS affects spermatids and spermatozoa whereas busulfan affects the prespermiogenic cells. These alkylating agents apparently attack the DNA of these cells with different repair mechanisms (Lee, 1983).

Spermatozoa may also be affected while being stored in epididymis. For example, the male antifertility agent α-chlorohydrin inhibits the fertilizing capacity of spermatozoa. Gossypol, another such agent that was extensively tried in China (Qian and Wang, 1984), probably acts through a similar mechanism.

The testis is hormonally regulated by the hypothalamus-pituitary-testis axis: follicle-stimulating hormone (FSH) is required in the initiation of spermatogenesis through the production of ABP in Sertoli cells, whereas luteinizing hormone (LH) acts on Leydig cells to synthesize testosterone. A toxicant may thus affect reproductive function via these endocrine hormones. An example is DBCP (dibromochloropropane), a fumigant used in agriculture. It has induced among occupational workers azoospermia and oligospermia, along with elevated serum concentrations of LH and FSH (Miller *et al.*, 1987).

Reproductive functions are also under the influence of the autonomic nervous system. Thus, the hypotensive drug losulazine, which acts by depleting norepinephrine, causes reversible infertility in male rats, probably through altered sexual behavior and ejaculatory disturbances (Mesfin *et al.*, 1989). Guanethidine, another hypotensive drug may cause/fail to induce pregnancy by interfering with seminal emission (Palmer, 1976).

Tumors may develop in the testis. For example, the herbicide linuron may induce Leydig cell tumors. The tumorigenesis is mediated through a sustained hypersecretion of LH (Cook *et al.*, 1993). In contrast to rats, which are likely to develop Leydig cell tumors, testicular tumors are more likely to arise from germ cells in men. Cadmium has been reported to induce prostate cancer in men (Waalkes and Rehm, 1994).

Female reproductive system

Oocytes may be damaged by chemotherapeutic agents such as nitrogen mustard and vinblastine, and polycyclic aromatic hydrocarbons (PAH) such as 3-methylcholanthrene and benzo[a]pyrene. Prostaglandin synthetase inhibitors, e.g., aspirin-like drugs, may block the release of ovulation. Oocytes before puberty are more resistant to the toxic effects of chemicals, evidently because they are dormant. Certain organochlorine pesticides such as methoxychlor, similar to estradiol, may increase the weight of the uterus (Eroschenko and Rourke, 1992).

Other reproductive functions may also be affected. Haloperidol prevents implantation. DDT and nicotine may affect the development and growth of the conceptus and thus lower the fetal weight (Fabro, 1978). Spironolactone may interfere with ovulation and implantation of the fertilized ovum; it may also retard the development of the sex organs of the offspring (Nagi and Virgo, 1982). Gossypol is also toxic in the female. It suppresses ovarian steroid hormone secretion, interrupts regular cyclicity and inhibits embryo implantation (Lin *et al.*, 1994). There is a relationship between the extent of cigarette smoking and the onset of menopause; menopause is an indication of oocyte depletion (Miller *et al.*, 1987). The toxic effects that are specifically related to the production of congenital anomalies are dealt with in Chapter 9.

Routine testing: multigeneration reproduction studies

Animals and doses

In general, rats are the animal of choice. A minimum of 20 females and 10 males are placed in each of three dose groups and a control group. OECD Guidelines (1995) recommend 10 animals of each sex. The doses are selected so that the high dose will produce some minimal toxic signs but will not result in a mortality greater than 10%. The low dose will not induce any observable effect.

Prior to breeding, the animals are dosed for 10 weeks prior to mating. However, because of the difference in the time required for maturation of the gametes, the males are dosed for 70 days, the period of spermatogenesis, and the females are dosed for 14 days, the length of the development of the ova. Dosing of the females is continued through the gestation and lactation periods. The test chemical should be administered by a route that most closely resembles the human exposure condition.

To determine the potential effect of the chemical on the reproductive function of the offspring (F_1), a second generation offspring (F_2) is bred and reared to reproductive maturity.

Observations and examinations

The adult animals are observed for the body weight, food consumption, general appearance, estrus cycle, and mating behavior. In addition, the fertility and nesting and nursing behaviors are also noted. Half of the maternal rats are killed on day 13 of gestation for examination of corpora lutea, implantations, and resorptions.

The other half of the pregnant rats are allowed to deliver their pups. The pups are examined for litter size, number of stillborn, gender distribution, and congenital anomalies. In addition, the viability and pup weight are recorded at birth, on day four, and at weaning, and preferably also on day 12 or 14. Auditory and visual functions and behavior are also examined for subtle congenital defects.

An appropriate number of males and females are randomly selected from all generations and examined by gross necropsy and histopathology, especially with respect to the reproductive organs. In the males, weights and histopathology of the testes, epididymides, seminal vesicles, prostate, and pituitary often provide useful information on the site of action of the toxicant under test. Other indicators of the effects are the sperm count, and its motility and morphology, as well as the levels of certain hormones, especially testosterone, FSH and LH. In the females, weights and histopathology of the vagina, uterus, oviduct, ovaries and pituitary should be assessed, along with the levels of the relevant hormones.

Additional details and references to the reproduction and fertility studies are provided in the EPA test guidelines (1994).

Evaluation

From these data, a number of disturbances of reproductive function can be deduced from the following indices:

1   Fertility index: the percentage of matings resulting in pregnancy.
2   Gestation index: the percentage of pregnancies resulting in the birth of live litters.
3   Viability index: the percentage of live pups that survive four days or longer.
4   Lactation index: the percentage of pups alive on day four that survive 21 days or longer.

Other indicators of effects include (1) mating index (the percentage of estrus cycles that had matings), (2) male fertility index (the percentage of males exposed to fertile nonpregnant females that resulted in pregnancies), (3) female fertility index (the percentage of females exposed to fertile males that resulted in pregnancies), and (4) 12- or 14-day survival indices.

Multigeneration reproductive study can reveal a variety of toxic effects on the reproductive function as well as on the *conceptus*. Examples are indices of gestation, viability, and survival. However, nonspecific response (e.g., nonpregnancy) is common. It may follow unusual routes of administering the chemical, such as inhalation, topical application to the eye or nose, and parenteral administration. Excessive handling may also disturb the normal reproductive function. A number of other interfering factors are discussed by Palmer (1976).

The pathologic examination may reveal suppression of spermatogenesis, advanced rates of follicle atresia, and ovulatory or meiotic failure.

Other tests

The effects revealed in multigeneration reproduction studies outlined above may result from paternal, maternal, or fetal exposure. Thus, additional tests are often conducted to establish the cause of the effect. A few such tests are outlined below.

Pathological examinations are useful in identifying a variety of toxic effects. The weight of testis is a simple but sensitive index of testicular damages. The extent and nature of such damages can often be assessed microscopically. The weights of prostate and seminal vesicle are often correlated with levels of testosterone. Similarly, gross and microscopic analysis of *semen* is useful in epidemiologic and animal studies. The sperm count and the motility, survival, and morphology of the spermatozoa often provide information on toxic effects on the testis (Eliasson, 1978). As noted above, certain toxicants affect the reproductive function through disturbances of *hormones*, especially testosterone, estrogens, FSH, and LH. Assays of their levels may indicate the mode of action of the toxicant.

The *perfused male reproductive tracts* have been shown to be useful models in studying the effects of chemicals on the secretion and accumulation of androgens (Bardin *et al.*, 1978).

Certain *biomarkers* have been used in a variety of tests for disorders of the reproductive system. For example, DNA probes have been used to detect gene mutation and massive deletion and translocations in meiotic, and postmeiotic germ cells as well as Sertoli and Leydig cells in the testis (Hecht, 1987).

CARDIOVASCULAR SYSTEM

General considerations

The cardiovascular system is composed of two parts: the heart and the blood vessels. The heart is a vital organ in the body. Although it is not a common target organ, it can be damaged by a variety of chemicals. They act either directly on the myocardium or indirectly through the nervous system or blood vessels. A list of such chemicals, as compiled by Van Stee (1980), is reproduced in Table 18.1.

The heart is mainly composed of myocardial cells, each measuring about $15 \times 80\,\mu m$. Unlike skeletal muscle cells, each of which is innervated, only some of the heart muscle cells are innervated. However, these cells are joined, at their ends, to each other by the nexus. It has low resistance and thus allows rapid transmission of electrical stimulus from one cell to the next. These characteristics are essential to the programmed sequence of contraction of different parts of the heart.

The myocardium is different from skeletal muscles also in that there is less contractile material (50% vs. 80%) but much more mitochondrial material (35% vs. 2%). Mitochondria evidently play an important role in the cardiac contractility and are a common subcellular target of cardiotoxicity.

Myocardial contraction involves the liberation of energy from oxidative

Table 18.1 Cardiotoxic drugs and chemicals

Cardiomyopathy:

Allylamine	Adrenergic agonists
Furazolidone	Methysergide
Ethanol	Vasodilators
Cobalt	

Interference with nucleic acid metabolism and protein synthesis:
Antineoplastic drugs

Electrophysiologic mechanisms:

Cardiotonic drugs	Local anesthetics
Phenytoin (diphenylhydantoin)	Emetine
Tricyclic antidepressants	Chlordimeform
Clofibrate	Contrast media
Lithium	Antimalarial drugs
Propylene glycol	Calcium antagonists

Nonspecific myocardial depression:

Lipid-soluble, organic compounds	Antimicrobial antibiotics
Myocardial depressant factor	Carbromide, carbromal

Involvement with lipid metabolism:

High cholesterol diet	Brominated vegetable oils
Rapeseed oil	

Miscellaneous:
Phenothiazines

Source: Van Stee, 1980.

metabolism, conservation of the energy by adenosine triphosphate and creatine phosphate, and utilization of the energy by contractile proteins. The most vulnerable mechanisms include the utilization of energy and intracellular movement of calcium ion, which is involved in the contractility of myocardium as well as regulating enzyme activities, transduction of hormonal information, etc.

The vascular system consists of arteries, arterioles, capillaries, venules, and veins. A toxicant may affect any of these vessels; the seriousness of the effect depends on the physiological role of the organ that is supplied by the affected blood vessel.

Toxic effects on the heart

Cardiomyopathy

The usual toxic effects of cobalt are polycythemia, goiter, and signs of gastrointestinal irritation such as vomiting and diarrhea. However, its inclusion in beer as a foam stabilizer caused a number of serious and fatal cases of cardiomyopathy. Subsequent studies showed that there is also intramitochondrial accumulation of calcium. The toxicity of cobalt on the heart was greatly enhanced by malnutrition, especially the deficiency of certain amino acids. Among the heavy beer drinkers, this condition existed because of the large caloric intake of beer. It was also noted that cobalt ions depressed oxygen uptake and interfered with cardiac energy metabolism in the tricarboxylic acid cycle, as thiamine deficiency does (Grice, 1972). As noted above, Ca^{2+} plays a vital role in various functions of myocardium. Cobalt may reduce the available myocardial Ca^{2+} by complexing with macromolecules and may also be antagonistic to endogenous Ca^{2+}.

Adrenergic β-receptor agonists, isoproterenol in particular, and vasodilating antihypertensive drugs, such as hydralazine are capable of inducing myocardial necrosis. The former chemicals have direct adrenergic effects, whereas the antihypertensive drugs exert adrenergic effects via the induced hypotension. These effects produce an augmented transmembrane calcium influx, which in turn causes an increase in the rate and force of contraction. This, along with the concomitant hypotension, results in cardiac hypoxia. The hypoxia and the calcium deposits in the mitochondria cause disintegration of organelles and sarcolemma (Balazs *et al.*, 1981).

Interference with nucleic acid synthesis

The anthracycline antibiotics doxorubicin and daunorubicin are effective antineoplastic drugs. However, they produce hypotension, tachycardia, and arrhythmias acutely. More prolonged administration causes degeneration and atrophy of cardiac muscle cells and interstitial edema and fibrosis. The likely mode of action is the binding of these antibiotics to mitochondrial and nuclear DNA, which in turn interferes with synthesis of RNA and protein. This effect on the heart is important because the half-life of the contractile proteins is short (12 weeks). Other possible mechanisms of action include peroxidation of membrane lipids, and hypotension resulting from release of cytokines (Van Stee, 1980).

Arrhythmias

A number of fluorocarbons are capable of producing cardiac arrhythmias. This effect is mediated by a sensitization of the heart to epinephrine, depression of contractility, reduction of coronary blood flow, and reflex increase in sympathetic and vagal impulses to the heart following irritation of mucosa in the respiratory tract (Aviado, 1978).

Tricyclic antidepressants can also cause cardiac arrhythmias. These effects are likely the result of imbalances within the autonomic regulatory system of the heart. Propylene glycol, a common solvent, can convert ventricular tachycardia induced by deslanoside into ventricular fibrillation (Keller et al., 1992).

Myocardial depression

A number of lipid-soluble organic compounds, such as general anesthetics, depress cardiac contractility. The probable mechanism of action is a nonspecific expansion of various cellular membranes by the insertion of chemically indifferent molecules in the hydrophobic regions of integral proteins and membrane phospholipids.

Antibiotics, such as amphotericin B, chloramphenical, streptomycin, and tetracycline cause hypotension through depression of cardiac contractility. The mechanism of action appears to be related to an inhibition of Ca^{2+} bound to superficial membrane sites (Keller et al., 1992).

Miscellaneous

Rapeseed oil, a common cooking oil in many parts of the world, causes accumulation of lipid globules in heart muscles in rats. This effect was attributed to the high content of erucic acid in rapeseed oil. Brominated vegetable oils, used in adjusting the density of flavoring oils and in enhancing cloudy stability in beverages, induce biochemical and morphologic changes in cardiac myofibrils. The coloring Brown F.K. also produces severe morphologic changes in the heart muscles (Grice, 1972).

Toxic effects on blood vessels

Increased capillary permeability

Lead, mercury, and several other toxicants damage endothelial cells of capillaries in the brain. This effect will result in brain edema and an impairment of the blood–brain barrier (Chapter 16). Inhalation of irritating gas induces pulmonary edema (Chapter 11).

Endothelial damage

Monocrotaline, a plant toxin, may cause pulmonary vascular damage. This chemical, after ingestion, is bioactivated in the liver, but sufficient amounts of the active metabolites leave the liver and cause cross-linking of DNA in the endothelial cells of the pulmonary vasculature. This effect may damage the repair capability of the endothelial cells leading to thrombosis and progressive pulmonary hypertension (Boor *et al.*, 1995). Arsenic has been suggested as the cause of the *black-foot* disease, a result of peripheral endarteritis (see p. 316).

Vasoconstriction and vasodilatation

Ingestion of ergot alkaloids (fungal contaminants in certain foods) may cause gangrene resulting from vasoconstriction. A clinical syndrome known as "black-foot disease" is endemic in certain areas in South America and Taiwan. It has been attributed to vasoconstriction following consumption of drinking water with high levels of arsenic (Chapter 18). Exposure to pure oxygen over a prolonged period may result in blindness especially among premature infants, evidently because of the associated vasoconstriction in the eye.

Occupational workers exposed to nitroglycerin on work days have been reported to have died suddenly of heart attack on weekends. Apparently the continued exposure to a coronary dilator has rendered the workers accustomed to a low level of coronary flow, and the sudden cessation of exposure to the coronary dilator precipitated coronary insufficiency.

The musculature of the coronary artery may be damaged by large doses of certain hypotensive drugs, such as minoxidil and hydralazine. The lesion may be a result of exaggerated pharmacodynamic changes (Boor *et al.*, 1995).

Others

Degenerative changes

Atherosclerosis is a complex degenerative disease affecting mainly large blood vessels such as the coronary and carotid arteries. Narrowing of these arteries may result in heart attacks and strokes, respectively. While the etiology of atherosclerosis is complex, certain toxicants may aggravate the pathological condition. CO may increase the permeability of capillaries surrounding these arteries and promote the degenerative process. So does CS_2 by damaging their endothelium. Ramos *et al.* (1994) observed that certain allylamines and aromatic hydrocarbons may contribute to the development of atherosclerosis. These toxicants may act through nitric oxide and endothelin on the smooth muscle and endothelium of arteries, and induce vascular lesions which may contribute to the development of atherosclerosis.

Fibrosis

Cadmium and lead may affect blood vessels in the kidney causing renal fibrosis. The impairment of blood supply may interfere with the "nonexcretory functions" of the kidney (Chapter 14), and indirectly cause hypertension.

Hypersensitivity reaction

Gold salts, penicillin, sulfonamides, and a number of other toxicants may induce vasculitis or exacerbate preexisting polyarteritis. The condition usually affects small vessels and is associated with infiltration of eosinophils and mononuclear cells indicating involvement of the immune system.

Tumors

Tumors of blood vessels may result from certain toxicants. For example, vinyl chloride has been shown to cause hemangiosarcoma in the liver in humans and animals (Chapter 7), and hemangioendothelioma has been reported to result from exposure to thorium dioxide.

Testing procedures

Cardiovascular toxicity can be studied in intact normal animals, in animals with specific pathologic conditions, or in isolated hearts and blood vessels.

Normal animals

A variety of examinations for cardiovascular toxicity can be performed on animals in conventional toxicity studies. These include blood pressure, heart rate, and electrocardiography. The rate of blood flow is a useful indicator of the functions of the cardiovascular systems, and can be measured using, among others, pulsed Doppler flowmeter (Haywood *et al.*, 1981). The status of the arteriole, capillaries and venules can be studied either at special site of organism (e.g., conjunctiva and retina), or through microvascular chamber which can be chronically placed on a laboratory animal (Smith *et al.*, 1994). Functional tests, such as swimming until exhaustion, have been suggested. At necropsy, the organ weight is often determined. Gross, light, and, in particular, electron microscopic examinations are valuable. Biochemical studies of the myocardium and of the blood are also useful.

Animals with pathologic conditions

The hearts of rabbits fed a diet containing 2% cholesterol become atherosclerotic. These hearts are more susceptible to myocardial ischemia (Lee *et al.*, 1978). Other models, such as infarcted myocardium, cardiomyopathic hamster, obesity, and drug interaction models, have been briefly described and referenced by Van Stee (1980).

Isolated heart

The isolated, perfused heart is a common model for studying the effects of drugs on the strength and rate of heart contractions and the rate of coronary flow. It has also been used to detect the cardiac effects of toxicants. For example, Toy *et al.* (1976) have shown that certain halogenated alkanes depressed the peak left ventricular pressure as well as the rate of increase of that pressure. The isolated atrium and cultured heart cells have also been used in the study of cardiotoxicity (Adams *et al.*, 1978; Sperelakis, 1978).

Evaluation

The cardiovascular toxicity of chemicals is not readily detected in conventional toxicity studies. For example, the toxic effects of cobalt and the anthracycline antibiotics on the heart were reproduced in animal experiments only after they were detected in humans first. Negative results therefore do not necessarily exclude potential cardiotoxicity.

To demonstrate such toxicity, specific testing procedures may be required. These procedures usually mimic the clinical conditions. For example, intermittent administration of the anthracycline antibiotics was necessary to elicit the cardiotoxicity; presumably continuous treatment caused the animals to die from other toxic effects before heart lesions developed. The toxicity of adrenergic β-receptor agonists is best detected in acute studies; the effects of prolonged treatment may be masked by tolerance development. The effect of cobalt on the heart is more readily revealed when the animals are on a protein- and vitamin-deficient diet (Balazs and Ferrans, 1978).

References

Adams, H. R., Parker, J. L., and Durrett, L. R. (1978) Cardiac toxicities of antibiotics. *Environ. Health Perspect.* 26:217–231.

Allmark, M. G., Grice, H. C., and Lu, F. C. (1955) Chronic toxicity studies on food colors: observations on the toxicity of FD&C Yellow No. 3 (Oil Yellow AB) and FD&C Yellow No. 4 (Oil Yellow OB) in rats. *J. Pharm. Pharmacol.* 7:591–603.

Aviado, D. M. (1978) Effects of fluorocarbons, chlorinated solvents, and inosine on the cardiopulmonary system. *Environ. Health Perspect.* 26:207–216.

Balazs, T. and Ferrans, V. J. (1978) Cardiac lesions induced by chemicals. *Environ. Health Perspect.* 26:181–191.

Balazs, T., Ferrans, V. J., El-Hage, A. *et al.* (1981) Study of the mechanism of hydralazine-induced myocardial necrosis in the rat. *Toxicol. Appl. Pharmacol.* 59:524–534.

Bardin, C. W., Baker, H. W. G., Jefferson, L. S., and Santen, R. J. (1978) Methods for perfusing male reproductive tract: models for studying drugs and hormone metabolism. *Environ. Health Perspect.* 24:51–59.

Boor, P. J., Gotlieb, A. I., Joseph, E. C., Kerns, W. D., Roth, R. A., and Tomaszewski, K. E. (1995) Chemical-induced vasculature injury. *Toxicol. Appl. Pharmacol.* 132:177–195.

Brusick, D. (1987) *Principles of Genetic Toxicology*, 2nd edn. New York, NY: Plenum Press.

Cook, J. C., Mullin, L. S., Frame, S. R., and Biegel, L. B. (1993) Investigation of a mechanism for Leydig cell tumorigenesis by linuron. *Toxicol. Appl. Pharmacol.* 119:195–204.

Eliasson, R. (1978) Semen analysis. *Environ. Health Perspect.* 24:81–85.

EPA (1994) *Health Effects Test Guidelines*. Washington, DC: U.S. Environmental Protection Agency.

Eroschenko, V. P. and Rourke, A. W. (1992) Stimulating influences of the technical grade methoxychlor and estradiol on protein synthesis in the uterus of the immature mouse. *J. Occup. Med. Toxicol.* 1:307–315.

Fabro, S. (1978) Penetration of chemicals into the oocyte, uterine fluid and preimplantation blastocyst. *Environ. Health Perspect.* 24:25–29.

Grice, H. C. (1972) The changing role of pathology in modern safety evaluation. *CRC Crit. Rev. Toxicol.* 1:119–152.

Haywood, J. R., Shaffer, R. A., Fink, G. D., and Brody, M. J. (1981) Regional blood flow measurements with pulsed Doppler flowmeter in conscious rat. *Am. J. Physiol.* 241:14273–14278.

Hecht, N. B. (1987) Detecting the effects of toxic agents on spermatogenesis using DNA probes. *Environ. Health Perspect.* 74:31–40.

Keller, R. S., Parker, J. L., and Adams, H. R. (1992) Cardiovascular toxicity of antibacterial antibiotics, in *Cardiovascular Toxicology*, D. Costa (ed.), New York, NY: Raven Press, pp. 165–195.

Lee, I. P. (1983) Adaptive biochemical repair response toward germ cell DNA damage. *Am. J. Ind. Med.* 4:135–147.

Lee, I. P. and Dixon, R. L. (1978) Factors influencing reproduction and genetic toxic effects on male gonads. *Environ. Health Perspect.* 24:117–127.

Lee, R. J., Zaidi, I. H., and Baky, S. H. (1978) Pathophysiology of the atherosclerotic rabbit. *Environ. Health Perspect.* 26:225–231.

Lin, Y. C., Coskun, S., and Sanbuissho, A. (1994) Effects of gossypol on *in vitro* bovine oocyte maturation and steroidogenesis in bovine granulosa cells. *Theriogenol.* 41:1601–1611.

Mesfin, G. M., Morris, D. F., Seaman, W. J., and Marks, T. A. (1989) Testicular lesions in rats treated with a sympatholytic hypotensive agent (losulazine). *J. Am. Coll. Toxicol.* 8:525–538.

Miller, R. K., Kellogg, C. K., and Saltzman, R. A. (1987) Reproductive and perinatal toxicology, in *Handbook of Toxicology*, T. J. Haley and W. O. Berndt (eds), Washington, DC: Hemisphere, pp. 195–309.

Nagi, S. and Virgo, B. B. (1982) The effects of spironolactone on reproductive functions in female rats and mice. *Toxicol. Appl. Pharmacol.* 66:221–228.

OECD (1995) *OECD guidelines for testing of chemicals: reproduction/developmental toxicity screening test.* Paris: Organization of Economic Development.

Palmer, A. K. (1976) Assessment of current test procedures. *Environ. Health Perspect.* 18:97–104.

Qian, S. and Wang, Z. (1984) Gossypol: a potential antifertility agent for males. *Annu. Rev. Pharmacol. Toxicol.* 24:329–360.

Ramos, K. S., Bowes, R. C., Ou, X. L., and Weber, T. J. (1994) Responses of vascular smooth cells to toxic insult: cellular and molecular perspectives for environmental toxicants. *J. Toxicol. Env. Health* 43:419–440.

Ramos, K. S., Chacon, E., and Acosta, D., Jr. (1996) Toxic responses of the heart and vascular system, in *Casarett and Doull's Toxicology*, C. D. Klaassen (ed.), New York, NY: McGraw-Hill, pp. 487–527.

Smith, T. L., Koman, L. A., and Mosberg, A. T. (1994) Cardiovascular physiology and methods for toxicology, in *Principles and Methods of Toxicology*, A. W. Hayes (ed.), New York, NY: Raven Press.

Sperelakis, N. (1978) Cultured heart cell reaggregate model for studying cardiac toxicology. *Environ. Health Perspect.* 26:243–267.

Toy, P. A., Van Stee, E. W., Harris, A. M., Horton, M. L., and Back, K. C. (1976) The effects of three halogenated alkanes on excitation and contraction in the isolated, perfused rabbit heart. *Toxicol. Appl. Pharmacol.* 38:7–17.

Van Stee, E. W. (1980) Myocardial toxicity, in *The Scientific Basis of Toxicity Assessment*, H. R. Witschi (ed.), New York, NY: Elsevier/North Holland.

Waalkes, M. P. and Rehm, S. (1994) Cadmium and prostate cancer. *J. Toxicol. Envir. Health* 43:251–269.

Part IV

Toxic substances and risk assessment

Chapter 19

Food additives and contaminants

Introduction

With the increasing world population, there has been a growing demand for more food. Various physical means and chemical substances have been developed and utilized to increase the food supply. However, the increased efficiency of farming reduced the number of farmers. In addition, with industrialization and urbanization, more and more people lived away from the farmland. These social changes have resulted in an ever-increasing demand for processed foods that can be transported from the farm to the city and that will retain their nutritive value and organoleptic properties. These demands have been met largely by the addition of chemicals known as food additives. These chemicals serve a variety of technological functions as described in the section "Functional Groups."

Legal definition of food additives

The following definition has been adopted by the Codex Alimentarius Commission, an intergovernmental agency consisting of more than 150 nations (FAO/WHO, 1994).

> *Food Additive* means any substance not normally consumed as a food by itself and not normally used as a typical ingredient of the food, whether or not it has nutritive value, the intentional addition of which to food for a technological (including organoleptic) purpose in the manufacture, processing, preparation, treatment, packing, packaging, transport or holding of such food results, or may be reasonably expected to result (directly or indirectly) in it or its by-products becoming a component of or otherwise affecting the characteristics of such foods. The term does not include "contaminants" or substances added to food for maintaining or improving nutritional qualities.

The U.S. legal definition appearing in the U.S. Federal Food, Drug and Cosmetic Act, as amended in October 1976 (1979), is different from the above in several aspects. The U.S. legislation excludes color additives and those substances that are to be added to food but are defined as "generally recognized as safe (GRAS)." On the other hand, the U.S. legislation considers nutritional supplements and irradiated foods as food additives.

Classification of food additives and contaminants

Functional groups of direct food additives

A number of chemicals are added to food to increase its shelf life, to render it more amenable to mass production, or to enhance its consumer appeal with respect to color, flavor, texture, and convenience. These chemicals are grouped according to their technological functions. Detailed listing of various groups of food additives and their uses is given in a Codex document (FAO/WHO, 1994). The major functional groups and some examples are listed in Appendix 19.1.

Indirect (unintentional) food additives

The substances described above are intentionally added to foods for specific technological purposes. Consequently they are considered "direct" or "intentional" food additives. However, a number of substances may become part of the foods as a result of their use during the production, processing, or storage of the foods. These include antibiotics and anabolic agents used during the raising of farm animals, residues from food processing machinery, and migrants from packaging materials.

Food contaminants

These substances are present in foods as a result of environmental pollution or faulty handling of the food. In other words, they serve no useful purpose either in the final food product or in its processing. Examples are mercury in fish harvested from contaminated waters, and mycotoxins found in improperly stored nuts and grains. Thus they differ from both the direct and indirect food additives.

International aspects

Food, raw and processed, is commonly traded internationally. The additives and contaminants (and residues of pesticides) must be considered acceptable for the protection of the health of consumers. But the food that was considered acceptable by the exporting country might not be considered acceptable by the importing country.

In an attempt to reduce such disputes, the World Health Organization (WHO) and the Food and Agriculture Organization of the United Nations (FAO), at the request of governments, established mechanisms to provide independent toxicological evaluation. The mechanisms created were the Joint FAO/WHO Expert Committee on Food Additives and Contaminants (JECFA) and the Joint FAO/WHO Meeting of Experts on Pesticide Residues (JMPR). Members of these committees were selected from a panel of internationally known experts acting independently.

Since their inception in the early 1960s, they have been convened annually. During these meetings, they have evaluated and re-evaluated many food additives, contaminants and pesticide residues. Acceptable daily intakes (ADIs) are allocated to those chemicals that the toxicological data so indicates. The ADIs are used by regulatory agencies in some countries.

More importantly, the ADIs are used by the Joint FAO/WHO Food Standard Program, the Codex Alimentarius Commission to establish international food standards. There are more than 150 nations that are members of the commission. Some details on the relationship among the national food regulatory agencies, national research facilities and the Codex Alimentarius Commission are given in Chapter 25. A comprehensive review of this subject is provided in a review (Lu, 1988).

Toxicological testing and evaluation

Categories of data required

Because these chemicals are added to foods to be consumed by large numbers of people, they are in general extensively tested and strictly evaluated. Furthermore, because of their low toxicity, precise LD_{50}s are as a rule not required. The studies required by JECFA are categorized as follows:

1   Biochemical studies, absorption, distribution, elimination (and storage), biotransformation, and effects on enzymes and other biochemical parameters.
2   Acute toxicity studies.
3   Short-term toxicity studies.
4   Long-term toxicity studies.
5   Reproductive toxicity studies.
6   Mutagenicity studies.
7   Carcinogenicity studies.
8   Teratogenicity (developmental) studies.
9   Observation in humans.

Brief description of these studies are given in Chapters 2, 3, 6, 7, 8, and 9.

Extent of testing

The Joint FAO/WHO Expert Committee on Food Additives considers, as a general rule, that the types of biological data listed above are required for proper evaluation of food additives. However, for certain groups of additives, depending on their chemical nature, source, and usage, much less data are required. These include:

1   components of food and closely related chemicals,
2   certain enzymes used in food processing,

3 certain food colors, and
4 certain metals (e.g., copper, iron, and zinc).

Detailed descriptions of the types of additives and the required data are given in several WHO reports (WHO, 1974, 1982a, 1986). These descriptions are summarized in a review article (Lu, 1988).

The U.S. Food and Drug Administration established a set of criteria to determine the "level of concern," which in turn dictates the extent of testing required (FDA, 1982a). The level of concern is determined by the chemical structure of the additive and concentration in food. Additives are placed in three categories according to their chemical structure: A, B, and C. Additives of low probable toxicity are assigned to category A. This category comprises nine types of chemicals, such as simple aliphatic, non-cyclic hydrocarbons with no unsaturation; sugars and polysaccharides; fats, fatty acids; and endogenous inorganic salts of alkali metals (Na, K) and alkaline earth metals (Mg, Ca). Additives with functional groups of high probable toxicity are assigned to category C. Additives of intermediate or unknown probable toxicity are assigned to category B.

Evaluation

As described in Chapter 25, toxicological evaluation of food additives follows the procedure of determining the adequacy of data, establishing an appropriate no-effect level, and selecting a proper safety factor to obtain the acceptable daily intake. This procedure is generally adopted by many national regulatory agencies including the U.S. Food and Drug Administration, as well as the international organizations WHO and FAO. The toxicological basis for drafting the provisions for food additives in the International Food Standards is provided by the Joint FAO/WHO Expert Committee on Food Additives. The interrelationship between the various national and international bodies is described in a review article (Lu, 1988).

GRAS

As noted above, the U.S. legislation considers certain chemicals as "generally recognized as safe." This was done originally in 1958, and that list included more than 600 direct additives with a variety of technological functions and some 2,000 indirect additives. Since then, the list of direct additives has been expanded mainly by the addition of more than 1,000 flavoring ingredients proposed by the Flavor and Extract Manufacturers' Association (FEMA).

On the basis of new toxicological information, the safety of a number of substances on the list has since been questioned. The most notable was the suspected carcinogenicity of the artificial sweetener cyclamate. As a result,

FDA in 1970 asked the Life Sciences Research Office of the Federation of American Societies for Experimental Biology to evaluate the safety of all the substances on the GRAS list. A Select Committee on GRAS Substances was formed and issued many reports containing its conclusion and summaries of the available information on 468 substances. A detailed account of the work of the committee is given by Carr (1987).

Additives of toxicological concern

Some 600 intentional food additives are being added to a variety of our foods. The toxicity of most of these additives has been evaluated according to prevailing procedure and found to be "safe." However, the use of some additives has been restricted, suspended, or requires label declaration because of toxicological concern.

Carcinogenicity

For example, the safety of *saccharin* has been questioned because of its reported carcinogenicity. In fact, the first study that revealed increased bladder tumors in rats involved the dosing of the animals with a combination of saccharin and cyclamate at the ratio of 1:9. Saccharin has been found to be excreted as such and non-mutagenic in most test systems. However, a large-scale experiment carried out in a Canadian government laboratory showed that rats fed saccharin at 7.5% in the diet developed bladder tumors (Arnold *et al.*, 1977). The significance of this finding is somewhat doubtful because of the excessively high dosage and because the tumors occurred mainly among the male rats of the second generation.

Cyclamates were considered innocuous and were used widely in foods and beverages for many years. However, doubt was cast on their safety because of the discovery that they are metabolizable by intestinal flora in animals and humans to cyclohexylamine, which appears to be more toxic (Classen *et al.*, 1968). Its use as a food additive was suspended in 1969 when it was discovered that a mixture of saccharin and cyclamate increased the incidence of bladder tumors in rats (Price *et al.*, 1970). Subsequent studies on cyclamate showed no carcinogenicity and the short-term mutagenicity tests yielded no consistent results. This is also true with cyclohexylamine. Summaries of the reports are included in two publications (IARC, 1980; WHO, 1982a). Its use has been restored in a number of countries, although it is still not permitted for use as an additive in the United States.

Nitrates and nitrites are useful preservatives and they impart a special color and flavor to treated meat such as ham and corned beef. However, they can form, with certain amines, a variety of nitrosamines, many of which are potent carcinogens. However, nitrates and nitrites are valuable in controlling toxin-forming microorganisms such as *Clostridium botulinum*. Furthermore, nitrites occur in the body, notably in the saliva, and it has been demonstrated that nitrosation of certain amines can occur in the stomach.

For these reasons, the use of these preservatives has not been suspended, but the amount used has reduced. On the other hand, the preservative *diethylpyrocarbonate* (DEPC) presents a distinctly different picture. It had been used in a variety of beverages, but its use was suspended. This decision was based on the finding that DEPC may combine with ammonium ion in beverages to form urethane, a wide-spectrum carcinogen in all animal species tested, and the fact that its use was not indispensable.

BHA (butylated hydroxyanisole) and *BHT* (butylated hydroxytoluene) are widely used antioxidants and have been investigated in several long-term studies without revealing any serious adverse effects. However, Ito *et al.* (1983) reported that BHA at very high dietary levels induced hyperplasia and tumors in the forestomach of rats. Since the tumors were only found in the forestomach, the relevance of this finding in terms of human health hazard was questioned. Additional studies using species without a forestomach were performed. The results were negative in the dog, and the increased mitotic rate in the esophagus of pigs was questionable (WHO, 1989). Olsen *et al.* (1983) reported an increase in the hepatocellular adenoma and carcinoma. However, several other studies yielded negative results. Furthermore, other studies on these antioxidants produced cancer-protective effects (Prochaska *et al.*, 1985). In light of these conflicting results, BHA and BHT are still being used.

Hypersensitivity reactions

A number of food additives are known to induce hypersensitivity reactions in susceptible individuals. Because they affect only a small proportion of the general population, and because their effects are usually mild and transitory, most regulatory agencies consider label declaration as sufficient to provide warning to these individuals. The following are the more commonly known ones.

Tartrazine, a widely used yellow color in a variety of processed foods, has been known to induce allergic reactions, especially among those who are allergic to aspirin (Juhlin, 1980).

Sulfur dioxide (SO_2) and related chemicals, such as bisulfites and metabisulfites, are used as preservatives in processed foods as well as salads. In the latter case, these chemicals help to preserve the freshness of the vegetables. Since it is difficult to provide warning labels, such use has been discouraged.

Monosodium glutamate (MSG) has been used as a flavor enhancer for many decades in China and Japan. No untoward effects have been reported. However, a "Chinese restaurant syndrome" has been reported (Schaumberg *et al.*, 1969). It usually appears after the individual had consumed a special Chinese soup, which contains relatively large amounts of MSG. The hypersensitivity reaction consists of a burning sensation, tingling in the face and neck, tightness in the chest, etc. Because of these findings, it is now possible, in many restaurants, to order soups and other dishes specifying "no MSG." For additional details, see Kenney (1986). The fact that adverse reactions to MSG have not been observed in the Far East is evidently related to the custom of consuming the soup as the last course, that is, on a full stomach, thereby delaying the absorption of this chemical and preventing a dramatic rise in blood level.

Other adverse effects

In addition to carcinogenicity and hypersensitivity reactions, the discovery of other adverse effects has prompted regulatory decisions or additional investigations. Examples are heart lesions in laboratory animals associated with brominated vegetable oils (BVO), a suspending agent in certain beverages, and liver lesions associated with Orange RN and Ponceau 2R, which were responsible for the suspension of their use. Other effects such as red blood cell damage (Orange RN), storage in tissues (BVO), and testicular atrophy (cyclohexylamine from cyclamate) were contributing factors to toxicological decisions on these additives (see Lu, 1979a).

Indirect additives and contaminants

Apart from direct food additives, there is a large number of indirect additives and some contaminants that pose toxicological problems and require different control measures. The problems are highlighted as follows.

Indirect food additives

The most important of these chemicals are (1) the constituents of packaging material, which may migrate into the food that is in contact with them, and (2) animal drug residues that are commonly used in raising food-producing animals.

Packaging materials

A number of substances may migrate from food containers, wrappers, etc. to the food that is packaged in them. Most of the chemicals that might migrate from the conventional types of packaging materials, such as paper and wood, had been considered safe and included in FDA's GRAS list. More recently, however, the packaging items are generally made of polymeric materials. The polymers per se are generally inert, but the components, the monomers, which are present to some extent, residual reactants, intermediates, manufacturing aids, solvents and plastic additives, as well as the products of side reaction and chemical degradation may migrate into the food that is in contact with them. Some of these chemicals have been shown to be toxic. For example, vinyl chloride has been shown to be a human carcinogen at high levels of exposure, and acrylonitrile is a probable human carcinogen. Both are carcinogenic in a number of animal species (Chapter 7). However, because of the exceedingly low levels of exposure from migration to food, their continued use has been provisionally approved.

Animal drug residues in human food

There are essentially three types of drugs used in food-producing animals that may leave residues in human food such as meat, milk, and eggs. The drugs present not only a problem related to the parent chemicals. It is also necessary to consider their metabolites, which are produced as a result of the metabolic processes, including bioactivation, in the animals, and which may possess different toxic properties (Hayes and Borzelleca, 1982).

Therapeutic drugs such as the anthelmintic agents febantel, fenbendazole, and oxfendazole, are generally used in individual animals for specific disease and only over short periods of times. Therefore they do not pose a widespread health concern. On the other hand, tranquilizing agents such as chlorpromazine and propylpromazine are used shortly before slaughter, and hence leave residues in the meat. Their use is therefore not allowed (WHO, 1995).

Antibiotics such as benzylpenicillin and oxytetracycline are usually incorporated in the animal feeds to prevent outbreaks of bacterial diseases and to promote growth. The residue levels are generally extremely low and not expected to induce toxic effects. The antibiotics can result in resistance in humans, which is a concern.

Anabolic agents are growth-promoting substances and are implanted subcutaneously in a part of the animal that is usually not eaten, such as the ear. Their residue levels in the meat are low enough to be essentially devoid of general toxic effects, except carcinogenicity. A carcinogen may be effective at extremely low dose levels. Diethylstilbestrol (DES) is no longer used as a growth promoter, because of the discovery that tumors of genital organs have developed in the offspring of mothers who had taken DES during the pregnancy in large doses for medical purposes.

The anabolic agents in use may be considered either "endogenous" or "exogenous." The former includes estradiol, progesterone, and testosterone. The latter includes porcine somatotropin and trenbolone acetate. The "endogenous" anabolic agents are considered indistinguishable from the endogenous hormones and the "erogenous" hormones leave very low levels of residues. Acceptable daily intakes have been allocated to their residues (WHO, 2000a).

Contaminants

There are three main types of food contaminants, mycotoxins, heavy metals, and synthetic chemicals. They contaminate food because of growing or harvesting from contaminated soil or water, improper handling, and accidental release from industrial sources.

Mycotoxins

Aflatoxins, produced by the mold *Aspergillus flavus*, occur in nuts and grains, especially when these commodities are stored in a humid and warm climate. These toxins exist as mixtures of aflatoxins B_1, B_2, G_1, and G_2. Among these aflatoxins, B_1 is the most potent carcinogen in most species of animals, especially the rat. In one experiment, rats fed a diet containing 1 ppb of aflatoxin B_1 had hyperplastic nodules and carcinoma of the liver (Wogan *et al.*, 1974). Aflatoxins G_1 and M_1 (a metabolite of B_1 and occurring in milk) are also carcinogenic but much less potent. Positive correlation was noted between aflatoxin intake and liver cancer incidence in certain regions in Africa and Thailand (IARC, 1976). Lu (2002) has provided a more extensive review on aflatoxins. As noted in Chapter 3, aflatoxin is bioactivated to aflatoxin-8,9-epoxide which may covalently bind to DNA, thus initiate carcinogenesis.

A number of other mycotoxins also occur in foods. Their characteristics are summarized in Table 19.1. Additional information on these and other mycotoxins may be found in two WHO publications (1990, 2000b).

Table 19.1 Source, occurrence, and toxicity of certain mycotoxins

Mycotoxin	Source	Occurrence	Toxic effects
Aflatoxins	Aspergillus	Nuts, grains	Cancers
Ergot	Claviceps purpura	Grains, especially rye	Ergotism (spasm, cramps, dry gangrene)
Fumonisin B_1	Fusarium	Maize	Esophageal cancer
Ochratoxins	Aspergillus Penicillium	Grains	Nephropathy
Trichothecenes	Fusarium trichoderma	Grains	Vomiting, diarrhea, skin inflammation, multiple hemorrhage
Zearalenone	Fusarium	Grains	Estrogenic effects

Source: WHO, 1990, 2000b.

Neurotoxins

Certain toxins are found in marine animals that are used as food. The notable ones are saxitoxin, which may be present in clams, and tetradotoxin, which is found in puffer fish, especially its ovaries. An important and extremely toxic substance is botulinum toxin. It is produced by the bacteria *Clostridium botulinum* in improperly canned food. The major toxic effects of these toxins are on the nervous system. Descriptions of these effects are provided in Chapter 17. Another toxin (ciguatoxin) is occasionally present in large coastal fishes in certain geographical areas, notably the Caribbean Sea. In addition to the nervous system, it often produces toxic effects on the G.I. system.

Metals

The toxic properties of a number of metals are described in Chapter 20, but human exposure via food is highlighted in this section. Among the metals that have caused the most concern are mercury, lead, and cadmium.

A number of acute and chronic poisoning episodes have resulted from improper application or consumption of alkyl *mercury* compounds used as fungicides to preserve seed grains. Others followed consumption of fish contaminated with methyl mercury. The compound can be formed via bioactivation (aided by microorganisms in the mud) of mercury discharged from factories (e.g., in Minamata and Niigata, Japan; Chapter 1, Appendix 1.2). Because of the biomagnification factor along the food chain, large carnivorous fishes generally contain much higher levels of methyl mercury (WHO, 1976).

Lead has been used as a fuel additive, in lead batteries, in paints, etc. Humans are exposed to this metal from air, water, and food. According to one analysis, daily intakes from these media amount to 15, 20, and 140 μg, respectively (NRC Canada, 1973). One unusual source of lead intake is improperly fired ceramic foodware, which may release large amounts of lead from the glaze and which has caused a number of

Table 19.2 Source, occurrence, and toxicity of certain neurotoxins

Toxins	Source	Occurrence	Toxic effects
Botulinum toxin	*Clostridium botulinum*	Improperly canned food	Impairing ACh release
Ciquatoxin	Blue-green algae	Large coastal fishes	Various effects on nervous and G.I. systems
Saxitoxin	*Gonyolax*	Clams	Blocking of nerve conduction
Tetrodotoxin	Uncertain	Puffer fish	Blocking of nerve conduction

poisonings. This fact has prompted the promulgation of limits in the extent of release of lead from various types of foodware (WHO, 1979). The estimated intake of lead from ceramic ware would be in the range of 30–80 μg per day if all the wares in use released this metal to the legal limit (Lu, 1979b). Among certain populations, ceramic foodware still constitutes an important source of lead (Rojas-Lopez *et al.*, 1994).

Cadmium is used as a pigment and occurs in the environment, especially through the refining of zinc ores, which contain varying concentrations of cadmium. It enters the food chain through pollution of soil and water. Itai-itai disease in Japan has been attributed to chronic exposure to cadmium, through long-term ingestion of contaminated rice. It may also be leached from decorated ceramic foodware.

Certain organic compounds

Among these chemicals are *organochlorine insecticides*, which had been widely used. Their use has been discontinued because of their persistence in the environment. However, they are still present in foods in trace amounts. Others include *polychlorinated biphenyls* (PCB), which are used in electrical capacitors and transformers, as plasticizers and heat exchangers, and in paper manufacturing. Through leakage and discharge of waste, they enter the environment. Because of their persistence and biomagnification properties, they enter the food chain. These chemicals attracted much attention because of the episode of consumption of a batch of rice oil contaminated with PCB through a leak in a heat exchanger in 1968. Thousands of consumers in Japan were affected (Chapter 1, Appendix 1.2). The main sign of toxicity was chloracne, although there were many other symptoms and signs (see p. 340). Similarly, an inadvertent addition of *polybrominated biphenyls* (PBB) to cattle feed in Michigan resulted in the contamination of a large amount of beef and milk.

The "action levels" for these and other contaminants have been established by the U.S. FDA to control their levels in food and feed. Some of them are listed in Table 19.3.

Table 19.3 Action levels for certain food contaminants

Contaminants	Commodity	Action level
Aflatoxin	Nuts	20 ppb
	Foods and feeds	20 ppb
	Milk*	0.5 ppb
Aldrin and dieldrin	Various foods	0.02–0.3 ppm
Cadmium, in leaching solution	Flat ware	0.5 µg/ml
from ceramic ware	Small hollowware	0.5 µg/ml
	Large hollowware	0.25 µg/ml
Lead, in leaching solution from	Flat ware	3.0 µg/ml
ceramic ware	Small hollowware	2.0 µg/ml
	Large hollowware	1.0 µg/ml
Mercury	Fish, shellfish, crustaceans	1.0 ppm
	Wheat	1.0 ppm
Polychlorinated biphenyls	Red meat (fat basis)	3 ppm

Source: FDA, 2000.

Note
*Aflatoxin M1.

References

Arnold, D. L., Moodie, C. A., Stavric, D., Soltz, D. R., Grice, H. C., and Munro, I. C. (1977) Canadian saccharin study. *Science* 197:320.

Carr, C. J. (1987) Food additives: A benefit/risk dilemma, in *Handbook of Toxicology*, T. J. Haley and W. O. Berndt (eds), Washington, DC: Hemisphere.

Classen, H. G., Marquardt, P., and Spath, M. (1968) Sympathomimetic effects of cyclohexylamine. *Arzneimittel-Forsch.* 18:590–594.

Eaton, D. L. and Gallagher, E. P. (1994) Mechanisms of alfatoxin carcinogenesis. *Ann. Rev. Pharmacol. Toxicol.* 34:135–172.

FAO/WHO (1994) Food Additives. *Codex Alimentarius*, vol. XIV. Rome: Food Agriculture Organization of the United Nations.

FDA (1982) *Toxicological Principles for the Safety Assessment of Direct Additives and Color Additives Used in Food*. U.S. Food and Drug Administration. Springfield, VA: National Technical Information Service, PB 83–170696.

FDA (2000) Action levels for poisonous or deleterious substances in human food and animal feed. Washington, DC: Food and Drug Administration.

Hayes, J. R. and Borzelleca, J. F. (1982) Biodisposition of xenobiotics in animals, in *Animal Products in Human Nutrition*, D. C. Beitz and R. Hanson (eds), New York, NY: Academic Press, pp. 225–259.

IARC (1976) *Evaluation of Carcinogenic Risk of Chemicals to Man, Vol. 10: Some Naturally Occurring Substances*. Lyon, France: International Agency for Research on Cancer.

IARC (1980) *Evaluation of the Carcinogenic Risk of Chemicals to Humans. Vol. 22: Some Non-Nutritive Sweetening Agents*. Lyon, France: International Agency for Research on Cancer.

Ito, N., Fukushima, S., Hagiwara, A., Shibata, M., and Ogiso, T. (1983) Carcinogenicity of butylated hydroxyanisole in F344 rats. *J. Natl. Cancer Inst.* 70:343–352.

Juhlin, L. (1980) Incidence of intolerance to food additives. *Int. J. Dermatol.* 19:548–551.

Kenney, R. A. (1986) The Chinese restaurant syndrome: an anecdote revisited. *Food Chem. Toxicol.* 24:351–354.

Lu, F. C. (1979a) The safety of food additives: the dynamics of the issue, in *Toxicology and Occupational Medicine*, W. B. Deichmann (ed.), New York, NY: Elsevier/North Holland.

Lu, F. C. (1979b) *Review of Total Intake of Lead from All Sources.* WHO: HCS/CER/79.5. Geneva: World Health Organization.

Lu, F. C. (1988) Acceptable daily intake: inception, evolution and application. *Regul. Toxicol.-Pharmacol.* 8:45–60.

Lu, F. C. (2002) Assessment of safety/risk vs. public health concerns. *Environ. Health Preventive Med.* 7(3): (in press).

NRC Canada (1973) *Lead in the Canadian Environment.* NRCC No. 13682. Ottawa: National Research Council of Canada.

Olsen, P., Bille, N., and Meyer, O. (1983) Hepatocellular neoplasms in rats induced by butylated hydroxytoluene (BHT). *Acta Pharmacol. Toxicol.* 54:433–434.

Price, J. M., Biava, C. G., Oser, B. L., Vogen, E. E., Steinfeld, J., and Ley, H. L. (1970) Bladder tumors in rats fed cyclohexylamine or high doses of a mixture of cyclamate and saccharin. *Science* 167:1131–1132.

Prochaska, H. J., DeLong, M. J., and Talalay, P. (1985) On the mechanisms of induction of cancer-protective enzymes: a unifying proposal. *Proc. Natl. Acad. Sci. USA* 82:8232–8236.

Rojas-Lopez, M., Santos-Burgoa, C., Rios, C., Hernandez-Avila, M., and Romieu, I. (1994) Use of lead-glazed ceramics is the main factor associated to high lead in blood levels in two Mexican rural communities. *J. Toxicol. Envir. Health* 42:45–52.

Schaumberg, H. H., Byck, R., Gerstl, R., and Marshman, J. H. (1969) Monosodium glutamate: its pharmacology and role in the Chinese restaurant syndrome. *Science* 163:826.

U.S. Federal Food, Drug, and Cosmetic Act, As Amended (1979) Washington, DC: U.S. Government Printing Office.

WHO (1974) *Toxicological Evaluation of Certain Food Additives with a Review of General Principles and of Specifications* (17th Report). Tech. Rep. Ser. 539. Geneva: World Health Organization.

WHO (1976) *Mercury.* Environmental Health Criteria 1. Geneva: World Health Organization.

WHO (1979) *Ceramic Foodware Safety. Report of a Meeting of Experts.* HCS/79.7. Geneva: World Health Organization.

WHO (1982a) *Evaluation of Certain Food Additives and Contaminants* (26th Report). Tech. Rep. Ser. 683. Geneva: World Health Organization.

WHO (1982b) *Evaluation of Certain Food Additives.* WHO Food Additives Series 17. Geneva: World Health Organization.

WHO (1986) *Evaluation of Certain Food Additives and Contaminants* (29th Report). Tech. Rep. Ser. 733. Geneva: World Health Organization.

WHO (1989) *Evaluation of Certain Food Additives and Contaminants.* WHO Food Additives Series 24. Geneva: World Health Organization.

WHO (1990) *Selected Mycotoxins: Ochratoxins, Trichothecene, Ergot.* Envir. Health Criteria No. 105. Geneva: World Health Organization.

WHO (1995) *Evaluation of Certain Veterinary Drug Residues in Food* (38th Report). Tech. Rep. Ser. 815. Geneva: World Health Organization.

WHO (2000a) *Toxicological Evaluation of Certain Veterinary Drug Residues in Food.* Food Additives Series No. 43. Geneva: World Health Organization.

WHO (2000b) *Fumonisin B$_1$.* Envir. Health Criteria No. 219. Geneva: World Health Organization.

Wogan, G. N., Paglialunga, S., and Newberne, P. M. (1974) Carcinogenic effects of low dietary levels of aflatoxin B in rats. *Food Cosmet. Toxicol.* 12:681–685.

Appendix 19.1 Major functional groups of direct food additives

1 Preservatives are added to prolong the shelf life of foods by preventing or inhibiting microbial growth. Examples are benzoic acid, propionic acid, and sorbic acid, their salts, nitrates and nitrites, and sulfur dioxide and related compounds.

2 Antioxidants are added to oils to prevent them from becoming rancid, which is a result of oxidative changes. Some are added to fruits and vegetables to prevent enzymatic browning. The commonly used ones include butylated hydroxyanisole (BHA), butylated hydroxytoluene (BHT), various gallates, ascorbic acid and its salts, and α-tocopherol.

3 Emulsifying, stabilizing, and thickening agents are added to improve the homogeneity, stability, and "body" of a variety of food products. These include mono- and diglycerides, sucrose esters of fatty acids, lecithin, salts of various types of phosphate, modified starches, calcium gluconate, calcium citrate, agar, alginic acid and its salts, various vegetable gums, and cellulose derivatives.

4 Colors are used to enhance visual appeal of food products. Some of these substances are derived from natural colors, such as carotene, chlorophyll, and cochineal. Others are synthetic, such as allura red, amaranth, azorubine, indigotine, and tartrazine.

5 Flavors and flavor enhancers. The flavors constitute the largest group of food additives. However, they are used, in general, at very low levels in foods. Some are synthetic (mainly esters, aldehydes, and ketones); others are derived from natural sources (such as oleoresins, plant extracts, and essential oils). Flavor enhancers, such as monosodium glutamate, enhance the flavor of the food to which it is added.

6 Artificial sweeteners have a strong sweet taste but little or no caloric value. They are therefore useful for diabetics and those who wish to enjoy the sweet taste without increasing the caloric intake. The notable ones are the cyclamates, saccharin, and aspartame.

7   Nutrients include vitamins, minerals, and essential amino acids. As noted above, national regulations in most countries, contrary to those of the United States, do not consider these as food additives. However, a food additive used for a technological reason may incidentally have certain nutritional values. For example, riboflavin may be used as a color but is also a vitamin.

8   Miscellaneous groups. These include (a) acidity regulators (acids and bases) which are used to adjust the pH of beverages and canned fruits and vegetables; (b) anticaking agents which are added to salt, sugar, etc. to maintain their free-flowing property; (c) antifoaming agents, which are added to liquids to prevent foaming; (d) flour treatment agents, which are added to flour to improve its baking qualities; (e) glazing agents; (f) propellants; and (g) raising agents.

Chapter 20

Toxicity of pesticides

CONTENTS

Introduction

Value of pesticides

Pesticides are substances that kill or control *pests*. There are various types of pests. The most common are insects. Some of them serve as vectors for diseases. The most important vector-borne diseases, malaria and onchocerciasis ("river blindness"), are transmitted to humans by mosquitoes and black flies. Both diseases are debilitating and affect millions of people in the tropical and subtropical regions. Other vector-borne diseases include filariasis, yellow fever, rickettsial pox, viral encephalitis, typhus, and bubonic plague. Insecticides have helped to control these diseases.

Insects are also detrimental to various *plants* and their products. Insecticides are therefore widely used to protect the farmer's products. Although most of the insecticides currently in use are synthetic chemicals, a number of natural substances have been used by farmers for a long time. These substances include nicotine from tobacco, pyrethrum from flowers of a species of chrysanthemum, and various compounds of lead, copper, and arsenic.

Aside from insects, *weeds* constitute a very important nuisance to the farmer. Before the introduction of herbicides, farmers used to spend much time to remove the weeds manually, a very time-consuming and back-breaking task. Other pesticides have also been developed to control other pests such as *fungi*, *rodents*, and others. The great variety of agricultural uses and chemical categories may be seen from a recent compilation of the 230 pesticides that have been evaluated and re-evaluated by the WHO Expert Committee on Pesticide Residues since 1965 (Lu, 1995).

A number of *household pesticide* products are also available to control household nuisance pests, such as flies and mosquitoes.

Adverse effects of pesticides

These may involve human health and/or the environment. The most dramatic of such effects on humans are the accidental acute poisonings. Several major outbreaks of poisoning with methyl and ethyl mercury compounds and hexachlorobenzene as fungicides and with parathion, an organophosphorus insecticide, have occurred in several parts of the world involving thousands of individuals and hundreds of deaths. A few examples are listed in Chapter 1, Appendix 1.2. Individual cases of acute poisoning have usually resulted from ingestion of large quantities of pesticides accidentally or with suicidal intent.

Occupational exposure to pesticides may involve workers engaged in the manufacturing, formulating, and application of pesticides. The pesticides enter the body generally through the respiratory tract and by dermal absorption, but small amounts may enter the gastrointestinal tract through the use of contaminated hands and utensils. This type of poisoning is more likely to happen with pesticides that are more toxic acutely. The major public health concern, however, is the ingestion of pesticide residues in foods, as this may involve large populations over long periods of time.

In addition to these human health hazards, pesticides may have a serious impact on the *environment*. Apart from large-scale accidental release to the environment, only minimal levels are found in various environmental media. However, the levels are likely to be higher with pesticides that are persistent and/or have a propensity for biomagnification. In the latter case, the concentration of a pesticide increases as it moves through the trophic chain. The organism with a high concentration may be adversely affected. For example, the bald eagle was nearly extinct, resulting from its fragile egg shells as a toxic effect of high levels of DDT bioaccumulated through the contaminated food chain of the bird. Such environmental pollution may also affect human health by virtue of the contaminated soil and water, which then result in the production of contaminated human food and drinking water.

Categories of pesticides

Pesticides are usually grouped according to their uses and their chemical nature. The major groups are the following.

Insecticides

As noted above, this is the largest group of pesticides and consists of a number of different chemical subgroups.

Organophosphorus insecticides

These are esters of phosphoric acid or thiophosphoric acid, represented by dichlorvos and parathion, respectively. They act by inhibiting acetyl-cholinesterase (AChE), resulting in an accumulation of acetylcholine (ACh). The excess ACh induces a variety of symptoms and signs (see also p. 291). The severity of the symptoms and signs is more or less correlated with the extent of the inhibition of cholinesterase in blood, but the precise relationship varies depending on the compound (Wills, 1972).

In addition to parathion and dichlorvos, other pesticides in this group include parathion-methyl, azinphos-methyl (Guthion), chlorfenvinphos, diazinon, dimethoate, disulfoton (Di-Syston), malathion, mevinphos, and trichlorfon (Dipterex). Their toxicities vary over a wide range (see Appendix 20.1).

Carbamate insecticides

These are esters of N-methylcarbamic acid. They also act by inhibiting AChE. However, their effects on the enzyme are much more readily reversible than those of the organophosphorus insecticides. Insecticides of this class include carbaryl (Sevin), aldicarb (Temik), carbofuran, methomyl, and propoxur (Baygon). In addition, with carbamates, signs of toxicity appear more promptly and, for many of them, there is a greater range from the doses that cause minor toxic effects and those that are lethal. For this reason, on an acute basis, the carbamates are safer than the organophosphorus insecticides. Appendix 19.1 also lists their toxicities.

Organochlorine insecticides

These include the chlorinated ethane derivatives, the cyclodienes, and the hexachlorocyclohexanes. Some of these chemicals (e.g., DDT) were introduced in the 1940s and were widely used in agricultural and health programs. This was because of their relatively low acute toxicity and their persistence, which reduced the need for repeated applications. However, the persistence has later been recognized as a liability rather than an asset.

Both DDT and methoxychlor are chlorinated ethane derivatives, but methoxychlor is much less toxic and less persistent than DDT. The cyclodiene insecticide endrin is extremely toxic, aldrin and dieldrin somewhat less toxic, and chlordane, heptachlor, and mirex even less toxic. Lindane is the gamma isomer of hexachlorocyclohexane (HCH) that is in use. It is highly toxic but less cumulative. Consequently, lindane is used much more widely than HCH.

Botanical and other insecticides

These include nicotine from tobacco. It is extremely toxic acutely and acts on the nervous system. Pyrethrum is obtained from the flowers of *Chrysanthemum cinerariaefolium*. An enzyme inhibitor, piperonyl butoxide, is often used in combination with this insecticide as a synergist. Pyrethrum has a low toxicity in mammals but is allergenic to sensitive individuals, causing contact dermatitis. It is also a neurotoxicant. The major active principles in pyrethrum are pyrethrin I and pyrethrin II. The former acts on the central nervous system and the latter on the peripheral nervous system. Both are synthesized and more stable than pyrethrum. Rotenone is extracted from roots of the plant *Derris elliptica*. It also has a low toxicity in mammals but is more toxic to insects and fish. Many microorganisms are known to be pathogenic to insects. The ones being used are *Bacillus thuringiensis* and certain insect baculoviruses. They are not known to be pathogenic to humans.

Herbicides

There are several types of herbicides. Some retard the growth of weeds by inhibiting photosynthesis, respiration, cell division or synthesis of protein or lipids. Others act as growth stimulants thereby disturbing the normal growth (Ecobichon, 1998).

Chlorophenoxy compounds are exemplified by 2,4-D (2,4-dichloro-phenoxyacetic acid) and 2,4,5-T (2,4,5-trichlorophenoxyacetic acid). They act in plants as growth hormones. Their toxicities in animals are relatively low. However, chloracne, the main toxic effect of 2,4,5-T in humans, seems attributable to the contaminant 2,3,7,8-tetrachlorobenzo-*p*-dioxin (TCDD). For additional information on this contaminant, see p. 53.

Bipyridyl herbicides, such as paraquat and diquat, have been widely used. They exert their toxicity via the formation of free radicals. The toxicity of paraquat is characterized by its pulmonary effects not only after exposure via inhalation but also by the oral route, as noted in Chapter 12.

Other herbicides include dinitro-*o*-cresol (DNOC), amitrole, the carbamates propham and chloropropham, and a number of other chemicals.

Fungicides

Mercury compounds such as methyl and ethyl mercury are very effective fungicides and had been widely used to preserve seed grains. However, several tragic accidents, involving numerous deaths and permanent neurologic damage, occurred with their use (Chapter 1, Appendix 1.2). This fact has deterred their further use.

Dicarboximides include the dimethylthiocarbamates (ferbam, thiram, and ziram) and the ethylenebisdithiocarbamates (maneb, nabam, and zineb). These compounds have relatively low acute toxicity and have hence been widely used in agriculture. However, there is concern about their carcinogenic potential (see p. 293).

Phthalimide derivatives such as captan and folpet have very low acute and chronic toxicity. However, captan has been shown to reduce body weight of pups of treated rats and folpet induced keratosis of the G.I. tract (FAO, 1990).

Substituted aromatics such as pentachlorophenol (PCP) have been widely used as wood preservatives. PCP increases metabolic rate through uncoupling of oxidative phosphorylation. It has a low LD_{50} but its technical grade is more toxic, indicating greater toxicity of its contaminants. Pentachloronitrobenzene (PCNB) has been used as a fungicide in treating soil. It is somewhat less toxic acutely than PCP, but may be carcinogenic.

Other fungicides include certain N-heterocyclic compounds such as benomyl and thiobendazole. These chemicals have very low toxicity and have been widely used in agriculture. Hexachlorobenzene has been used as a seed treatment agent but has caused mass poisoning (Chapter 1, Appendix 1.2).

Rodenticides

Warfarin is an anticoagulant by acting as an antimetabolite to vitamin K, thereby inhibiting the formation of prothrombin. It has been widely used because its toxicity is observed only after repeated ingestion, a circumstance unlikely to occur among children and pets.

Thioureas such as ANTU (α-naphthylthiourea) are extremely toxic to rats but only moderately toxic to humans. Their main toxicity is pulmonary edema and pleural effusion.

Sodium fluoroacetate ("1080") and fluoroacetamide ("1081") are extremely toxic and their use has hence been restricted to licensed personnel. They exert toxic effect through blockage of the citric acid cycle as described in Chapter 4 under "Lethal Synthesis."

Other rodenticides include botanical products such as the alkaloid strychnine, a potent CNS stimulant, and red squill, which contains the glycosides scillaren-A and -B. These glycosides, similar to digitalis, have cardiotonic and central emetic effects. Because of the latter effect, these substances are relatively nontoxic to most mammals but are potent poisons to rats, which do not vomit. Inorganic rodenticides include zinc phosphide, thallium sulfate, arsenic trioxide, and elemental phosphorus, acting through different mechanisms.

Fumigants

As the name implies, this group of pesticides includes a number of gases, liquids that readily vaporize, and solids that release gases by chemical reactions. In the gaseous form, they permeate storage areas and soil to control insects, rodents, and soil nematodes. Many fumigants, such as acrylonitrile, chloropicrin, and ethylene dibromide, are reactive chemicals and are also used widely in the chemical industry; some of them will be described in Chapter 24.

Toxicological properties

Toxicity on the nervous system

The organochlorine (OC) insecticides stimulate the nervous system and induce paresthesia, susceptibility to stimulation, irritability, disturbed equilibrium, tremor, and convulsions. The precise mode of action is not known. However, some of these chemicals, such as aldrin, dieldrin and lindane, induce facilitation and hyperexcitation at synaptic and neuromuscular junctions, resulting in repetitive discharge in central, sensory, and motor neurons. Whereas DDT may exert its toxic effect in the nervous system by adversely affecting the axon membrane (Doherty, 1979; Narahashi, 1980).

The organophosphate (OP) and carbamate insecticides inhibit acetylcholinesterase. Normally, the neurotransmitter acetylcholine (ACh) is released at the synapses. Once the nerve impulse is transmitted, the released ACh is hydrolyzed to acetic acid and choline by the acetylcholinesterase (AChE) at the site. Upon exposure to OP and carbamate insecticides, AChE is inhibited, resulting in an accumulation of ACh. The accumulated ACh in the CNS will induce tremor, incoordination, convulsion, etc. In the autonomic nervous system it will cause diarrhea, involuntary urination, bronchoconstriction, miosis, etc. Its accumulation at the neuromuscular junction will lead to contraction of the muscles, followed by weakness, loss of reflexes, and paralysis. The inhibition of AChE induced by the carbamate is readily reversible, whereas that following exposure to OP compounds is generally less readily so. In fact, certain OP compounds, such as DFP (diisopropyl fluorophosphate), cause irreversible inhibition; recovery only follows synthesis of new AChE.

Several OP compounds, including DFP, TOCP, leptophos, mipafox, and trichlorofon, cause a "delayed neurotoxicity." For the mechanism of action and testing procedures, see Chapter 16.

As noted above, pyrethrin I and II act on different parts of the nervous system.

Interactions

The most notable type of interaction is the *potentiation* observed between certain organophosphorus insecticides. Frawley and co-workers (1957) reported marked potentiation of the toxicity of the EPN [o-ethyl-o-(4-nitrophenyl) phenyl phosphonothioate] and malathion. Combinations of a number of OP insecticides have since been tested. Some showed additive effects, others were less than additive, and still others were synergistic. The most pronounced potentiation (about 100-fold increase) was observed between malathion and TOCP (tri-o-cresyl phosphate). The mechanism of the potentiation has been attributed to the inhibition of enzymes, such as carboxylesterase and amidases, which are responsible for the detoxication of certain OP compounds such as malathion and its more toxic metabolite malaoxon (Murphy, 1969).

Carcinogenicity

The organophosphate insecticides are in general not carcinogenic, with the exception of compounds that contain halogens such as tetrachlorvinphos. These chemicals evidently possess this property of the organochlorine insecticides (see below). The carbamate insecticides per se are not carcinogenic either. But carbaryl has been shown to form, in the presence of nitrous acid, nitrosocarbaryl, which is carcinogenic. A number of other pesticides are also nitrosatable under extreme conditions, and their products are carcinogenic and mutagenic (IARC, 1983). However, because of the unrealistic conditions required for such nitrosation to take place, the health concern arising from this type of reaction is questionable.

On the other hand, the organochlorine insecticides tested have all been shown to induce hepatoma in mice (IARC, 1983). The pesticide that has aroused most controversy has been DDT. It showed no carcinogenicity in rats, nor in hamsters and several other species of animals. Furthermore, epidemiological findings are essentially negative, and so are the short-term mutagenesis tests. For these reasons the WHO Expert Committee on Pesticide Residues reaffirmed in 1984 the ADI for DDT and several other organochlorine insecticides. A comprehensive review of the toxicological data and their interpretations on DDT was provided by Coulston (1985). Nevertheless, its use has been restricted or suspended in several nations based partly on this potential health hazard and partly on its ecological impact. The only pesticide on which there is some epidemiological evidence of carcinogenicity is hexachlorocyclohexane (Wang et al., 1988).

The fumigants EDB (ethylene dibromide) and DBCP (1,2-dibromo-3-chloropropane) have been found to produce highly malignant squamous-cell carcinoma in the stomach of rats and mice (IARC, 1977). However, their use has not been restricted or suspended, because the fumigated foods, upon aeration, contain negligible residue.

Amitrole (aminotriazole), a herbicide, produces thyroid tumors apparently through an indirect mechanism (Steinhoff et al., 1983). Thyroid peroxidase normally oxidizes iodine to an oxidized form, which then conjugates with tyrosine to form thyroxine. Amitrole inhibits this enzyme, thus lowering the thyroxine level. This lowered level, through a biofeedback mechanism, stimulates pituitary gland to release more thyroid-stimulating hormone (TSH). TSH in turn stimulates thyroid gland to become hyperplastic and eventually to form tumors. Amitrole is thus a "secondary carcinogen." Similarly, the ethylenebisdithiocarbamates fumigants (mancozeb, maneb, nabam, and zineb) have also been reported to produce thyroid tumors. This action is evidently mediated through the major breakdown and metabolic product ethylenethiourea.

Teratogenicity and effects on reproductive functions

In the late 1960s, several articles appeared reporting a variety of teratogenic and reproductive effects of carbaryl in dogs. Summaries of these reports have been included in a monograph (WHO, 1970). A comprehensive study in rats, given carbaryl in the diet at doses of 100 mg/kg and 200 mg/kg showed no effect on various reproductive functions and no teratogenic effects. Some effects were observed in rats given carbaryl by gavage (Weil et al., 1972). The authors attributed the effects in rats to the gavage method of administering the pesticide and the effects in the dog to its routes of biotransformation of cabaryl being different from those in humans and several other species.

Other pesticides reported as having teratogenic effects include the dithiocarbamate fungicides. Such effects are likely due, at least partly, to their breakdown product ETU (WHO, 1974). In addition, abamectin, dinocap, glyphosate, and procymidone induced cleft palate, defects in the neural tube, renal defects, and hypospadia respectively (see Lu, 1995).

Other adverse effects

Certain *renal* effects of carbaryl were reported in a group of human volunteers ingesting carbaryl at a daily dose of 0.12 mg/kg for six weeks. There was an increase in the ratio of urinary amino acid nitrogen to creatinine, compared to those taking placebo. This was interpreted as an indication of a decrease in the ability of the proximal convoluted tubules to reabsorb amino acids. This effect was not observed in individuals taking carbaryl at 0.06 mg/kg daily (Wills et al., 1968).

Paraquat produces *pulmonary* edema, hemorrhage, and fibrosis (Smith and Heath, 1976) following either inhalation or ingestion, but the closely related herbicide diquat does not (see also Chapter 12). However, both chemicals are toxic to cultured lung cells. Since paraquat is retained in the lung whereas diquat is not, it is evident that the difference between those two herbicides in their pulmonary toxicity is related to the special affinity of paraquat for certain pulmonary cells (type II cells).

Hypersensitivity reactions to pyrethrum have been reported. The most common form is contact dermatitis. Asthma has also been reported. Anaphylactic reactions are very rare (Hayes, 1982).

Organochlorine insecticides, such as DDT, chlordecone, and mirex, are hepatotoxic, inducing *liver* enlargement and centrolobular necrosis. They are also inducers of microsomal monooxygenases, thereby affecting the toxicity of other chemicals.

A number of organophosphorus, carbamate, and organochlorine insecticides, the dithiocarbamate fungicides, and herbicides alter various *immune functions*. For example, malathion, methylparathion, carbaryl, DDT, paraquat, and diquat have been shown to depress antibody formation, impair leukocyte phagocytosis, and reduce the germinal centers in spleen, thymus, and lymph nodes (Koller, 1979; Street, 1981).

Bioaccumulation and biomagnification

These properties per se do not necessarily represent adverse biological effects. They are generally associated with substances that are lipophilic and resistant to breakdown. The organochlorine pesticides in general are more persistent in the environment and tend to be stored in the fat depot. However, the bioaccumulation is more marked with some chemicals than others. For example, DDT is stored in the body fat for a much longer time than methoxychlor. The half-lives of these insecticides in rats are 6–12 months and 12 weeks, respectively.

Their persistence in the environment may create ecological problems. DDT and related chemicals in the environment enhance the metabolism of estrogens in birds. In the egg-laying and nestling cycle of certain birds, this disturbance of hormones adversely affects reproduction and survival of the young (Peakall, 1970).

Biomagnification is the result of bioaccumulation in the organism alone or in conjunction with persistence in the environment. For example, DDT is lipophilic, and thus occurs in the fat portion of body fluids including milk. While a mother's daily intake of DDT may be 0.5 μg/kg, her breast-fed baby's might be 11.2 μg/kg. This magnification results from the fact that DDT is stored in the human body at 10- to 20-fold chronic daily intake level and the baby consumes essentially only the milk. Furthermore, the caloric intake per kilogram body weight is higher in babies compared to adults. The significance of the much greater intake of DDT by babies is not clear because of the relatively short duration of this greater level of intake and the remarkable insensitivity of the young versus the adult (Lu *et al.*, 1965).

The biomagnification is even more marked in carnivorous animals. DDT and methyl mercury can accumulate through a series of plankton, small fish, large fish, and birds, and result in a magnification of the concentration amounting to several hundredfold (Woodwell, 1967). The decision to suspend the use of DDT was partly based on its adverse ecological impact, as noted above.

Testing, evaluation, and control

Categories of data required

Various categories of data are required in the evaluation of pesticides. The basic data required are essentially the same as those listed for food additives (see Chapter 18). However, a number of specific toxicological problems have been encountered with pesticides as outlined in the preceding section. The additional studies for certain pesticides include the following.

LD_{50} and short-term toxicity

Because of the greater acute toxicity of most pesticides, the LD_{50} is usually determined more precisely. Furthermore, in view of the fact that certain occupational workers, such as manufacturers, formulators, and applicators, may be exposed through the skin and respiratory tract, the dermal LD_{50} and the LC_{50} by inhalation are generally required. As occupational workers are likely to be exposed for some length of time, the toxicity of repeated exposure through dermal and inhalation is generally ascertained (see Chapters 12 and 15).

Delayed neurotoxicity (peripheral axonopathy)

This type of toxicity has been observed with a number of organophosphorus insecticides. The appropriate test is performed on new chemicals of this group to exclude this potential hazard (see Chapter 17).

Interaction

Marked interaction exists between certain pairs of organophosphorus insecticides. The potential health hazard is assessed using LD_{50}s of the individual chemicals alone and in combination.

Toxicological evaluation

The assessment of an acceptable daily intake (ADI) involves assessing the database for completeness and relevance, determining a no-observed adverse-effect level in terms of mg/kg body weight (NOAEL), and selecting an appropriate safety factor to extrapolate to an acceptable daily intake for humans, also in terms of mg/kg body weight. A list of the ADIs of the 230 pesticides that have been evaluated and re-evaluated by the WHO Expert Committee on Pesticide Residues since 1965, along with the NOAELs, safety factors, and critical effects is included in a review article (Lu, 1995).

While all pesticides are toxic, they vary in the nature and magnitude of toxicity. Certain pesticides have an inherent potential for specific toxic effects. The presence of such properties must be assessed by conducting appropriate tests as discussed above (p.295), before determining a NOAEL. The size of the safety factor will depend on a number of factors, as discussed in Chapter 24.

Standards

Tolerances

To protect the health of the consumer, standards are formulated. The standards, in the form of "tolerances" (also known as "maximum residue limits"), are established. The standards provide maximum permitted levels in each food commodity in which the pesticide may leave residues following its use. A pesticide may be used during any one or more stages of the preplanting, growth, harvesting, handling, and storage of the food crop.

Dietary intakes

Several procedures are used to ensure that the total intake of each pesticide from its residues in all food commodities does not exceed its ADI. One procedure involves chemical analysis of the residue levels in food represented in the "total diet" and the calculation of the "dietary intake" of each pesticide by adding the products of the residue levels and the per capita consumption of each of these foods. The latest survey by the U.S. FDA shows the dietary intakes of all the pesticides analyzed were considerably lower than the corresponding ADIs (FDA, 1987).

The other procedure, which is much simpler, involves calculating the "potential daily intake" and comparing it with the corresponding ADI. The former figure is obtained by adding the products of the tolerance levels in each of the foods and the per capita consumption of these foods. Evidently the potential daily intake represents an overestimation. First, a pesticide is not necessarily used in all the food commodities in which there are tolerances. Furthermore, in a vast majority of the cases, the actual residue levels are much lower than the tolerances. Nevertheless, this procedure offers distinct advantages. Apart from a few industrialized countries, figures for dietary intakes of pesticides are not available; for them the potential daily intakes provide a ready yardstick for assessing the health hazards to the consumer posed by the dietary intake of pesticides. The overestimation may also compensate for differences in dietary habits in different parts of the world and for variations in the levels of pesticide residues in certain foods. According to actual analysis, the residue levels may, although infrequently, exceed the tolerances (see also Chapter 25).

Apart from assessing the potential hazard of pesticides, the dietary intake figures, obtained by analysis or calculation, are also used in assessing, and possibly in recommending modification of the agricultural use of these chemicals. Where the residue levels appear too high, they may be lowered, for example, by a reduction of the rate of application or by an increase of the interval between the last application and harvesting of the food crop.

Gulf War Syndrome

Between August 1990 to April 1991 there were over 750,000 military personnel from the U.S., Canada, and the United Kingdom that participated in the air, sea, and ground war in the Persian Gulf region. During this war, service personnel were concurrently exposed to certain biological, chemical, and psychological environments. In particular amongst some veterans there was an increased frequency of chronic symptoms including headache, loss of memory, fatigue, muscle and joint pain, ataxia, skin rash, respiratory difficulties, and gastrointestinal disturbances. Potential exposure was to fumes and smoke from the following: military operations, oil well fires, diesel exhaust, toxic paints, pesticides, fire sand, depleted uranium, chemoprophylactic agents, and multiple immunizations. The variety of symptoms reported by veterans make it unlikely that a single etiologic cause was responsible for producing the Gulf War illnesses.

It was suggested by the news media that chemical interactions among pyridostigmine bromide (PB), permethrin, and N_1N-diethyl-m-toluamide (DEET) might contribute to Gulf War illnesses. This reported mixture served to protect the military personnel against insect-borne diseases. Furthermore, PB protected against potential nerve gas attack. However, heavy use of DEET by 1%–5% of the Persian Gulf War veterans (7,000–35,000 persons) may be related to the unexpected increase in the number of complaints of some of the veterans, which included fatigue, joint pain, ataxia, and rash (Institute of Medicine, 1995). Other complaints reported by "heavy users" of DEET were stumbling, weakness, and muscle cramps. The fact that these complaints occurred with excess frequency within this subpopulation can be deemed that exposure to contaminants in the Persian Gulf was responsible for this illness.

Pyridostigmine bromide (PB) is a quaternary ammonium carbamate that has been approved by the Food and Drug Administration (FDA) as a treatment for myasthenia gravis and the reversal of nondepolarizing neuromuscular blocking agents. PB was used in the Gulf War at a dose of one 30 mg tablet every 8 h (90 mg/d). PB was taken for about two weeks at the start of the air war in mid January and again at the start of the ground war in mid February. The majority of service members in the theater of operations took some PB during these periods. Toxicity from an overdose of PB results from the accumulation of acetylcholine at nicotinic and muscarinic acetylcholine receptors in the peripheral nervous system (PNS). The resultant effect is exaggerated cholinergic response such as muscle fasciculations, cramps, weakness, muscle twitching, respiratory difficulty, tremor, gastrointestinal tract disturbances, and paralysis (Abou-Donia *et al.*, 1996). Finally, death occurs from asphyxia. It should be clearly noted that a therapeutic oral dose of PB for myasthenia gravis is 200–1,400 mg/d but that much less was taken in the Persian Gulf.

Permethrin, a third-generation synthetic pyrethroid, has been approved for use as an insecticide by the U.S. Environmental Protection Agency (EPA). This compound has also been used to impregnate army battle-dress uniforms (BDUs) in the field. Formulations for application include a 0.5% aerosol and a 40% solution applied either with a 2 gal. compressed air sprayer or via a passive absorption method in a plastic bag (for uniform impregnation). The impregnation method available to soldiers prior to and during the Gulf War was the aerosol spray can method. The aerosol spray cans received only limited distribution within the war theater (less than 5% of deployed units had distributional access) (McCain *et al.*, 1997). Permethrin modifies sodium channels to open longer during a depolarizing pulse, evoking repetitive after-discharges by a single stimulus. This repetitive nerve action is associated with hyperactivity, tremor, ataxia, convulsion, and eventually paralysis.

DEET is an aromatic amide used as a personal insect repellent against mosquitoes, biting flies and ticks, among other insects. It has been used since 1946 by the U.S. Army and since 1957 by the general population. Approximately 30% of the U.S. population uses DEET as a lotion, stick, or spray at concentrations between 10% and 100% active ingredient. DEET is an EPA-approved insect repellant that is widely used commercially. Several formulations using various concentrations of DEET are available. It is the active ingredient in products such as Deep Woods Off and Cutter Insect Repellent. Formulations prepared for the U.S. Army include 75% DEET in ethanol, 33% extended duration formulation, and 19% in stick. Entomologists assigned in the Persian Gulf during the conflict indicated a very low usage of personal repellents, including DEET, even at times and in areas where mosquitos were present and biting. The cool seasonal climatic conditions that prevailed at the time of the war (January and February 1991) resulted in the near absence of biting insects. Extensive and repeated topical applications of DEET resulted in human poisoning including two deaths (de Garbino and Laborde, 1983; Roland *et al.*, 1985). Symptoms of poisoning are characterized by tremor, restlessness, slurred speech, seizures, impaired cognitive functions, and coma (Institute of Medicine, 1995). The exact mechanism underlying DEET toxicity is unknown. Pathological findings, following DEET administration, indicate that this compound is a demyelinating agent that causes spongiform myelinopathy, primarily of the cerebellar roof nuclei.

In light of the established safety of PB, it was surprising that approximately half of all military personnel seen in health care facilities during the Gulf War complained of PB side effects consistent with muscarinic stimulation (Institute of Medicine, 1995). One of the conclusions reached by the Committee to Review the Health Consequences of Service during the Persian Gulf War was that "studies are needed to resolve uncertainties about whether PB, DEET, and permethrin have additive effects" (Institute of Medicine, 1995). The Committee also recommended for immediate action that "appropriate laboratory animal studies of interactions between DEET, PB, and permethrin should be conducted." Regardless of the need for further studies, it is clear that contaminant mixture exposure produced a Gulf War syndrome in humans.

References

Abou-Donia, M. B., Wilmarth, K. R., Jensen, K. F., Oehme, F. W., and Kurt, T. L. (1996) Neurotoxicity resulting from coexposure to pyridostigmine bromide, DEET, and permethrin: implications of Gulf War chemical exposures. *J. Toxicol. Environ. Health* 48:35–56.

Coulston, F. (1985) Reconsideration of the dilemma of DDT for the establishment of an acceptable daily intake. *Regul. Toxicol. Pharmacol.* 5:332–383.

de Garbino, J. P. and Laborde, A. (1983) Toxicity of an insect repellent: N., N-diethyltoluamide. *Vet. Human Toxicol.* 25:422–423.

Doherty, J. D. (1979) Insecticides affecting ion transport. *Pharmacol. Therap.* 7:123–151.

Ecobichon, D. J. (1998) Toxic effects of pesticides, in *Casarett and Doull's Toxicology*, C. D. Klaassen (ed.), New York, NY: McGraw-Hill, Inc.

FAO (1990) Pesticide Residues in Food – 1990. *Report of the FAO and WHO Groups of Experts on Pesticide Residues.* FAO Plant Production and Protection Paper No. 102. Rome: Food and Agricultural Organization of the United States.

FAO (1993) *Pesticide Residues in Food – 1993.* FAO Plant Production and Protection Paper No. 122. Rome: Food and Agriculture Organization of the United Nations.

FDA (1987) *Residues in Foods, 1987.* Washington, DC: Food and Drug Administration.

Frawley, J. P., Fuyat, H. N., Hagen, E. C., Blake, J. R., and Fitzhugh, O. G. (1957) Marked potentiation in mammalian toxicity from simultaneous administration of two anticholinesterase compounds. *J. Pharmacol. Exp. Ther.* 121:96–106.

Hayes, W. J., Jr. (1982) *Pesticides Studied in Man.* Baltimore, MD: Williams & Wilkins.

IARC (1977) *Monographs on the Evaluation of Carcinogenic Risk of Chemicals to Man, Vol. 15. Some Fumigants, the Herbicides 2,4-D and 2,4,5-T, Chlorinated Dibenzodioxins and Miscellaneous Industrial Chemicals.* Lyon, France: International Agency for Research in Cancer.

IARC (1983) *Monographs on the Evaluation of Carcinogenic Risk of Chemicals to Man, Vol. 30. Miscellaneous Pesticides.* Lyon, France: International Agency for Research in Cancer.

Institute of Medicine (1995) *Health Consequences of Service During the Persian Gulf War: Initial Findings and Recommendations for Immediate Action.* Washington, DC: National Academy Press.

Koller, L. D. (1979) Effects of environmental contaminants on the immune system. *Adv. Vet. Sci. Com. Med.* 23:267–295.

Lu, F. C. (1995) A review of the acceptable daily intakes of pesticides assessed by WHO. *Regul. Toxicol. Pharmacol.* 21:352–364.

Lu, F. C., Jessup, D. C., and Lavallée, A. (1965) Toxicity of pesticides to young versus adult rats. *Food Cosmet. Toxicol.* 5:591–596.

McCain, W. C., Lee, R., Johnson, M. S., Whaley, J. G., Ferguson, J. W., Beall, P., and Leach, G. (1997) Acute oral toxicity study of pyridostigmine bromide, permethrin, and DEET in the laboratory rat. *J. Toxicol. Environ. Health* 50:113–124.

Murphy, S. D. (1969) Mechanisms of pesticide interactions in vertebrates. *Residue Rev.* 25:201–221.

Narahashi, T. (1980) Nerve membrane as a target of environmental toxicants, in *Neurotoxicology*, P. Spencer and H. H. Schaumberg (eds), Baltimore, MD: Williams & Wilkins.

Peakall, D. B. (1970) Pesticides and the reproduction of birds. *Sci. Am.* 222:72–78.

Roland, E. H., Jan, J. E., and Rigg, J. M. (1985) Toxic encephalopathy in a child after brief exposure to insect repellents. *Can. Med. Assoc. J.* 132:155–156.

Smith, P. and Heath, D. (1976) Paraquat. *CRC Crit. Rev. Toxicol.* 4:411–445.

Steinhoff, D., Weber, H., Mohr, U., and Boehme, K. (1983) Evaluation of amitrole (aminotriazole) for potential carcinogenicity in orally dosed rats, mice and golden hamster. *Toxicol. Appl. Pharmacol.* 69:161–169.

Street, J. C. (1981) Pesticides and the immune system, in *Immunologic Considerations in Toxicology*, R. P. Sharma (ed.), Boca Raton, FL: CRC Press.

Wang, X. Q., Gas, P. Y., Lin, Y. Z., and Chen, C. (1988) Studies on hexachlorocyclohexane and DDT contents in human cerumen and their relationship to cancer mortality. *Biomed. Environ. Sci.* 1:138–151.

Weil, C. S., Woodside, M. D., Carpenter, C. P., and Smyth, H. F., Jr. (1972) Current status of tests of carbaryl for reproductive and teratogenic effects. *Toxicol. Appl. Pharmacol.* 21:390–404.

Wills, J. H. (1972) The measurement and significance of changes in the cholinesterase of erythrocytes and plasma in man and animals. *CRC Crit. Rev. Toxicol.* 2:153–202.

Wills, J. H., Jameson, E., and Coulston, F. (1968) Effects of oral doses of carbaryl on man. *Clin. Toxicol.* 1:265–271.

Woodwell, G. M. (1967) Toxic substances and ecological cycles. *Sci. Am.* 216:24.

World Health Organization (1970) Pesticide Residues in Food. *WHO Tech. Rep. Ser.* 458. Geneva: WHO.

World Health Organization (1974) Pesticide Residues in Food. Report of the 1973 Joint FAO/WHO Meeting. *Tech. Rep. Ser.* 545. Geneva: WHO.

Appendix 20.1 Toxicological findings and evaluation on certain insecticides

Pesticides	LD_{50} (mg/kg)	NOAEL (mg/kg) Rat	NOAEL (mg/kg) Dog	NOAEL (mg/kg) Human	ADI (mg/kg)
Azinphosmethyl	13	0.45	0.74	0.3	0.005
Chlorfenvinphos	15	0.05	0.05		0.002
Diazinon	108	0.02	0.02	0.025	0.002
Dichlorvos	80			0.04	0.004
Dimethoate	215	0.4		0.2	0.02
Disulfoton	6.8	0.06	0.03	0.01	0.0003
Malathion	1,375	5.0		0.2	0.02
Mevinphos	6.1	0.02	0.025	0.014	0.0015
Parathion	13			0.05	0.005
Parathion-methyl	14	0.1	0.375	0.3	0.02
Trichlorfon	630	2.5	1.25		0.01
Aldicarb	0.8	0.125	0.25	0.025	0.003
Carbaryl	850	10		0.06	0.01
Propoxur	83	12.5	50		0.02
DDT	113	0.05			0.01
Aldrin/dieldrin	40	0.025	0.025		0.0001
Chlordane	335	0.25	0.05		0.0005
Endrin	18	0.05	0.025		0.002
Heptacholor	100	0.25	0.025		0.0001
Lindane	88	1.25	1.75		0.008
Methoxychlor	6,000	10			0.1

Source: LD_{50}s from Gaines (1969), other data from various WHO reports, summarized in Lu (1995).

Chapter 21

Toxicity of metals

CONTENTS

Introduction

Metals are a unique class of toxicants. They occur and persist in nature, but their chemical form may be changed because of physicochemical, biological, or anthropogenic activities. Their toxicity may be drastically altered as they assume different chemical forms. Most of them have some value to humans because of their uses in industry, agriculture, or medicine. Some are essential elements, required in various biochemical/physiological functions. On the other hand, they may pose health hazards to the public because of their presence in food, water, or air, and to workers engaged in mining, smelting, and a variety of industrial activities.

Occurrence

Most of the metals and "metalloids" occur in nature, dispersed in rocks, ores, soil, water, and air. However, their distribution is grossly uneven. In general, their levels are relatively low in soil, water, and air. These levels may be increased by such geological activities as degassing, which releases, for example, 25,000–125,000 tons of mercury a year. Anthropogenic activities such as mining of mercury contribute about 10,000 tons a year. It must be noted that anthropogenic activities may be more significant in relation to human exposure because they increase the levels of the metals at the site of the human activities.

Uses and human exposure

In ancient times, certain metals such as copper, iron, and tin were used to make utensils, machinery, and weapons. Mining and smelting were undertaken to supply such demands. These activities increased their environmental levels. In addition, as the ores often contain other metals, such as lead and arsenic, the levels of these "contaminants" were also increased.

In later years, a greater variety of metals has found uses in industry, agriculture, and medicine. For example, mercury is used extensively in the chlor-alkali industry as the cathode in the electrolysis of salt in water to produce chlorine and sodium hydroxide, both of which are important raw materials in the chemical industry. Lead is used in storage batteries and the cable industry. However, the use of various lead compounds as insecticides, fuel additives, and pigments in paints has gradually been discontinued.

More recently, the aerospace industry and medico-dental profession require materials that have strength, resistance to corrosion, and nonirritant properties. Alloys of titanium and other metals are becoming even more important.

These human activities have increased the extent of exposure not only to occupational workers but also to the consumers of these products. In addition, the toxicity of a metal may be significantly altered by changes of its chemical form. For example, inorganic mercury compounds are toxic primarily to the kidney, whereas methyl mercury is a CNS toxicant.

Certain common features

Metals have a wide range of toxicity. Some, such as lead and mercury, are very toxic; others are almost nontoxic, such as titanium. They also possess a variety of toxic properties. Nevertheless, there are a number of toxicological features that are shared to some extent by many metals.

Site of action

Enzymes

A major action of toxic metals is the inhibition of enzymes. This action usually occurs as a result of the interaction between the metal and the SH group of the enzyme. An enzyme may also be inhibited by a toxic metal through displacement of an essential metal cofactor of the enzyme. For example, lead may displace zinc in the zinc-dependent enzyme δ-aminolevulinic acid hydratase (ALAD).

Another mechanism by which metals interfere with the functions of enzymes is by inhibiting their synthesis. For example, nickel and platinum inhibit the δ-aminolevulinic acid synthetase (ALAS), thereby interfere with the synthesis of heme, which is an important component of hemoglobin and cytochrome (Maines and Kappas, 1977). The enzymes can be protected from toxic metals by the administration of "chelating agents," such as dimercaprol (BAL), that form stable bonds with the metals.

Enzymes differ in their susceptibility to metals. Figure 21.1 depicts the synthesis of heme and the various enzymes involved, most of which may be inhibited by lead. However, they differ in susceptibility (see the section on lead, p. 313). Inhibition of ALAD occurs at a blood lead level (Bl–Pb) of 10 µg/dl or lower. As a result, ALA will not be processed to become porphobilinogen and thus will be spilled over into urine at a Bl–Pb of 40 µg/dl, and anemia will only occur at a Bl–Pb of about 50 µ/dl (WHO, 1977).

Subcellular organelles

In general, the toxic effects of metals result from reactions between them and intracellular components. For a metal to exert its toxic effect on a cell, it must enter the cell. The entry across the membrane is facilitated if it is lipophilic such as methyl mercury. When it is bound to a protein, it is absorbed by endocytosis. Passive diffusion is another form of entry of metals such as lead.

After their entry into the cell, metals may affect different organelles. For example, the endoplasmic reticulum contains a variety of enzymes. These microsomal enzymes are inhibited by many metals, such as cadmium,

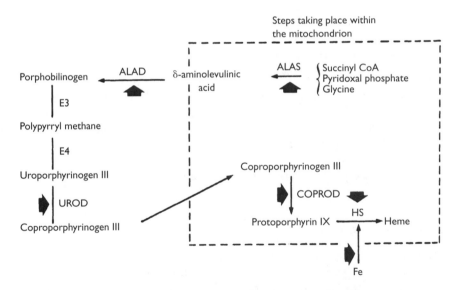

Figure 21.1 Schematic diagram representing the reactions involved in heme synthesis. Large arrows indicate steps that are inhibited by Pb. ALAS: δ-aminolevulinic acid synthetase; ALAD: δ-aminolevulinic acid dehydratase; UROD: uroporphyrinogen decarboxylase; COPROD: coproporphyrinogen oxidase; and HS: heme synthetase.

Source: Adapted from Jaworski, 1978. For further explanation, see section on Lead, p. 000.

cobalt, methyl mercury, and tin. Toxic metals also disrupt the structure of the endoplasmic reticulum. The lysosomes are another site of action of metals such as cadmium (as conjugate of metallothionein). Cadmium is accumulated in the lysosomes of renal proximal tubular cells. In the lysosomes, the cadmium complex degrades and releases Cd^{2+}. The cadmium ion inhibits the proteolytic enzymes in the lysosomes and causes cell injury. The mitochondria, because of their high metabolic activity and rapid membrane transport, are also a common target of metals. The respiratory enzymes in these organelles are readily inhibited by metals. A number of metals enter the nucleus and may form inclusion bodies. For example, chronic exposure to lead can induce inclusion bodies in the nuclei of renal proximal tubular cells. It also stimulates DNA, RNA, and protein synthesis. The lead-induced renal adenocarcinoma has been attributed to this mechanism (Goering et al., 1987).

It is therefore evident that the subcellular organelles either enhance or impede the movement of metals across these biological membranes, thereby affecting their toxicity. In addition, certain proteins in cytosol, lysosomes, and nuclei may bind with toxic metals, such as Cd, Pb, and Hg, thereby reducing their availability for toxic effects on sensitive organelles and metabolic sites (Fowler et al., 1984).

Factors affecting toxicity

Levels and duration of exposure

As with other toxicants, the toxic effects of metals are related to the level and duration of exposure. In general, the higher the level and the longer the duration, the greater the toxic effects. However, apart from these quantitative differences, changes in the level and duration of exposure may alter the nature of the toxic effects. For example, ingestion of a single, large dose of cadmium induces gastrointestinal (G.I.) disturbances. Repeated intakes of smaller amounts of Cd result in renal dysfunction.

Chemical form

A notable example is mercury. Its inorganic compounds are essentially renal toxicants, while methyl mercury and ethyl mercury compounds are more toxic to the nervous system. The latter type of mercury compounds are lipophilic and thus readily cross the blood–brain barrier. Similarly, tetraethyllead readily enters the myelin sheath and affects the nervous system. Organic compounds of metals are generally excreted in the bile, while their inorganic compounds are excreted in the urine. Furthermore, the former are biodegradable and the latter are not (Furst, 1987).

Metal–protein complexes

Perhaps as protective mechanisms, various metal–protein complexes are formed in the body. For example, the complexes formed with lead, bismuth, and mercury-selenium are microscopically visible as "inclusion bodies" in the affected cells. Iron may combine with protein to form ferritin, which is water soluble, or hemosiderin, which is not. Cadmium and several other metals (e.g., zinc) combine with metallothionein, a low-molecular-weight protein. The Cd complex is less toxic than Cd^{2+}. However, in the renal tubule cells, the cadmium-metallothionein is broken down by the cysteine protease in lysosomes to release Cd^{2+} and causes toxic effects (Squibb and Fowler, 1984; Min et al., 1992).

Host factors

As with most other toxicants, the young and the old animals are in general more susceptible than young adults to metals (Chapter 5). Young children appear to be especially susceptible to lead because of the generally greater sensitivity and the greater extent of G.I. absorption. Furthermore, they have, on a unit body weight basis, a greater intake of food, which is the main source of lead.

Dietary factors such as deficiencies of protein and vitamins C and D enhance the toxicity of lead and cadmium. Certain metals, such as lead and mercury, can cross the placenta, thus affecting the fetus. There is evidence that prenatally exposed children are affected more severely than their mothers: it was found in a study that the median dose that caused ataxia in the mothers was $2.7 \pm 0.18\,mg/kg$, whereas that in the prenatally exposed children was 1.23 ± 0.87 (Clarkson, 1981).

Biological indicators/biomarkers

Exposure to metals can usually be quantitatively assessed. Some of the indicators reveal the extent and the approximate time of exposure. Others are early signs of biological effects.

The presence and level of the metal in blood and urine are often used as indicators of recent exposure. As the metal compounds are distributed, stored, or excreted, the levels in blood and urine will diminish.

Many metals are accumulated in hair and nail. Their levels generally bear a relationship with those in blood at the time when the hair and nails are formed. Therefore hair, which grows at a relatively constant rate, has been used to determine the level of exposure at various times in the past. For example, this procedure has been used extensively to ascertain the intake of methyl mercury among the inhabitants in the areas where methyl mercury poisoning was reported. Using different approaches, a fairly reliable conversion factor has been established. Thus the level of methyl mercury in hair is about 250 times of that in blood, and their relation to the daily intake, after a steady state is reached, is as follows: $0.2 \mu g/g$ in blood $= 50 \mu g/g$ in hair $= 3 \mu g/kg$ body weight per day (WHO, 1976).

Such biological indicators are also useful in assessing the average blood level of selenium of inhabitants. In areas where there was selenosis it was $3.2 mg/L$; where there was Se deficiency syndrome, it was $0.021 mg/L$; and in an area where there was neither overexposure nor deficiency, it was $0.095 mg/L$ (WHO, 1987).

Minimal inhibition of δ-aminolevulinic acid dehydrase by lead represents a special type of "indicator of exposure" in that this biological effect does not seem to indicate an adverse effect.

Common toxic effects

Carcinogenicity

A number of metals have been shown to be carcinogenic in humans or animals or both. As listed in Appendix 7.1, arsenic and its compounds, cadmium, certain chromium compounds, and nickel and its compounds have been shown to be human carcinogens. Beryllium, cadmium, and cis-platin are probable human carcinogens. Certain other metals may be carcinogenic, but the available information is insufficient to confirm this suggestion.

The aforementioned metals as well as several others might be carcinogenic through multiple mechanisms of action such as the substitution of Ni^{2+}, Co^{2+}, or Cd^{2+} for Zn^{2+} in finger-loops of transforming proteins (Sunderman and Barber, 1988) and injury to cytoskeleton by certain metals (Chou, 1989) that affects fidelity of the polymerase involved in DNA biosynthesis.

Immune function

Exposure to certain metals may result in inhibition of immune functions (Chapter 11, Immunodysfunction, p. 163). Other metals such as beryllium, chromium, nickel, gold, mercury, platinum and zirconium may induce hypersensitivity reactions. The clinical manifestations and mechanism of action are listed in Table 21.1.

Nervous system

Because of its susceptibility, the nervous system is a common target of toxic metals. However, even with the same metal, its physicochemical form often determines the nature of the toxicity. As noted above, metallic

Table 21.1 Hypersensitivity reactions to metals

Metal	Type of reaction*	Clinical features	Mechanism of reactions
Platinum, beryllium	I	Asthma, conjunctivitis, urticaria, anaphylaxis	IgE reacts with antigen on mast cell/basophil to release vasoreactive amines
Gold, salts of mercury	II	Thrombocytopenia	IgG binds to complement and antigen on cells, resulting in their destruction
Mercury vapor, gold	III	Glomerular nephritis, proteinuria	Antigen, antibody and complement deposit on epithelial surface of glomerular basement
Chromium, nickel	IV	Contact dermatitis	Sensitized T cells react with antigen to cause delayed hypersensitivity reaction
Beryllium, zirconium		Granuloma formation	

Note
*For descriptions see section on Hypersensitivity and Allergy, Chapter 11, p. 161.

mercury vapor and methyl mercury readily enter the NS and induce toxic effects. Inorganic mercury compounds are unlikely to enter the NS in significant amounts and thus usually are not neurotoxic. Similarly, the organic compounds of lead are mainly neurotoxic, whereas inorganic lead compounds affect the synthesis of heme first. But at much higher levels of exposure, they may induce encephalopathy, and in young children a moderate level of exposure to these compounds may result in a deficit of mental functions. Other neurotoxic metals include copper, triethyltin, gold, lithium, and manganese. For additional information, see Bondy and Prasad (1988).

Kidney

The kidney, as the main excretory organ in the body, is also a common target organ. Cadmium affects the renal proximal tubular cells, causing urinary excretion of small-molecule proteins, amino acids, and glucose. In addition, inorganic mercury compounds, lead, chromium and platinum, also induce kidney damage, mainly in the proximal tubules (see Chapter 14).

Respiratory system

The respiratory system is the primary target organ of most metals following occupational exposure. There are several types of responses. Many cause irritation and inflammation of the respiratory tract; the parts affected depend on the metal and the duration of exposure. With acute exposures, chromium affects the nasal passage, arsenic the bronchi, and beryllium the lungs. Prolonged exposure may cause fibrosis (aluminum, iron), carcinoma (arsenic, chromium, nickel), or granuloma (beryllium). These effects are included in Appendix 12.1 and Table 24.2.

Metals of major toxicological concern

Lead, mercury, and cadmium are metals of major health concern because of their impact on large numbers of people resulting from environmental pollution as well as the serious nature of their toxic effects. Several other metals also pose serious toxicological problems.

Mercury

General considerations

The elemental form of mercury (Hg) exists in liquid form. It is released from the earth's crust through degassing. It is also present in the environment as inorganic and organic compounds. Elemental Hg may become inorganic compounds by oxidation and revert to elemental Hg by reduction. Inorganic Hg may become organic Hg through the action of certain anaerobic bacteria, and degrade to inorganic Hg slowly.

A variety of anthropogenic activities may raise its levels in the environment. Among these are mining, smelting (to produce metals from their sulfide ores), burning of fossil fuel, and production of steel, cement, and phosphate. Its principal users include the chlor-alkali plants, paper-pulp industry, and electrical equipment manufacturers. These uses fortunately have decreased in recent years.

The Hg level in the ambient air is extremely low. The level in water in unpolluted areas is about 0.1 µg/L, but it may be as high as 80 µg/L near Hg ore deposits. Its level in food, except fish, is very low, generally in the range of 5–20 µg/kg. Most fishes contain higher levels; the levels in tuna and swordfish usually range from 200 to 1,000 µg/kg.

Toxicity

Because of the massive outbreaks of poisoning from consuming grain treated with mercury fungicide or fish contaminated with methyl mercury (Chapter 1, Appendix 1.2), extensive investigations have been carried out. The populations studied ranged from "normal" subjects to those fatally poisoned. Table 21.2 lists some of these population groups. The "fishermen" were exposed to higher than normal levels but showed no signs of

Table 21.2 Daily intake of methyl mercury by certain populations

Population	Daily intake (µg) Average	Range
"Normal"	–	1–20
Fisherman	300	Up to 1,000
Niigata	1,500	250–5,000
Iraq	4,500	Up to 12,000

poisoning. Those involved in the Niigata episode were exposed to smaller intakes than those in the Iraq episode, and hence the latency in Niigata was generally two to three years whereas those in Iraq was two to three months.

These studies have revealed that the toxic effects are related to the nervous system, which is extremely sensitive to this toxicant and readily invaded by it. Paresthesia is usually the earliest symptom. Constricted visual field is pathognomonic. At higher levels of exposure, ataxia, dysarthria, deafness, and eventually death occur. Figure 21.2 shows graphically the dose–response and dose–effect relationships. Pathologically the major damage is atrophy in the occipital lobe, the cerebellar folia, and calcarine cortex. There are also degenerative changes in the axons and myelin sheaths of peripheral nerves.

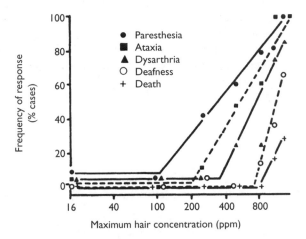

Figure 21.2 The frequency of signs and symptoms of methyl mercury poisoning in adult victims in Iraq plotted according to the estimated maximum hair concentration. Hair samples were not available for all patients and are estimated based on the patient's history of exposure, observed blood levels, and blood half-times and a hair-to-blood concentration ratio of 250 to 1.

Source: Clarkson, 1987.

From these studies it was concluded that methyl mercury poisoning would be unlikely if the daily intake corresponds to a blood level of $20\,\mu g/dl$ and a hair level of $50\,\mu g/g$ (WHO, 1976). More recent studies indicate that fetal brain is much more susceptible to methyl mercury than that of adults. This difference is due to the ease of transport across the placenta, the preferential uptake by the fetal brain, and the inhibitory action on cell division and cell migration, both of which are essential in the proper development of fetal brain (Clarkson, 1991).

Elemental Hg vapor constitutes a hazard virtually only in occupational settings. Its target organ is also the CNS. The usual symptoms are tremors and mental disturbances. Among workers exposed to Hg vapor the triad of excitability, tremors, and gingivitis have long been observed (Goldwater, 1972). After a continual exposure to a time-weighted air concentration of $0.05\,mg\,Hg/m^3$, sensitive workers may exhibit nonspecific (neurasthenic) symptoms, and at a concentration of $0.1\text{--}0.2\,mg/m^3$, they may have tremors (WHO, 1976).

Inorganic Hg salts are either monovalent or divalent. The divalent mercuric chloride, the "corrosive sublimate," is corrosive on contact. After ingestion, it causes abdominal cramps and bloody diarrhea, with corrosive ulceration, bleeding, and necrosis of the G.I. tract. These effects are followed by *renal* damage, mainly necrosis and sloughing off of the proximal tubular cells, thereby blocking the tubules and causing oliguria, anuria, and uremia. It may also damage the glomerulus, possibly as a result of disturbed immune function. The monovalent salt calomel, the mercurous chloride, is less corrosive and less toxic. But mercurous chloride may cause the "pink disease," characterized by *dermal* vasodilation, hyperkeratosis, and hypersecretion of the sweat glands. This effect is probably a hypersensitivity reaction, since it is not dose-related.

Lead

General considerations

Lead is more ubiquitous than most other toxic metals. The environmental levels have been increasing because of lead mining, smelting, refining, and various industrial uses.

Generally the Pb levels in soil range from 5 to $25\,mg/kg$, in ground water from 1 to $60\,\mu g/L$ and somewhat lower in natural surface water, and in air under $1\,\mu g/m^3$, but may be much higher in certain workplaces and areas with heavy motor traffic.

The major industrial uses, such as fuel additives, and lead pigments in paints, which contributed greatly to the Pb levels in the environment, have been gradually phased out. However, its uses in storage batteries and cables have not been significantly reduced. Drinking water may be appreciably contaminated by Pb from the use of lead and PVC pipes. Glazed ceramic foodware is another source of Pb, as noted in Chapter 19. For most people, the major source of their Pb intake is food, which contributes generally 100–300 µg per day.

Infants and young children are likely exposed to a greater extent than adults, because of their habit of licking, chewing, or eating foreign objects, such as soil and flakes of old paints from the wall.

Toxicity

The *hematopoietic system* is extremely sensitive to the effect of Pb. The main component of hemoglobin is heme. It is synthesized from glycine and succinyl coenzyme A (CoA), with pyridoxal phosphate as cofactor. After a number of steps, it finally combines with iron to form heme. The initial and final steps take place in the mitochondria, with the intermediate steps in the cytoplasm, as shown in Figure 21.1. Among the seven enzymes involved in these steps, five are susceptible to the inhibitory effect of Pb. δ-Aminolevulinic acid dehydratase (ALAD) and heme synthetase (HS) are the most susceptible, whereas δ-aminolevulinic acid synthetase (ALAS), uroporphyrinogen decarboxylase (UROD), and coproporphyrinogen oxidase (COPROD) are less sensitive to inhibition by Pb. Only two of them are not affected, namely, porphobilinogen deaminase and uroporphyrinogen cosynthetase.

While clinical anemia is evident only when there is moderate exposure to Pb, with its level in blood around 50 µg/dl, a number of other effects may be observed at much lower levels of exposure. For example, ALAD inhibition becomes perceptible at a blood Pb level just over 10 µg/dl and free erythrocyte porphyrins (FEP) at 20–25 µg/dl. ALAD inhibition, and possibly FEP, may be considered as an indicator of exposure rather than an indicator of toxicity. The impaired heme synthesis may result in anemia that is hypochromatic and microcytic. The anemia may be due partly to the greater fragility of the erythrocyte membrane (WHO, 1977).

The *nervous system* is also a main target organ of Pb. After high levels of exposure, with blood Pb level over 80 µg/dl, encephalopathy may occur. There are damages to the arterioles and capillaries, resulting in cerebral edema, increased cerebrospinal fluid pressure, neuronal degeneration, and glial proliferation. Clinically this condition is associated with ataxia, stupor, coma, and convulsion. In children, this clinical syndrome may occur with a blood Pb level of 70 µg/dl. At still lower levels (40–50 µg/dl), children may exhibit hyperactivity, decreased attention span, and a slight lowering of IQ scores (Ernhardt *et al.*, 1981). These subtle manifestations may be a result of impairment of the function of neurotransmitters and calcium ion. Peripheral neuropathy is characterized by wrist-drop and foot-drop, signs of damage to the motor nerves. Lead causes degeneration of Schwann cells followed by demyelination and possibly axonal degeneration. This syndrome occurs mainly among occupational workers.

Lead generally affects the kidney insidiously, resulting in chronic renal failure after long-term exposure. The proximal tubule is the main target. An early sign of lead toxicity on the kidney is the excretion of the lysosomal enzyme N-acetyl-β-D-glucosaminidase (Verschoor et al., 1987). One characteristic of lead poisoning is the presence of lead "inclusion bodies" in the nucleus of tubular cells. These bodies consist of fibrillary lead-protein complexes.

Other effects

Carcinogenicity of Pb has been demonstrated in kidneys of rodents, but there is little human data in this respect (IARC, 1980). Pb also adversely affects reproductive functions, mainly through its gametotoxicity in both male and female animals, resulting in low sperm counts, decreased sperm motility, sterility, abortion, and neonatal deaths. Young children are likely to be exposed to higher levels of Pb, as noted above. Furthermore, they and unborn fetuses are also more sensitive to the toxicity of this metal.

Organic lead compounds such as tetraethyllead and tetramethyllead are readily absorbed after inhalation and dermal exposures, and rapidly enter the CNS with ensuing encaphalopathy. This hazard concerns essentially occupational workers, but not the general public, because the small amounts emitted from automobile exhaust readily degrade.

Cadmium

General considerations

Cadmium occurs in nature mainly in lead and zinc ores. It is thus released near the mines and smelters of these metals. It is used as a pigment (such as in ceramics), in electroplating, and in making alloys and alkali storage batteries. Its level in the air is usually in the range of nanograms per cubic meter, but may amount to several milligrams per cubic meter in certain workplaces. The level in water is very low (around 1 μg/L) except in contaminated areas. Most foods contain trace amounts of cadmium. Grains and cereal products usually constitute the main source of Cd.

While meat, poultry, and fish have relatively low levels of Cd, liver, kidney, and shellfish have much higher levels. The environmental levels are raised by smelting and industrial uses. An additional source is the use of sludge as a food crop fertilizer.

Apart from these environmental sources, humans may be exposed to Cd through cigarette smoking: a pack a day may double the Cd intake. Extensively decorated and improperly fired ceramic foodware is another source of Cd (see Chapter 19). Occupational exposure occurs mainly in smelteries.

Toxicity

The *acute* effects of Cd exposure result mainly from local irritation. After ingestion, the clinical manifestations are nausea, vomiting, and abdominal pain; after inhalation, the lesions include pulmonary edema and chemical pneumonitis.

Cadmium is very slowly excreted, with a half-life of about 15–30 years. After long-term exposure, *kidney* lesions predominate. The primary site of action is the proximal tubules. Damages to these tubules generally occurs when the Cd level in the kidney reaches $200\,\mu g/g$, the "critical concentration." These tubular damages result in their inability to reabsorb small-molecular proteins, the major one of which is β_2-microglobulin. Other proteins include retinol-binding protein, lysozyme, ribonuclease, and immunoglobulin light chains (Lauwerys *et al.*, 1979). Similarly, aminoaciduria is another result of damage to tubular cells that normally reabsorb the amino acids filtered through the glomeruli. Other related effects are glycosuria and decreased tubular reabsorption of phosphate.

At later stages, there may be hypercalcinuria, which, probably in conjunction with altered bone metabolism, may lead to *osteomalacia*. However, the connection between Cd and itai-itai disease, characterized by chronic renal disease and bone deformity, reported in Toyama, Japan where the Cd level in rice was high (see Appendix 1.2), has not been firmly established (Nomiyama, 1980).

Effects on the *respiratory system* result from inhalation exposure. Chronic bronchitis, progressive fibrosis of the lower airway, and rupture of septae between alveoli lead to emphysema.

Other effects include *hypertension*, which may be the result of sodium retention, vasoconstriction, and hyperreninemia. *Carcinoma* of the prostate has been reported among occupational workers (Kipling and Waterhause, 1967).

Other metals

Arsenic

Although arsenic is a ubiquitous metalloid, its levels in water and ambient air are generally low. The major source of human exposure is food, which contains somewhat less than 1 mg/kg. However, its level in seafood may reach 5 mg/kg.

In certain parts of Taiwan, South America, and Bangladesh, the water may contain hundreds of milligrams per liter. In these areas, the inhabitants may suffer from dermal hyperkeratosis and hyperpigmentation. A more serious condition is gangrene of lower extremities, the *black-foot disease*, resulting from peripheral endarteritis (Tseng, 1977; Chowdhury *et al.*, 2000).

Cancer of the skin is also observed in those areas, as well as among patients who had been taking Fowler's solution ($KAsO_2$) as a therapy for leukemia. Cancer of the lung may occur among workers exposed to As in copper smelteries and plants that manufacture As-containing pesticide (Pinto *et al.*, 1978; Enterline *et al.*, 1987; Viren and Silvers, 1994). Unlike other human carcinogens, As has not been shown to be carcinogenic to laboratory animals. Furthermore, mutagenesis tests have been essentially negative.

Other effects include toxicity to *liver* parenchyma, resulting clinically in jaundice in early stages and in cirrhosis and ascites later. *Acutely*, very large doses of As compounds induce G.I. damage with vomiting and bloody diarrhea, muscular cramps, and cardiac abnormality (WHO, 1981). Exposure to excessive amounts of As may interfere with heme formation as evidenced by the increased urinary excretion of porphyrins (Xie *et al.*, 2001).

Beryllium

Beryllium is released into the environment mainly through combustion of fossil fuel. It is used in ceramic plants and in making alloys. Beryllium and its alloys have a number of applications in nuclear, space, and other industries.

The major toxic effect is *berylliosis*, resulting from long-term inhalation exposures. This disease of the lung is characterized by granulomas, which in time become fibrotic tissues. These lesions reduce the number of alveoli and consequently pulmonary function.

After dermal contact, beryllium produces *hypersensitivity reactions* of the skin. The reaction is cell-mediated, and therefore delayed (type IV allergy). The soluble compounds of Be induce papillovesicular lesions, whereas the insoluble compounds induce granulomatous lesions.

Beryllium has been shown to be carcinogenic to several species of animals. Epidemiological data suggest that Be is a human carcinogen (IARC, 1994).

Chromium

Chromium occurs in ores. Mining, smelting, and industrial uses tend to increase its environmental levels. It is used in making stainless steel, various alloys, and pigments. Fossil-fuel-powered plants and cement-producing plants are also sources of environmental pollution. However, its levels in air, water, and food are generally very low. The major human exposure is occupational.

Chromium is a human carcinogen, inducing lung cancers among workers exposed to it. The carcinogenicity is generally attributed to the hexavalent Cr^{6+}, which is corrosive and water insoluble. It has been suggested that Cr^{6+}, which is more readily taken up by cells, converts to Cr^{3+} intracellularly. The trivalent Cr ion, which is more active biologically, binds with nucleic acid and initiates the carcinogenesis process. The Cr^{6+} is corrosive and causes *ulceration* of the nasal passages and skin. It also induces *hypersensitivity reactions* of the skin. Acutely, it induces *renal tubular necrosis*.

Nickel

Nickel occurs in ores. Smelting and industrial uses tend to increase its levels in the environment. Its many industrial uses include storage batteries, electrical contacts and similar devices, electroplating, and as catalysts. It is also emitted from coal gasification.

Nickel is a human carcinogen among occupational workers. Nasal cancer appears to be the predominant type of neoplasm. But Ni also induces cancer of the lung, larynx, stomach, and possibly also the kidney.

It is one of the most common causative agents of dermal hypersensitivity reactions among the general public. The reactions usually follow contact with Ni-containing metal objects such as coins and jewelry.

Risk/benefit considerations

The metals discussed in the previous section offer certain benefits because of their industrial and minor medical uses. However, they pose serious toxicological risks either to the population at large or specific occupational workers. On the other hand, there are two groups of metals that are more valuable. One group, the essential metals, is required in certain physiological functions, and the other is used for a variety of medical purposes. These three groups of metals are different in risk/benefit considerations.

Toxic metals

The general population is at risk to these metals mainly through *food*. Tolerances, or equivalents, are established for various foodstuffs to ensure that the total intake will not exceed the amount that is considered acceptable from a toxicological point of view.

However, more targeted action is taken in certain cases. For example, the main source of methyl mercury is fish. The levels in swordfish range from about 0.5 to 1.2 ppm, and in tuna from 0.2 to 0.5 ppm, whereas those in most other kinds of fish are 0.1 ppm or lower. The permissible levels for methyl mercury set by most nations range from 0.4 to 1.0 ppm. Assuming a daily consumption of 200 g fish, the intake of methyl mercury would not exceed 0.2 mg. An intake at this level is considered unlikely to induce methyl mercury toxicity (WHO, 1976). The safety is provided by the fact that most of the fish samples contain much less methyl mercury than the 1.0 ppm permitted. The Joint FAO/WHO Expert Committee on Food Additives and Contaminants established a "tolerable intake" of 0.2 mg/week, thus allowing a safety factor of 7, which the Committee considered adequate in this case (WHO, 1972). The rationale was the availability of the exceptionally extensive data obtained from populations exposed to the full gamut of intake levels, ranging from "normal" to questionably poisoned, minimally poisoned, seriously poisoned, and fatally poisoned (Table 21.2), as well as the fact that most of the investigations were thoroughly conducted and properly reported. Second, fish was considered as an important source of nutrients, which should not be discarded for minimal or nonexistent risks. The intake was set on a weekly basis because fish is consumed, in many parts of the world, once a week.

Similarly, targeted action has been taken with respect to Cd in rice in Japan, where rice is the main source of this contaminant. Permissible levels of release of Pb and Cd from ceramic foodware have been established internationally (WHO, 1979) and in many nations. See also Chapter 19.

There are also tolerances for toxic metals such as As, Cd, and Pb in water and foods for the protection of the health of consumers.

Occupational workers are likely exposed to higher levels of toxic metals in mining, smelting, manufacture, and similar occupations. The main routes of entry to the body are the skin and respiratory tract. For their protection, threshold limit values of toxicants in air are established. For additional information, see Chapter 23.

Essential metals

Selenium is a typical element that is toxic at high levels of intake and induces a deficiency syndrome when the intake is too low.

Human *overexposure* to Se has been observed in China as well as in a few isolated regions in the Americas. The clinical manifestations include hair loss, nail pathology, and tooth decay. In animals overexposure induces more severe ill effects including retarded growth, liver necrosis, enlargement of spleen and pancreas, anemia, and various disorders of reproductive function.

Deficiency of Se results in muscular dystrophy in sheep and cattle, exudative diathesis in chicken, and liver necrosis in swine and rats. In rats it may also cause reproductive failures, vascular changes, and cataracts.

Selenium is a component of glutathione peroxidase, which is responsible for the destruction of H_2O_2 and lipid peroxides. Its function is therefore closely related to that of vitamin E, the biological antioxidant. This close relation is reflected in the fact that the minimal intake of Se in rats is 0.01 mg/kg, but if there is also a vitamin E deficiency, an intake of 0.05 mg/kg will be needed.

It was only in the late 1970s that Se was recognized as an essential element in humans. In certain regions in China, where the Se levels were low in soil and food, a special type of *cardiomyopathy* was noted. It was known as Keshan disease because it was first observed there. The Se levels in the blood, urine, and hair of the inhabitants were low. As expected, the blood glutathione peroxidase activity was also low. When they were given a sodium selenite supplement, the incidence of this endemic cardiopathy dropped sharply. There is also an endemic *osteoarthropathy* observed in China. It is known as Kashin–Beck disease, and is believed to be due to Se deficiency. But the evidence on its etiology is not as strong. Selenium deficiency associated with muscular pain has been reported from New Zealand.

For the general population, the Se exposure is essentially from food, especially cereals. The average daily intake of Se of inhabitants in areas where there were cases of Keshan disease was about 0.011 mg, whereas in areas where there were cases of selenosis it was about 5 mg (Yang *et al.*, 1983). It has been estimated that there is about a 100-fold margin between the highest no-toxic-effect level and the lowest level at which deficiency syndrome is avoided. However, this margin is subject to the influence of various modifying factors. For example, vitamin E deficiency increases the toxicity as well as the physiological requirements of Se, thus effectively reducing the margin. Methyl mercury increases the effect of Se deficiency, whereas inorganic mercury increases the toxicity of methylated Se compounds. A hypothetical dose–response (all effects) relationship of Se is depicted in Figure 4.1 which shows that ill effects are induced when the dose is too low (curve A), whereas other ill effects are induced when the dose is too high (curve B). Furthermore, because of the great individual variations in susceptibility resulting from host and environmental factors, it is not clear whether there is a dose that can be considered as devoid of deficiency as well as toxic effect on a population basis. Additional details on various aspects of the Se problem and reference citations may be found in a WHO document (WHO, 1987).

Cobalt, copper, and *iron* are all essential metal elements required in the proper development of erythrocytes. Iron is a component of hemoglobin, and Cu facilitates the utilization of Fe in the synthesis of hemoglobin. Thus deficiency of either metal results in hypochromatic, microcytic anemia. Cobalt is a component of vitamin B_{12}, which is required in the development of erythrocyte. Its deficiency results in pernicious anemia.

Excessive intake of Co results in polycythemia, an overproduction of erythrocytes, and cardiomyopathy. The heart lesion was observed under special conditions, as discussed in Chapter 25. Excess Cu storage in the body is not a result of overexposure to Cu but rather a genetic disorder (Wilson's disease). Copper is accumulated in brain, liver, kidney, and cornea. Clinical manifestations are thus related to disorders of these organs. Overexposure to Fe may result from excessive intake of Fe or frequent blood transfusion. The excess Fe is deposited as hemosiderin mainly in liver, causing liver dysfunction.

Occupational exposure to Co induces respiratory irritation and dermal hypersensitivity reactions. Certain Fe industry workers have been reported as having pneumoconiosis and increased lung cancer incidence. Acute oral poisonings have been reported after consuming improperly canned vegetable juices containing excessive amounts of Cu and after taking large doses of Fe supplement medications. The clinical manifestations relate mainly to G.I. irritation.

Other essential metals include manganese and molybdenum, which are cofactors in a number of enzyme systems such as phosphorylase, xanthine oxidase, and aldehyde oxidase. However, these metals are so plentiful in the human diet that no cases of deficiency syndrome have been reported. These metals have a variety of industrial uses, notably in making high-temperature-resistant steel alloys. Occupational exposure to Mn results in pneumonitis acutely, and encephalopathy chronically. Overexposure to Mn in animals orally induces G.I. disturbances followed by fatty degeneration of liver and kidney.

Zinc is the cofactor in scores of metalloenzymes and is therefore an essential element. Deficiency of Zn thus induces a great variety of effects on the nervous system, hematopoietic system, skin, liver, eye, testis, etc. Zinc is readily excreted, and excessive intake by the oral route is thus unlikely to induce toxic effects. Occupational exposure to Zn_2O_3 fume results in "metal fume fever" (Goyer, 1996).

Metals used in medicine

Therapeutic agents

A number of metal compounds have been used in medicine. For example, compounds of Hg have been used as diuretics. Because of their toxicity, their uses have been discontinued. Those that are less toxic include compounds of aluminum as antacid, bismuth as astringent, gold for rheumatoid arthritis, lithium for mental depression, platinum complexes as anti-tumor agents and thallium as depilatory. They may produce toxic effects on the nervous system (e.g., Al, Bi, Li, Th), kidneys (e.g., Bi, Au, Li), skin (e.g., Au, Pl), and cardiovascular and gastrointestinal systems (e.g., Li, Th). Although used as antitumor agents, Pl complexes may induce tumors.

Other uses

Aluminum in hemodialysis for chronic renal failure has resulted in fatal neurologic syndrome. The use of barium and gallium, in conjunction with X-ray, as a radiopaque agent and radioactive tracer has proved to be relatively safe. However, accidental ingestion of soluble Ba salts has resulted in serious gastrointestinal, muscular, and cardiovascular disturbances. Therapeutic use of radiogallium has resulted in disease conditions related to radioactivity. Of special interest is titanium. It is inert and resistant to corrosion and thus has been used widely in surgical and dental implants. It is present in trace amounts in a variety of foods of plant origin, and titanium dioxide has been used as a color additive because of its low toxicity.

References

Bondy, S. C. and Prasad, K. N. (1988) *Metal Neurotoxicity*. Boca Raton, FL: CRC Press.

Chiou, H. Y., Hsueh, Y. M., Liow, K. F. *et al.* (1995) Incidence of internal cancers and ingested inorganic arsenic: a seven-year follow-up study in Taiwan. *Cancer Res.* 55:1296–1300.

Chou, I. N. (1989) Distinct cytoskeletal injuries induced by As, Cd, Co, Cr, and Ni compounds. *Biomed. Environ. Sci.* 2:358–365.

Chowdhury, U. K., Biswas, B. K., and Chowdhury, R. T. *et al.* (2000) Groundwater arsenic contamination in Bangladesh and West Bengal. *Environ. Health Persp.* 108:393–397.

Clarkson, T. W. (1981) Dose–response relationships for adult and prenatal exposures to methyl mercury, in *Measurements of Risk*, G. G. Bery and H. D. Maillie (eds), New York, NY: Plenum Press, pp. 111–130.

Clarkson, T. W. (1987) Metal toxicity in the central nervous system. *Environ. Health Perspect.* 75:59–64.

Clarkson, T. W. (1991) Methyl mercury. *Funda. Appl. Toxicol.* 16:20–21.

Enterline, P. E., Henderson, V. L., and Marsh, G. M. (1987) Exposure to arsenic and respiratory cancer: a reanalysis. *Am. J. Epidemiol.* 125:929–938.

Ernhardt, C. B., Landa, B., and Schnell, N. B. (1981) Subclinical levels of lead and developmental deficits: a multivariate follow-up reassessment. *Pediatrics* 67:911–919.

Fowler, B. A., Abel, J., Elinder, C. G. *et al.* (1984) Structure, mechanism and toxicity, in *Changing Metal Cycles and Human Health*, J. Nriagu (ed.), New York, NY: Springer-Verlag.

Furst, A. (1987) Relationships of toxicological effects to chemical forms of inorganic compounds, in *Toxicology of Metals*, S. S. Brown and Y. Kodama (eds), Chichester, U.K.: Halstead Press.

Goering, P. L., Mistry, P., and Fowler, B. A. (1987) Mechanism of metal toxicity, in *Handbook of Toxicology*, T. J. Haley and W. O. Berndt (eds), New York, NY: Hemisphere.

Goldwater, L. J. (1972) *Mercury: A History of Quicksilver*. Baltimore, MD: York Press.

Goyer, R. A. (1996) Toxic effects of metals, in *Casarett and Doull's Toxicology*, C. D. Klaassen (ed.), New York, NY: McGraw-Hill, pp. 691–736.

IARC (1980) *Monograph on the Evaluation of the Carcinogenic Risks of Chemicals to Humans. Some Metals and Metallic Compounds*, vol. 23. Lyon, France: International Agency for Research on Cancer.

IARC (1994) *Monograph on the Evaluation of Risks to Humans. Cadmium, Mercury, Benyllium and the Glass Industry*, vol. 58. Lyons, France: International Agency for Research on Cancer.

Jaworski, J. K. (1978) *The Effects of Lead in the Canadian Environment*. Ottawa, Canada: National Research Council Canada.

Kipling, M. and Waterhause, J. (1967) Cadmium and prostatic carcinoma. *Lancet* i:730–731.

Kuschner, M. (1981) The carcinogenicity of beryllium. *Environ. Health Perspect.* 40:101–106.

Lauwerys, R. R., Roels, H. A., Poncket, J. P., Bernard, A., and Stanerscu, D. (1979) Investigations on the lung and kidney function in workers exposed to cadmium. *Environ. Health Perspect.* 28:137–146.

Maines, M. D. and Kappas, A. (1977) Metals as regulators of heme metabolism. *Science* 198:1215–1221.

Min, K. S., Nakatsubo, T., Fujita, Y., Onosaka, S., and Tanaka, K. (1992) Degradation of cadmium metallothionein *in vitro* by lysosomal proteases. *Toxicol. Appl. Pharmacol.* 113:299–305.

Nomiyama, K. (1980) Recent progress and perspectives in cadmium health effects studies. *Sci. Total Environ.* 14:199–232.

Pinto, S. S., Henderson, V., and Enterline, P. E. (1978) Mortality experience of arsenic exposed workers. *Arch. Environ. Health* 33:325–331.

Squibb, K. S. and Fowler, B. A. (1984) Intracellular metabolism of circulating cadmium–metallothionein in the kidney. *Environ. Health Perspect.* 54:31–35.

Sunderman, F. W., Jr. and Barber, A. M. (1988) Fingerloops, oncogenes and metals. *Ann. Clin. Lab. Sci.* 18:267–288.

Tseng, W. P. (1977) Effects and dose–response relationships of skin cancer and Blackfoot disease with arsenic. *Environ. Health Perspect.* 19:109–119.

Verschoor, M., Wibowo, A., Herber, R., Van Hammen, J., and Zielhuis, R. (1987) Influence of occupational low-level lead exposure on renal parameters. *Am. J. Ind. Med.* 12:341–351.

Viren, J. R. and Silvers, A. (1994) Unit risk estimates for airborne arsenic exposure: an updated view based on recent data from two copper smelter cohorts. *Regul. Toxicol. Pharmacol.* 20:125–138.

WHO (1972) *Evaluation of Certain Food Additives and the Contaminants Mercury, Lead and Cadmium*. Tech. Rep. Ser. 505. Geneva: World Health Organization.

WHO (1976) *Mercury*. Environmental Health Criteria 1. Geneva: World Health Organization.

WHO (1977) *Lead*. Environmental Health Criteria 3. Geneva: World Health Organization.

WHO (1979) *Ceramic Foodware Safety*. Document HCS/79.7. Geneva: World Health Organization.

WHO (1981) *Arsenic*. Environmental Health Criteria 18. Geneva: World Health Organization.

WHO (1987) *Selenium*. Environmental Health Criteria 58. Geneva: World Health Organization.

Xie, Y., Kondo, M., Koga, H., Miyamoto, H., and Chiba, M. (2001) Urinary porphyrins in patients with endemic chronic arsenic poisoning caused by burning coal in China. *Environ. Health Prevent. Med.* 5:180–185.

Yang, G., Wang, S., Zhou, R., and Sun, S. (1983) Endemic selenium intoxication of humans in China. *Am. J. Clin. Nutr.* 37:872–881.

Chapter 22

Over-the-counter preparations

CONTENTS

General remarks

Pharmaceutical agents required by law to be prescribed to patients are called prescription drugs. However, over the years there has been an escalating number of products available to treat various ailments for which a written prescription is not necessary. This latter group of compounds are termed over-the-counter (OTC) drugs. The OTC drugs are believed to be relatively safe and effective in the view of the general public simply because the regulatory agencies allow these drugs to be sold without medical advice. It is the popular belief that if a drug needs to be prescribed then it must be regulated, as there are inherent adverse effects. However, the public does not know that many of these OTC products have not undergone extensive clinical testing. Although it may be laudable to treat serious illnesses and make available the compounds that are prescribed and required for these purposes, one must question the trend toward easy access of an uneducated public to more OTC drugs that are self-administered and have not undergone proper testing.

It is safe to assume with respect to OTC drugs that the public:

i   is generally overwhelmed and confused by the wide array of products available;
ii   will probably use those that are most heavily advertised;

iii will use these drugs inadvertently and inappropriately in some cases; and

iv may be subjected to adverse effects.

(Kacew, 1999)

A paradox exists with respect to public awareness and drug use. De Jong-van den Berg *et al.* (1992, 1993) found increased awareness of adverse drug effects led to a decrease in the use of prescription drugs during pregnancy. However, because of the perception that OTC drugs are safe, there was a disproportionate rise in the quantity of OTC medications such as laxatives and vitamins which were self-administered. From an epidemiological point of view, the population most at risk for adverse effects from OTC drugs are children, resulting from absence of safety caps, attractive packages, administration of overdoses by parents, etc. It is worthwhile to note that Kacew (1992, 1997) clearly demonstrated that pharmacokinetics and pharmacodynamics are different between children and adults, which consequently was associated with differences in responsiveness to drugs. Thus, prediction of therapeutic effectiveness based on adult data can lead to grave consequences in the child (Kogan *et al.*, 1994; Smith and Kogan, 1997).

Prevalence in society

In 1989, the American public spent approximately $10 billion on an estimated 300,000 OTC products to medicate themselves for self-diagnosed ailments ranging from acne to warts, colds, headaches, upset stomach, constipation, etc. (Koda-Kimble, 1992). These 300,000 products represent about 700 active ingredients in various forms and combinations. It is thus apparent that many are no more than "me too" products advertised to the public in ways that suggest that there are significant differences between them. Almost $2 billion per year is spent by the American public on cough and cold remedies (Rosendahl, 1998). There are more than 800 OTC preparations for the common cold (Lowenstein and Parrino, 1987), over 100 for treatment of diarrhea (Dukes, 1990) over 200 different systemic analgesic products, almost all of which contain aspirin (acetylsalicylic acid), paracetamol (acetaminophen), salicylamide, phenacetin, ibuprofen or a combination of these agents as primary ingredients (Leist and Banwell, 1974). OTC drugs can be made different from one another in the following ways:

i the addition of questionable ingredients such as caffeine or antihistamines;

ii creation of an identity by brand names chosen to suggest a specific use of strength ("feminine pain," "arthritis," "maximum," "extra"); or

iii indication of their special dosage form (enteric-coated tablets, liquids, sustained-release products, powder, seltzers).

Hence, the consumer could utilize a product without the realization that an analgesic agent was being ingested (Kacew, 1994).

OTC preparations also contain excipients and/or inactive ingredients such as dyes, sweeteners, flavorings or preservatives. The so-called "hidden ingredients" in OTC products may on their own initiate adverse effects or potentiate the actions of the active components (Golightly et al., 1988; Kumar et al., 1993). The findings that excipients cause adverse effects, including skin disorders, gastrointestinal upset and cardiovascular abnormalities, clearly indicates that OTC drugs should not be used merely due to the improper perception of safety from adverse effects.

The enormity and severity of OTC drug usage in our society has received little, if any, attention. In addition to the economics, it has been estimated that 70% of illnesses, predominantly in the adult population, are treated with OTC agents (Knapp and Knapp, 1972; Conn, 1991; Chrischelles et al., 1992). However, of greater concern is the fact that 48% to 63% of children, a population known to be far more susceptible to drug-induced adverse effects (Lock and Kacew, 1988; Kacew, 1997) received OTC drugs during a two-week period (Dunnell and Cartwright, 1972; Kovar, 1994) and that approximately 40% of these children received at least two preparations (Kogan et al., 1994; Smith and Kogan, 1997).

It is worthwhile noting that during pregnancy, both mother and fetus are equally exposed to a chemical but the risk of fetal toxicity far exceeds that of the mother or neonate (Kacew, 1997, 1999). Hence, the presumption of safety for the mother cannot be applied with certainty to the fetus. The hair cream Le Kair contains estrogens (Koda-Kimble, 1992) and presumably, if used appropriately does not produce toxicity. However, there have been reports that the use of estrogenic cosmetics resulted in gynecomastia in the child (Kacew, 1999). Although a correlation between estrogenic OTC products and fetal toxicity has not been examined, it is known that estrogens are teratogenic (Lock and Kacew, 1988; Safe, 1998). It should be noted that various foods are estrogenic (Safe, 1998) and thus the combination of certain foods and OTC products may potentially affect fetal development. This latter scenario is further compounded as there are numerous environmental estrogenic contaminants to which a pregnant mother is inadvertently exposed on a daily basis (Shore et al., 1993). Since estrogens are lipophilic and accumulate in tissue fat, the potential for fetal exposure to excess estrogens is dependent on diet and environment. These compounds can certainly convert a relatively safe OTC into a toxic agent.

Adverse consequences

As a general rule, all drugs, including OTC preparations, should be avoided whenever possible. High risk subpopulations have been identified, including children and geriatrics. Of even greater risk is the use of OTC in pregnancy where the fetus is the target (Hays and Pagliaro, 1987; Karboski, 1992). Although it is falsely perceived that OTC preparations are virtually without any adverse fetal consequences, the reverse may be the case. Palatnick and Tenenbein (1998) recently reported a case of fetal death in a 17-year-old, 37-week-pregnant girl who had ingested aspirin daily for one month. Autopsy of the fetus revealed petechiae of lungs, heart, thymus, and kidneys. Clearly, the amount of aspirin taken was excessive but the drug was also readily available. Aspirin is not contraindicated for the treatment of headaches during pregnancy (Underhill, 1994), but it is stressed that aspirin and other nonsteroidal anti-inflammatory products should be avoided during the third trimester (Bonati et al., 1990; Koren et al., 1998). It is of interest that ingestion of aspirin during the first 20 weeks of gestation does not significantly affect IQ at four years of age (Klebanoff and Berendes, 1988). These confusing messages are relayed to the public with the recommendation that even though aspirin can be taken safely during pregnancy, paracetamol should be used as the drug of choice.

Under pressure from the pharmaceutical industry, a number of prescribed drugs have been switched to OTC status (Fletcher et al., 1995). Although the effects of the antidiarrheal agent loperamide on fetal outcome have not been established, administration of this drug to infants produced paralytic ileus and persistent drowsiness in 20% of cases (Motala et al., 1990). The recent inclusion of the antiulcerogenic histamine blocker cimetidine in the OTC list is a further example of a drug with potential effects on the fetus and easy public accessibility. The finding that cimetidine concentrations in neonatal plasma exceeded those in the mothers suggested that there was substantial uptake by the fetus (Somogi and Gugler, 1983). The fact that cimetidine is known to inhibit hepatic microsomal enzymes and was reported to produce fetal liver toxicity when used in late pregnancy (Glode et al., 1980) indicates that self-administration of this drug for reflux esophagitis during pregnancy could have adverse consequences. This could be of particular concern if a pregnant epileptic mother with impaired liver function were to ingest cimetidine; plasma concentrations of anticonvulsants would be increased, with adverse consequences for the fetus. In patients that are utilizing tricyclic antidepressants for treatment of depression, cimetidine potentiates the actions of the antidepressant resulting in cardiovascular abnormalities, hallucinations, vomiting, and hypotension. In the elderly, cimetidine causes confusion, which could have dire consequences as this population tends to be more forgetful.

A number of current OTC products are associated with adverse consequences. Industry has applied pressure to make certain drugs more accessible and, because of a presumed history of safety and the public perception that self-administered therapies will hasten recovery, even more compounds will be transferred from prescription to nonprescription status (Splinter *et al.*, 1997). Consequently, a larger assortment of OTC drugs will be available to the pregnant mother and geriatric populations. Indeed, Rubin *et al.* (1993) reported that OTC preparations were used 1.5 times more often than prescription drugs during pregnancy; this figure is presumably underestimated because they failed to include vitamins in their study. It is disturbing to note that approximately 50% of products taken during pregnancy are OTC medications (Rayburn *et al.*, 1982). With aging, there is also an increased use of drugs.

Clearly, some pregnant women are self-medicating themselves during a period of fetal vulnerability. Although it is stressed that pregnant women should not drink or smoke, these activities still occur during pregnancy. Indeed, the maternal characteristics associated with increased OTC medication use were Caucasian, smoking more than 20 cigarettes per day and drinking alcohol (Buitendijk and Bracken, 1991). Hence, it is likely that despite warnings to the contrary, pregnant women will also use OTC medications, the choice of which is expanding. An example of this problem arises with the use of imidazolines as topical vasoconstrictors for nasal decongestion. These compounds are used for sinusitis, colds, and allergic rhinitis and are known to produce CNS depression, bradycardia, hypotension and miosis (Liebelt and Shannon, 1993). There is a lack of clinical data regarding the use of these compounds in high risk subpopulations yet the potential for adverse effects is quite serious as these drugs produce vasoconstriction.

The misconception that frequent bowel movements are essential has resulted in the misuse of cathartics amongst some women, especially the geriatric populations. Saline cathartic magnesium sulfate induces hypotonia, CNS, and respiratory depression. Bulk forming laxatives can produce cramping, nausea, and result in fluid loss and electrolyte imbalance. In patients with congestive heart failure, this type of OTC product is contraindicated.

Ingestion of a proper diet is sufficient to provide the necessary requirement for vitamins and iron. However, the erroneous belief that vitamin supplements provide extra energy and create a feeling of "well-being" has resulted in the ingestion of quantities of vitamins vastly in excess of the recommended dietary allowance. This widespread nutritional self-medication promoted through effective massive advertising can have dire consequences in susceptible populations. Vitamin A in the fetus is associated with spontaneous abortion, hydrocephalus and cardiac anomalies, while in the adult there are menstrual irregularities, exophthalmos and skin hyperpigmentation. With vitamin D, hypercalcemia occurs in the adult and is manifested as anorexia, fatigue, kidney dysfunction, and aortic stenosis. In the fetus, hypervitaminosis D results in elfin facies mental retardation and aortic stenosis. Liver dysfunction, jaundice, and hemorrhage occur as a result of excessive vitamin K intake. Excessive iron intake results in vomiting, cyanosis, and circulatory collapse. In the fetus, there are congenital anomalies and gastrointestinal upset. This reiterates the fact that essential nutritional OTC in excess are not safe. The use of OTC mixtures of vitamins and minerals is not effective in abolishing iron deficiency anemia and this practice should be discouraged. Although there is an increased demand for iron in pregnancy, the prophylactic use of iron to correct any deficiency should be carried out with caution.

An issue which still remains to be considered is the interaction between two OTC preparations or between a prescribed medication and an OTC preparation. In a situation where a mother is being treated for a peptic ulcer with cimetidine, it is conceivable that there is simultaneous consumption of large quantities of tea (theophylline). Cimetidine, by preventing the metabolism of theophylline, results in increased theophylline concentrations and potentially a higher risk of toxicity. Aspirin displaces oral hypoglycemic agents from protein binding sites which can lead to severe manifestations in diabetes. Another example is the ingestion of iron to correct iron deficiency anemia. If the mother is ingesting iron plus a multivitamin preparation, the latter preparation interferes with iron absorption. Consequently, less iron is available and the hematological response is impaired.

The omnipresence of OTC preparations and concerted advertising may be a fact of life; however, increased awareness of the dangers associated with the use of self-medication must be stressed. Table 22.1 lists examples of OTC preparations that have been reported to cause adverse effects.

Table 22.1 Select OTC preparations: their adverse effects and susceptible populations

Susceptible populations	OTC preparation	Adverse effects
Pregnant women	Aspirin	Fetal death with internal hemorrhage
	Cimetidine	Liver toxicity
	Imidazolines	Mental depression, hypertension, miosis
	Vitamin A	Spontaneous abortion, hydrocephalus, cardiac anomalies
	Vitamin D	Mental retardation, hemorrhage
	Vitamin K	Liver dysfunction
Infants	Loperamide	Paralytic ileus, persistent drowsiness
Geriatrics	Saline laxatives	Hypotonia, CNS and respiratory depression
	Bulk laxatives	Cramping, nausea, fluid loss, electrolyte imbalance
General	Hyperglycemic drugs and aspirin	Aggravation of diabetes
	Multi-vitamin preparation + Fe	Interference of Fe absorption
	Cimetidine + tea	Cimetidine interferes with metabolism of theophylline

References

Bonati, M., Bortolus, R., Machetti, F. *et al.* (1990) Drug use in pregnancy: an overview of epidemiological (drug utilization) studies. *Eur. J. Clin. Pharmacol.* 38:325–328.

Buitendijk, S. and Bracken, M. B. (1991) Medication in early pregnancy: prevalence of use and relationship to maternal characteristics. *Am. J. Obstet. Gynecol.* 165:33–40.

Chrischelles, E. A., Foley, D. J., Wallace, R. B. *et al.* (1992) Use of medications by persons 65 and over; data from the established populations for epidemiologic studies of the elderly. *J. Gerontol.* 47:M137–144.

Conn, V. S. (1991) Older adults: factors that predict the use of over-the-counter medication. *J. Adv. Nurs.* 16:1190–1196.

De Jong-van den Berg, L. T. W., van den Berg, P. B., Haaijer-Ruskamp, F. M. *et al.* (1992) Handling of risk-bearing drugs during pregnancy: do we choose less risky alternatives? *Pharm. Weekbl. Sci.* 14:38–45.

De Jong-van den Berg, L. T. W., Waardenburg, C. M., Haaijer-Ruskamp, F. M. *et al.* (1993) Drug use in pregnancy: a comparative appraisal of data collecting methods. *Eur. J. Clin. Pharmacol.* 45:9–14.

Dukes, G. E. (1990) Over-the-counter antidiarrheal medications used for the self-treatment of acute non-specific diarrhea. *Am. J. Med.* 88:24S–26S.

Dunnell, K. and Cartwright, A. (eds) (1972) *Medicine Takers, Prescribers and Hoarders.* New York, NY: Routledge and Kegan Paul.

Fletcher, P., Stephen, R., and Du Pont, H. (1995) Benefit/risk considerations with respect to OTC descheduling of loperamide. *Arzeimittelforschung* 45:608–613.

Glode, G., Saccar, C. L., and Pereira, G. R. (1980) Cimetidine in pregnancy and apparent transient liver impairment in the newborn. *Am. J. Dis. Child* 134:87–88.

Golightly, L. K., Smolinske, S. S., Bennett, M. L. *et al.* (1998) Pharmaceutical excipients: adverse effects associated with "inactive" ingredients in drug products (part II). *Concepts Toxicol. Rev.* 3:209–240.

Hays, D. P. and Pagliaro, L. A. (1987) Human teratogens, in *Problems in Pediatric Drug Therapy*, L. A. Pagliaro and A. M. Pagliaro (eds), Hamilton, IL: Drug Intelligence Publications, 51–191.

Hill, L. M. and Kleinberg, F. (1984) Effects of drug and chemicals on the fetus and newborn. *Mayo Clin. Proc.* 59:707–716.

Kacew, S. (1992) General principles in pharmacology and toxicology applicable to children, in *Similarities and Differences Between Children and Adults*, P. S. Guzelian, C. J. Henry, and S. S. Olin (eds), Washington, DC: ILSI Press.

Kacew, S. (1994) Fetal consequences and risks attributed to the use of over-the-counter (OTC) preparations during pregnancy. *Int. J. Clin. Pharmacol. Ther.* 32:335–343.

Kacew, S. (1997) General principles in pediatric pharmacology and toxicology, in *Environmental Toxicology and Pharmacology of Human Development*, S. Kacew and G. H. Lambert (eds), Washington, DC: Taylor & Francis.

Kacew, S. (1999) Effect of over-the-counter drugs on the unborn child. *Pediatr. Drugs* 1:75–80.

Karboski, J. A. (1992) Medication selection for pregnant women. *Drug Ther.* 22:53–61.

Klebanoff, M. A. and Berendes, H. W. (1988) Aspirin exposure during the first 20 weeks of gestation and IQ at four years of age. *Teratology* 37:249–255.

Knapp, D. A. and Knapp, D. E. (1972) Decision-making and self-medication between medication and preliminary findings. *Am. J. Hosp. Pharm.* 29:1004–1012.

Koda-Kimble, M. A. (1992) Therapeutic and toxic potential of over-the-counter agents, in *Basic and Clinical Pharmacology*, B. G. Katzung (ed.), Norwalk, CT: Appleton and Lange.

Kogan, M. D., Pappas, G., Yu, S. M., and Kotelchuck, M. (1994) Over-the-counter medication use among preschool aged children in the United States. *J. Am. Med. Assoc.* 272:1025–1030.

Koren, G., Pastuszak, A., and Ito, S. (1998) Drugs in pregnancy. *New Engl. J. Med.* 338:1128–1137.

Kovar, M. G. (1994) Use of medications and vitamin–mineral supplements by children and youths. *Public Health Rep.* 100:470–473.

Kumar, A., Rawlings, R. D., and Bearman, DC (1993) The mystery ingredients: sweeteners, flavorings, dyes, and preservatives in analgesic/antipyretic, antihistamine/decongestant, liquid theophylline preparations. *Pediatrics* 91: 927–933.

Leist, E. R. and Banwell, J. G. (1974) Products containing aspirin. *N. Engl. J. Med.* 291:710–712.

Liebelt, E. L. and Shannon, M. (1993) Small doses, big problems: a selected review of highly toxic common medications. *Pediatr. Emerg. Care* 9:292–297.

Lock, S. and Kacew, S. (1988) General principles, in pediatric pharmacology and toxicology, in *Toxicologic and Pharmacologic Principles in Pediatrics*, S. Kacew and S. Lock (eds), Washington, DC: Hemisphere Publishing, pp. 1–15.

Lowenstein, S. R. and Parrino, T. A. (1987) Management of common cold. *Adv. Intern. Med.* 32:207–234.

Motala, C., Hill, I. D., Mann, M. D. *et al.* (1990) Effect of loperamide on stool output and duration of acute infectious diarrhea in infants. *J. Pediatr.* 117:467–471.

Palatnick, W. and Tenenbein, M. (1998) Aspirin poisoning during pregnancy: increased fetal sensitivity. *Am. J. Perinatol.* 15:39–41.

Rayburn, W., Wible-Kaut, J., and Bledsoe, P. (1982) Changing trends in drug use during pregnancy. *J. Reprod. Med.* 27:569–575.

Rosendahl, I. (1998) Expense of physician care spurs OTC, self-care market. *Drug Topics* 132:62–63.

Rubin, J. P., Ferencz, C., and Loffredo, C. (1993) Use of prescription and non-prescription drugs in pregnancy. *J. Clin. Epidemiol.* 46:581–589.

Safe, S. (1998) Dietary estrogens: an overview (abstract). *J. Toxicol. Sci.* 42:352.

Shore, L. S., Gurevitz, M., and Shemesh, M. (1993) Estrogen, an environmental pollutant. *Bull. Environ. Contam. Toxicol.* 51:361–366.

Smith, M. B. H. and Kogan, M. D. (1997) Over-the-counter medication use and toxicity in children, in *Environmental Toxicology and Pharmacology of Human Development*, S. Kacew and G. H. Lambert (eds), Washington, DC: Taylor & Francis.

Somogi, A. and Gugler, R. (1983) Clinical pharmacokinetics of cimetidine. *Clin. Pharmacokinet.* 8:463–495.

Splinter, M., Sagraves, R., Nightengale, B. *et al.* (1997) Prenatal use of medications by women giving birth at a university hospital. *South Med. J.* 90:498–502.

Underhill, R. (1994) OTC products (correspondence). *Pharm. J.* 253:112.

Chapter 23

Environmental pollutants

CONTENTS

General remarks

The environment consists of air, water and soil; biota is sometimes included as one of the environmental media. Toxic substances may originate from any one medium; however, they are generally transported to other media. Humans are exposed to environmental pollutants from a variety of pathways. Figure 23.1 illustrates the transportation of lead to humans, via air, water, food, dusts, etc. The lead that entered the human bodies is returned to the environment via excreta, refuse, dumps, incinerators, etc. Many other pollutants also have complex routes of environmental transport and affect humans. A number of more important pollutants are briefly described in this chapter.

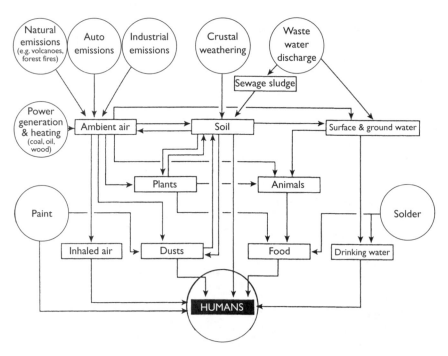

Figure 23.1 Environmental pathways of human exposure to lead.

Source: Risk Reduction Monograph No. 1, © OECD, 1993.

Air pollutants

Introduction

Past disasters

Several episodes of severe air pollution affecting the health and lives of large numbers of people have been reported. The notable ones occurred in Mense Valley, Belgium (December 1930); Donora, Pennsylvania (October 1948); London, England (December 1952); Los Angeles, California (August or September 1942, 1952, 1955); and Piscataway, New Jersey (September 1971). These episodes fell into two categories. One type occurred in winters, especially during the night, when domestic burning of coal was an important source of pollution, and the other occurred in summers, during daytime, when photooxidation of automobile exhaust was the major source of pollutants. In either case, the meteorological conditions, low wind and high barometric pressure, kept the pollutants at the ground level. The major effects were related to distress of respiratory and, to a lesser extent, cardiovascular systems. A number of deaths were reported, mainly from strains on preexisting diseases or deficiencies in these systems (Waldbott, 1978).

Current condition

As a result of these tragic events, measures have been taken to reduce the extent of air pollution. Nevertheless, the health problem remains, although somewhat abated. For example, Mar et al. (2000) reported that elevated levels of CO and NO_2 in Phoenix were associated with increased total non-accidental mortality, and increased cardiovascular mortality was associated with higher levels of CO, NO_2, SO_2 and PMs. Similar observations in other cities are cited in a review (Oehme et al., 1996).

The most important anthropogenic sources in many developed nations are automobiles. Other sources include combustion (coal, natural gas, fuel oil, incineration of refuse), metallurgical industry (see Chapter 21), and chemical industry (solvents, chemical intermediates, etc.).

Outdoor pollutants

Reducing-type of pollutants

COMPOSITION AND SOURCES

The major pollutants are sulfur oxides and suspended particulate matter. The former include sulfur dioxide, sulfuric acid, and sulfates; the latter includes finely divided solids and liquids. Particles of 0.1–10 μm in diameter settle very slowly, with a velocity of 8×10^{-7} to 3×10^{-3} m/s, while larger particles (1,000 μm in diameter) settle at a velocity of 3.9 m/s (Fuchs, 1964). Thus, particles smaller than 10 μm are suspended in air and are inhalable, as noted in Chapter 2.

The main sources of these pollutants are domestic burning of coal and other fuel for heating and cooking and industrial combustion of these fuels to generate energy. Smelting of ores also generates these and other pollutants.

TOXIC EFFECTS

SO_2 is very soluble, hence it is readily absorbed in the nose and upper respiratory tract, where it induces irritation. This is followed with thickening of the mucus layer in trachea and hypertrophy of goblet cells.

The irritation causes cough, expectoration, dyspnea, and bronchoconstriction. Respiratory functions are impaired, manifesting as decreased tidal volume, increased pulmonary resistance, and increased respiratory rate. Among exposed individuals, there is an increase of the incidence of respiratory tract infections, which may be attributable in part to an interference of the respiratory tract clearance mechanism. Under normal conditions, this mechanism is responsible for removing bacteria and other particles from the tract. Aerosols of sulfuric acid, formed from SO_3, are even more irritant than sulfur dioxide, which forms sulfurous acid (Costa and Amdur, 1996).

The effects of these sulfur pollutants are enhanced by the presence of suspended sulfur dioxide and smoke (suspended particulate matter) and can cause deaths, especially among the elderly and those with preexisting diseases of the respiratory tract and heart, as those in Belgium (1930), Pennsylvania (1948), and London (1952).

Even at lower concentrations (e.g. $SO_2 \geq 500$ μg/m^3 and smoke ≥ 500 μg/m^3), there is likely to be excess mortality among the elderly and the chronically sick. When exposure to these pollutants takes place at half of these concentrations, there is likely to be a worsening of existing respiratory disease (WHO, 1979).

Photochemical oxidants

COMPOSITION AND SOURCES

This group of air pollutants consists of nitrogen dioxide (NO_2), ozone, and a number of other oxides of nitrogen (N_2O, NO, NO_2, N_2O_3, N_2O_4, and N_2O_5). N_2O is the most abundant among these chemicals, but it is generated by anaerobic processes in the soil and in the surface layer of the oceans, and hence is not an important air pollutant, as far as human health is concerned. The last three oxides of nitrogen can be formed from NO and/or NO_2. However, their levels are very low and are not known to produce any harmful effects.

NO is the main oxide formed from man-made sources. However, after its discharge from the sources to the atmosphere, it reacts with O_2 to form NO_2. This reaction is facilitated in the presence of ozone.

Ozone is the most ubiquitous photochemical oxidant. At times, it constitutes as much as 90% of the oxidants in smog. Ozone is also a natural constituent of the upper atmosphere, formed by the photolysis of oxygen. Atmospheric circulation carries some to the lower levels.

The main sources of photochemical oxidants are automobiles and industrial combustion. Domestic heating and power stations also generate significant amounts. Ozone is also produced by a variety of high-voltage electrical equipment. Formaldehyde, which is one of the photochemical oxidants, will be discussed under "Indoor Air Pollutants" (below).

TOXIC EFFECTS

In contrast to CO_2, NO_2 is not very water soluble. It therefore passes through the upper respiratory tract to the terminal bronchioles and alveoli, where it forms nitric and nitrous acids. These acids are irritant and corrosive. Acute exposure causes pulmonary edema and congestion. It damages ciliated epithelium and type I cells (see Chapter 12), which are then replaced by the less sensitive nonciliated epithelial cells and cuboidal type II cells. Chronic exposure causes emphysema. Resistance to bacterial and viral infections is decreased (WHO, 1977).

After inhalation exposure, ozone reacts with organic matter in the respiratory tract. Similar to NO_2, its main effects are on the epithelial cells of the terminal bronchioles and alveoli, affecting the more susceptible ciliated epithelial cells and type I cells. The endothelia surrounding these structures are also damaged, resulting in pulmonary edema. Chronic exposure results in emphysema, atelectasis, focal necrosis, and sometimes bronchopneumonia. Resistance to bacterial and viral infection is decreased. Because of the oxidative activity of ozone, vitamin C decreases its toxicity whereas vitamin E deficiency has the opposite effect (WHO, 1978).

Apart from their toxic effects on the respiratory tract, these air pollutants also cause eye irritation (see Chapter 16).

Indoor air pollutants/"Sick Building Syndrome"

In recent years, the importance of indoor pollutants has become increasingly appreciated. The more efficient insulation of modern buildings, resulting in inadequate ventilation and in the use of certain insulation materials, has intensified the problem. Some of the more important pollutants and reactions are described below. Additional details are provided in articles by Karol (1991) and Samet (1993).

Formaldehyde

This organic chemical is a product of photooxidation of natural and man-made hydrocarbons. But it is more important as a component of urea formaldehyde foam insulation material, which has been widely used in mobile homes and, to a lesser extent, in conventional houses. Because of its volatility and toxicity, it has been a significant indoor air pollutant.

Formaldehyde is water soluble, and irritates the eyes, nose, and upper respiratory tract. At higher concentrations, it also affects the bronchioles and alveoli, and induces pulmonary edema and pneumonia. The dose–effect relationship is listed in Table 23.1. In addition, it has been reported to cause nasal cancers in rodents (Albert *et al.*, 1982). For a more detailed discussion on formaldehyde, see WHO (1989a).

Asbestos

Asbestos is a naturally occurring silicate fiber. Because of its heat and electrical insulation properties, it has been widely used in houses, ships, automobiles, etc. Workers in certain occupations are the main population at risk. However, the general public may also be exposed to it through the air and, to a lesser extent, the drinking water because it is used as a water filter (WHO, 1986).

After inhalation, it enters the alveoli and produces parenchymal asbestosis consisting of fibrosis and asbestos bodies. It may pierce the alveoli and

Table 23.1 Acute human health effects of formaldehyde at various concentrations

Reported effects (ppm)	Formaldehyde concentration
None reported	0.0–0.05
Neurophysiologic effects	0.05–1.5
Odor threshold	0.05–1.0
Eye irritation*	0.1–2.0
Upper airway irritation	0.10–25
Lower airway and pulmonary effects	5–30
Pulmonary edema, inflammation, pneumonia	50–100
Death	>100

Source: Adapted from NRC, Committee on Aldehydes (1981).

Note
*As measured by determination of optical chronaxy, electroencephalography, and sensitivity of dark-adapted eyes to light. The low concentration (0.01 ppm) was observed in the presence of other pollutants that may have been acting synergistically.

cause pleural asbestosis. It also causes lung carcinoma, the incidence of which is significantly higher among cigarette smokers (see Chapter 5). Mesothelioma is a rare type of malignant tumor. It may originate from the pleural and peritoneal surfaces after inhalation and ingestion respectively.

The asbestos fibrosis appears to result from its entering the cells (macrophages and lymphocytes) breaking the lysosomal membrane and releasing hydroxylases. It produces tumors either by carrying carcinogenic hydrocarbons into the body or by acting as cocarcinogen (Selikoff and Hammond, 1979).

CO, NO₂, SO₂ and suspended particle matters

These substances exist indoors as well as outdoors. In fact, this type of indoor air pollution may be more important than that which exists outdoors. This is because people in general spend more time indoors and because domestic heating may involve burning coal or other fuel without adequate ventilation, as shown by a study carried out under the sponsorship of WHO and the United Nations Environment Program (Wang *et al.*, 1988).

Others

Various volatile organic compounds are present in offices and homes, arising from paints, adhesives, cleaners, cosmetics, furnishings, and printed materials. In addition, there are many types of biological material such as bacteria, viruses, fungi, fungal spores, and dandruff. These substances may induce allergic reactions. The mixture of pollutants produces a gamet of reactions which has been named "Sick Building Syndrome." The common symptoms of this syndrome include irritation of eyes, nose and throat, headaches, fatigue, and nasal congestion (Samet *et al.*, 1988).

Water and soil pollutants

General considerations

Various pollutants are discharged into environmental media. Those that predominate in the air are described in the preceding section. Others are discharged in wastewater as effluent, or stored in dump sites. Generally these will contaminate both the water and soil.

Water and soil contaminants include pesticides and metals, which have been discussed in Chapters 21 and 22. Asbestos is also an important environmental pollutant. Its major health hazard is related to inhalation exposure as outlined in the preceding section. It is also present in water because of various mining, milling, and industrial uses as well as its use in filter pads for wine, beer, etc.

A great variety of organic chemicals, including some solvents and pesticides, have been detected in water, and most of these are present at extremely low levels. However, some of them are more persistent. In addition, a number of inorganic ions may also present health hazards. Both of these groups are described below (pp. 340–343). Drugs are released into water from human urine. Hormonal steroids are released into water from livestock and produce endocrine disruption.

Synthetic persistent chemicals

PCB

Polychlorinated biphenyls (PCB) are manufactured by the progressive chlorination of biphenyl. Commercial products are mixtures of biphenyl with a different degree of chlorine substitution. These products have a variety of uses in electric insulators, and rubber and paper industries, as plasticizers. It is stable, and hence persistent in the environment. Its levels in water range from 0.5 to 500 ppb, depending on the extent of contamination. It is lipophilic, and thus it bioaccumulates in aquatic organisms; fish caught from certain lakes containing 520 ppm PCB. Because of extreme persistence and toxicity, many nations have suspended or restricted its use. However, it will remain in the environment for a long time.

PCB, being lipophilic, is stored in adipose tissue and is secreted in milk. It is a potent inducer of microsomal enzymes. As a result, it enhances the metabolism of steroids such as estradiol and androsterone, a fact that may account for some of its effects on reproductive function. Because of this effect on enzymes, it can modify the toxicity of other chemicals and act as a promoter of carcinogenesis.

It has a variety of toxic effects in animals. For example, it induces hepatic adenoma and carcinoma. Among the *reproductive functions* affected are lengthened estrus cycles and decreased frequency of implanted ova in mice, lowered fertility in mink and rhesus monkey, and reduced hatchability of eggs in birds. On the *immune system*, it causes atrophy of lymphoid tissue in chickens and in rabbits. It suppresses a variety of humoral and cell-mediated immunity.

An outbreak of poisoning occurred in Japan in 1968, resulting from consumption of rice oil contaminated with PCB. It affected more than 1,000 people. The major clinical manifestations were chloracne hyperkeratosis and darkening of skin. Immunosuppression was also noted. Various subjective symptoms were reported, such as numbness of the limbs, coughing, expectoration, general fatigue, and eye discharge. There may also be an increase of liver and lung cancer among the male patients. Additional information and references to these topics are compiled in publications such as WHO (1993) and Japan–U.S. Joint Seminar (1985).

PBB

Polybrominated biphenyls are used as fire retardants. They gained notoriety because of a large-scale contamination of cattle feed in Michigan in 1973. The beef was contaminated with PBB (Fries, 1985). They are similar to PCB in many aspects, such as biotransformation, storage, and effects on reproduction, carcinogenesis, immune system, and skin (chloracne).

TCDD

2,3,7,8-Tetrachlorodibenzo-p-dioxin attracted wide attention after its accidental release from a factory in Seveso, Italy in 1976. While its level in water is low, it is important toxicologically because of its extreme potency. Furthermore, it is a contaminant of other chemicals, notably the herbicide 2,4,5-T, which was extensively used as a defoliant in Vietnam during the war there. It is extremely toxic, with LD_{50}s ranging from 0.0006 to 0.115 mg/kg in different species of animals (NRC, 1977).

TCDD is a potent inducer of microsomal enzymes, by binding to a specific receptor as described in Chapter 4. It is a potent carcinogen (2 ppb in rats), inducing cancers in a variety of organs such as liver, respiratory tract, and oral cavity (Kociba *et al.*, 1977). At somewhat higher doses, it is hepatotoxic, immunosuppressive, teratogenic, and fetotoxic. In humans, the predominant effect of TCDD is chloracne. It has not been reported to be carcinogenic in humans in spite of its extremely potent carcinogenicity in rats (Zack and Suskind, 1980; WHO, 1989b).

Other organic chemicals

Phthalate esters are extensively used in plastics, and are widely distributed in the environment, especially water. Their acute toxicity is low, but DEHP [di(2-ethylhexyl) phthalate] has been shown to be carcinogenic and to adversely affect reproductive functions in animals (Conference on Phthalates, 1982). *Trihalomethanes* are formed through the chlorination of water. These chemicals comprise chloroform, bromodichloromethane, dibromochloromethane, and bromoform. They are found in drinking water from less than 0.1 to 311 ppb. Among them, chloroform had the highest concentration. At high doses, these chemicals are hepatotoxic and may be carcinogenic (WHO, 2000).

Inorganic ions

Nitrates

The increase of nitrates in soil and water results mainly from intensive application of fertilizers, but also from wastes (excreta) of humans and farm animals. They are converted to nitrites in soil, water, and the G.I. tract through microbial action. Nitrites can induce methemoglobinemia, thus reducing the oxygen-carrying capacity of hemoglobin as noted in Chapter 4. Furthermore, they may react with certain amines to form nitrosamines, most of which are carcinogenic (Chapters 7 and 19).

Phosphates

These substances arise mainly from fertilizers and detergents. They have very low toxicity, but their presence in a body of stagnant water results in excessive growth of algae. The algae reduce the oxygenation of the water, resulting in fish kill. Certain "algae," the cyanobacteria, contain hepato-toxins and neurotoxins (see next section, pp. 342–343).

Fluoride

The natural level of fluoride in water varies greatly, depending on the location. Industrial activities may also raise its level. While fluoride has been added to water to about 1 ppm to reduce dental cavity formation, excessive levels in water (10 ppm) are likely to cause fluorosis. The enamel on the teeth is weakened, resulting in surface pitting. Changes in the bones, including osteosclerosis and exostoses, usually affect the spine and cause the knee deformity known as genu valgum. At lower levels of fluoride intake, chalky-white patches appear on the surface of the dental enamel. These patches are then stained yellow or brown and give rise to the characteristic "mottled" appearance (Dean, 1942).

Arsenic

In certain areas of Taiwan, South America, and Bangladesh, high levels of arsenic have been reported to be associated with a variety of skin lesions and possibly visceral cancers (see Chapter 21).

Cyanotoxins/eutrification

Eutrification occurs in lakes and ponds when there are excessive amounts of phosphorus. In general, this results from runoffs contaminated with fertilizers and detergents. Algae tend to thrive in such waters. Some of the algae produce cyanotoxins. There are two types of such toxins: one affects the nervous system and the other, the liver (Carmichael, 1997).

Neurotoxins

The most important among them is saxitoxin, also known as paralytic shellfish poison. Human exposure to saxitoxin is through consumption of contaminated shellfish. The toxin acts by blocking conduction of nerve impulse thereby inducing muscle paralysis (see Chapters 17 and 19).

Microcystins

The other type comprises microcystins and nodulins. These toxins are hepatotoxic to wild and domestic animals (Farrell, 1994). In an epidemiological study in several areas in China, Yu (1989) found a positive correlation between the use of surface water and high rates of primary liver cancer. Subsequently, Wang and Zhu (1996) showed that an extract of *microcystis aeruginosa* (a major species of cyanobacteria) promoted cell transformation of Syrian hamster embryo cells which had been exposed to a genotoxic carcinogen. It is thus evident that the extract is a carcinogen promoter. Carmichael (1997) has provided a comprehensive review of the literature on cyanotoxins. More recently, Gilroy *et al.* (2000) showed that a "health food product," made of blue-green algae, was contaminated with microcystins, more than 70% of the samples tested contained ≥ 1 mg/kg.

In 1996 in Caruaru, Brazil, 100 patients suffered acute liver failure from the use of partially treated municipal water for kidney dialysis. More than half of the patients died. The cause of the outbreak has now been attributed to certain cyanotoxins (Carmichael, 2001).

References

Albert, R. E. *et al.* (1982) Gaseous formaldehyde and hydrogen chloride induction of nasal cancer in the rat. *J. Natl. Cancer Inst.* 68:597–603.

Amdur, M. O. (1993) Air pollutants, in *Casarett and Doull's Toxicology*, M. O. Amdur, J. Doull, and C. D. Klaassen (eds), New York, NY: McGraw-Hill.

Brooks, B. O. and Davis, W. F. (1992) *Understanding Indoor Air Quality*. Boca Raton, FL: CRC Press.

Carmichael, W. W. (1997) *The Cyanotoxins*. Advances Botanical Res. 27:211–256.

Carmichael, W. W. (2001) Health effects of toxin producing cyanobacteria: "The Cyano HABs." 7:1393–1407.

Chiou, H. Y., Hsueh, Y. M., Liaw, K. F. *et al.* (1995) Incidence of internal cancers and ingested arsenic: a seven-year follow-up study in Taiwan. *Cancer Res.* 55:1296–1300.

Conferences on Phthalates (1982) Proceedings of the Conference. *Environ. Health Perspect.* 45:11–51.

Costa, D. L. and Amdur, M. O. (1996) Air pollution, in *Casarett and Doull's Toxicology*, C. D. Klaassen (ed.), New York, NY: McGraw-Hill, pp. 857–882.

Dean, H. T. (1942) The investigation of physiological effects by the epidemiological method. *Am. Assoc. Adv. Sci.* 19:23–31.

Ding, W. X., Shen, H. M., and Ong, C. N. (2000) Microcystic cyanobacteria extract induces cytosketal disruption and intracellular glutathione alteration in hepatocytes. *Environ. Health Persp.* 108:605–609.

Farrell, G. C. (1994) *Drug-induced Liver Diseases.* Edinburgh: Churchill Livingston.

Fries, G. F. (1985) The PBB episode in Michigan: an overall appraisal. *C.R.C. Crit. Rev. Toxicol.* 16:105–156.

Fuchs, N. A. (1964) *The Mechanisms of Aerosol.* Oxford: Pergamon Press, p. 28.

Gibson, J. E. (1983) *Formaldehyde.* Washington, DC: Hemisphere.

Gilroy, D. J., Kauffman, K. W., Hall, R. A. *et al.* (2000) Assessing potential health risks from microcystin toxins in blue-green algae dietary supplement. *Environ. Health Perspect.* 10:435–449.

Japan–U.S. Joint Seminar (1985) Toxicity of chlorinated biphenyls, dibenzhofurans, dibenzodioxins and related compounds. *Environ. Health Perspect.* 59:11–81.

Karol, M. H. (1991) Allergic reactions to indoor air pollutants. *Environ. Health Persp.* 95:45–51.

Kociba, R. J., Keyes, D. G., Beyer, J. E. *et al.* (1977) Results of a two-year chronic toxicity and oncogenicity study of 2,3,7,8-tetrachlorodibenzo-*p*-dioxin in rats. *Toxicol. Appl. Pharmacol.* 46:279–303.

Mar, T. F., Norris, G. A., Koenig, J. Q., and Larson, T. V. (2000) Associations between air pollution and mortality in Phoenix, 1995–1997. *Environ. Health Perspect.* 108:347–353.

NRC (1977) *Drinking Water and Health.* Washington, DC: National Research Council, National Academy of Sciences.

NRC, Committee on Aldehydes (1981) *Formaldehyde and Other Aldehydes.* Washington, DC: National Academy Press.

OECD (1993) *Risk Reduction Monograph No. 1: Lead Background and National Experience with Reducing Risk.* Paris: Organization for Economic Cooperation.

Oehme, F. W., Coppoch, R. W., Mostrom, M. S., and Khan, A. A. (1996) A review of the toxicology of air pollutants: toxicology of chemical mixtures. *Vet. Human Toxicol.* 38:371–377.

Samet, J. M. (1993) Indoor air pollution: a public health perspective. *Indoor Air* 3:219–226.

Samet, J. M., Marbury, M. C., and Spengler, J. D. (1988) Health effects and sources of indoor air pollution. Part II. *Am. Rev. Respir. Dis.* 137:221–242.

Selikoff, I. J. and Hammond, E. C. (1979) Health hazards of asbestos exposure. *Am. N.Y. Acad. Sci.* 330:1–814.

Waldbott, G. K. (1978) *Health Effects of Environmental Pollutants.* St. Louis, MO: C.V. Mosby.

Wang, H. B. and Zhu, H. G. (1996) Promoting activity of microcystins extracted from waterbloom in SHE cell transformation assay. *Biomed. Environ. Sci.* 9:46–51.

Wang, J. N., Cao, S. R., Li, Z., Zhang, Y., and Li, S. M. (1988) Human exposure to carbon monoxide and inhalable particulate in Beijing, China. *Biomed. Environ. Sci.* 1:5–12.

WHO (1964) *Seventh Report of the FAO/WHO Expert Committee on Food Additives.* Tech. Rep. Ser. 281. Geneva: World Health Organization.

WHO (1977) *Oxides of Nitrogen.* Environ. Health Criteria 4. Geneva: World Health Organization.

WHO (1978) *Photochemical Oxidants*. Environ. Health Criteria 7. Geneva: World Health Organization.

WHO (1979) *Sulfur Oxides and Suspended Particulate Matter*. Environ. Health Criteria 8. Geneva: World Health Organization.

WHO (1986) *Asbestos and Other Natural Mineral Fibers*. Environ. Health Criteria 53. Geneva: World Health Organization.

WHO (1989a) *Formaldehyde*. Environ. Health Criteria 89. Geneva: World Health Organization.

WHO (1989b) *Polychlorinated dibenzo-p-dioxins and dibenzoflurans*. Environ. Health Criteria 88. Geneva: World Health Organization.

WHO (1993) *Polychlorinated Biphenyls and Terphenyls*. Second Edition. Environ. Health Criteria 140. Geneva: World Health Organization.

WHO (2000) *Disinfectants and Disinfectant By-Products*. Environ. Health Criteria 216. Geneva: World Health Organization.

Yu, S. H. (1989) Drinking water and primary liver cancer, in *Primary Liver Cancer*, Y. Tang, M. C. Wu, and S. S. Xia (eds), Berlin: China Academic Publishers, Springer-Verlag.

Zack, J. A. and Suskind, R. R. (1980) The mortality experience of workers exposed to tetrachlorodibenzodioxin in a trichlorophenol process accident. *J. Occup. Med.* 22:1–114.

Chapter 24

Occupational toxicology

General remarks

As noted in previous chapters, humans are exposed to a variety of substances, by ingestion, inhalation, and dermal contact. Unlike the general populations, however, workers are often exposed to much higher levels of specific toxicants. Such exposures may well result in adverse effects. In fact, as early as 1775, Pott observed that chimney sweeps having been exposed to soot, developed cancer of the scrotum. Rehn discovered in 1895 that bladder tumors occurred among workers in aniline dye factories.

In the late nineteenth century, certain societal changes prompted the development of a variety of new occupations. One of the changes was the introduction of powerful machinery to facilitate many mining activities. While the machinery increased the output of mining, it also increased the airborne dusts to which miners were exposed.

Another major change was the invention of internal combustion machines, which increased air pollution from motor vehicles. To fuel these vehicles, large amounts of petroleum was produced. In fact, the excess petroleum became an excellent source of new chemicals. These petrochemicals, along with other raw materials, have found uses in the production of clothing, furniture, construction material, household and office commodities, as well as paints, pesticides, solvents, pharmaceuticals, etc. These and other changes in society increased the number of occupational workers as well as the variety of substances to which the workers are exposed.

Workers engaged in the production, processing or utilization of these substances are thus exposed to some chemical hazards. The severity of the adverse effects, however, depends not only on the nature of the substance but also on the level and duration of the exposure. Occupational toxicology is thus intended to assess the "permissible" levels of exposure, for a specified duration, to the toxicants encountered in workplaces. For the protection of the workers, the concentrations of the toxicants in the workplaces are to be maintained at or below their corresponding permissible levels. It should be noted that occupational exposure is not in a vacuum. A worker can be exposed to more than a single chemical, leading to mixture effects. Furthermore, a worker who smokes or drinks may be more susceptible than the non-smoking worker to the same chemical.

Exposure limits

Unlike food additives and most medications which, if too toxic, may be readily prohibited for use, occupational toxicants, in general, cannot be eliminated. To protect the health of occupational workers, permissible ("safe") limits of exposure are assessed.

Definitions

Permissible limits of exposure are existent in many countries. In the United States, a yearly booklet listing the threshold limit values (TLV) is published by the American Conference of Governmental Industrial Hygienists since 1946 (ACGIH, 2000). The limits refer to airborne concentrations of substances. They represent conditions under which "nearly all workers may be repeatedly exposed day after day without adverse effects." The list includes solvents, metals and their compounds, pesticides and others. There are three categories of TLV:

1   TLV-TWA (time-weighted average) refers to the time-weighted average concentration for a normal eight-hour workday and a 40-hour work week.
2   TLV-STEL (short-term exposure limit) refers to the short-term exposure limit to which workers may be exposed. It is defined as a 15-minute time-weighted average exposure. This limit is set mostly to avoid irritation and narcosis, but also to avoid chronic or irreversible tissue damage. The short-term exposure is acceptable provided that the TLV-TWA is not exceeded.
3   TLV-C refers to the ceiling that should not be exceeded during any part of the working exposure.

These limits are expressed in terms of ppm and/or milligrams per cubic meter. Since 1 mole of an ideal gas at 25 °C and 760 mm Hg occupies 24.45 liters, the following equation can be used to convert the limits: parts of vapor/million parts air (ppm) = (mg/m^3) × 24.45/(molecular weight of the solvents).

The Occupational Safety and Health Administration (OSHA) has published a list of "permissible exposure limits" (PELs) which are essentially similar to the TLVs of ACGIH. There are other occupational exposure limits such as the maximum allowable concentration (MAC). However, the TLVs published by ACGIH have been widely accepted, even outside of the U.S.A.

Scientific basis

The permissible levels of exposure are assessed on the basis of relevant test results in experimental animals as well as clinical observations and epidemiological studies in humans.

Tests in animals

These include the various types of tests described in previous chapters. However, with occupational toxicants, the major routes of exposure are the respiratory tract and the skin. After inhalation, gases and vapors may exert effects locally, and may also be absorbed. Large particulate matters and liquid droplets (>10 μm) do not enter the respiratory tract; very small particles (<0.01 μm) are likely to be exhaled. Those within the range of 0.01–10 μm may be absorbed from the respiratory tract and exert systemic effects and may also induce local effects, in the lungs.

Skin is relatively impermeable to most chemicals, but some may be absorbed in sufficient quantities to induce systemic effects. Some toxicants may cause local irritation and hypersensitization.

After absorption, a toxicant is distributed to various parts of the body. Depending on its nature, a small or large portion of it may be stored. In general, it is excreted as it is or after undergoing biotransformation. In general, this process renders the toxicant more water-soluble, hence more excretable. However, some chemicals undergo bioactivation and become more toxic. For additional information on bioactivation, see Chapter 3.

Although all organs and systems may be adversely affected by occupational toxicants, the most commonly affected targets, apart from the respiratory tract and skin, are the nervous system, the liver, and kidney. In addition, potential adverse effects on the immune system, reproductive function, and fetal development merit special attention.

Human data

To obtain relevant data from humans, a variety of studies may be used. The *case-controlled study* is generally used to unravel the etiology of a specific adverse effect. For example, Cole *et al.* (1972) observed a higher rate of lower urinary tract cancer among workers engaged in the manufacture of dyestuff, rubber, and leather. This observation provided a basis for further confirmatory studies.

Epidemiological studies are more elaborate, and usually provide more precise information. Prospective studies are usually carried out to confirm a suspected cause–effect relationship, and/or to provide more precise quantitative data. Retrospective studies involve analysis of clinical data obtained in exposed workers versus a group of unexposed cohort, matched for age, gender and such lifestyle as smoking and alcohol consumption.

Assessment of permissibility

With adequate and relevant animal and human data, a "No Observed Adverse Effect Level" (NOAEL) can generally be assessed. The permissible exposure level can be obtained by applying an appropriate "safety factor" to the NOAEL. A detailed description of the procedure used in Europe to assess the permissible levels of exposure to pesticides has been described by de Raat *et al.* (1997). Procedures used in the U.S.A., Canada, Germany, and the Czech Republic are outlined in a WHO document (WHO, 2000).

Occupational toxicants

Organic solvents

Solvents comprise a variety of organic chemicals such as aromatic hydro-carbons (e.g. chloroform, CCl_4), alcohols, or glycols and their ethers. These chemicals are used extensively in paints, inks, thinners, adhesives, pharmaceuticals, cosmetics, etc. Some solvents are used mainly for dry-cleaning clothes and degreasing machinery. Their manufacture and use in industry may pose health hazards to occupational workers. In addition, some of them become components of household products, thereby consti-tuting potential health hazards to the consumer. Their toxic effects are outlined below, and summarized along with their TLV-TWAs in Table 24.1.

Table 24.1 Toxic effects and TLV-TWAs of certain organic solvents

Organic solvents	Toxic effects	TWA, ppm
Benzene	Leukemia	0.5
Carbon disulfide	CNS, neuropathy	10
Carbon tetrachloride	Liver	5
Chloroform	CVS, liver, kidney CNS	10
Dioxane	Skin	20
n-hexane	Neuropathy, CNS irritation	50
Methanol	Neuropathy, vision CNS	200
Methyl n-butyl ketone	Neuropathy	5
Methylene chloride	CNS, anoxia	50
Toluene	CNS, skin	50
Trichloroethylene	CNS, liver	50

Source: ACGIH (2000).

General effects

Most of the solvents exert certain nonspecific effects. These include irritation at the site of contact, and depression of CNS.

IRRITATION

At room temperature solvents are in the liquid form. When they are in contact with skin, irritation may occur. As they are volatile, inhalation of their vapors may cause irritation of the respiratory tract, and they may also cause eye irritation.

CNS DEPRESSION

At sufficiently high levels of exposure, a consistent effect of solvents is CNS depression. The clinical manifestation begins with disorientation, giddiness, and euphoria. The last-named effect is responsible for abuse of some of these chemicals. The syndrome may progress to paralysis, unconsciousness, and convulsions. Death may ensue.

The mechanism of action is not clear, but well over half a century ago, Meyer (1937) observed that the narcosis (CNS depression) was related to the solubility of these substances in lipid and not related to their chemical structure, and hence suggested that narcosis resulted from CNS cell dysfunction following solubilizing of the solvents in the cell membrane.

INTERACTION

As noted above, most solvents may undergo biotransformation and may elevate the activities of cytochrome P-450 isozymes. Since solvents are often present in mixtures, interaction between them may occur. For example, a solvent, such as benzene, may potentiate the toxic effects of others by enhancing their bioactivation. On the other hand, the toxicity may also be decreased with certain mixtures. For example, toluene may reduce the toxicity of benzene by competitively inhibiting the bioactivation enzyme systems (Andrews *et al.*, 1977). These effects are dependent on normal liver function but become skewed in an alcoholic. The presence of drugs will also affect solvent biotransformation.

Specific effects

Apart from the general effects described above, a variety of specific effects may follow exposure to solvents. The diversity of these effects is a result of different reactive metabolites being formed. Some of the specific effects are described below.

LIVER

As noted in Chapter 13, ethanol is a common cause of fatty liver and liver cirrhosis. These effects likely result from the direct toxicity of ethanol plus nutritional deficiency commonly present among alcoholics. Various chlorinated hydrocarbons may cause a variety of liver damages. These include fatty liver as well as liver necrosis, cirrhosis, and cancer. The liver lesions are induced by reactive metabolites of these solvents. For example, the likely metabolite of carbon tetrachloride is tricholoromethyl radical, that of chloroform is phosgene, and those of halogenated aromatic hydrocarbons, such as bromobenzene, are their epoxides (Reid and Krishna, 1973). However, the recurrent cytotoxicity and chronic tissue regeneration may be the cause of the carcinogenicity.

KIDNEYS

As noted in Chapter 14, certain chlorinated hydrocarbons, such as chloroform and carbon tetrachloride, are nephrotoxic in addition to being hepatotoxic. At lower levels of exposure, the renal effects are related to tubular functions, such as glycosuria, amino aciduria, and polyuria. At higher levels, there may be cell death along with elevated BUN and anuria. In humans, CCl_4 affects mainly kidney when the route of exposure is inhalation, whereas liver is the major target organ when the chemical is ingested. Ethylene glycol is nephrotoxic because of its direct cytotoxicity as well as the blocking of the proximal tubules by the crystals of its metabolite, calcium oxalate.

NERVOUS SYSTEM

Apart from their effects on CNS, as noted above, aliphatic hydrocarbons and certain ketones such as n-hexane and methyl n-butyl ketone affect also the peripheral nervous system. The clinical manifestation of this polyneuropathy begins with numbness and paresthesia, as well as motor weakness of both hands and feet. These effects then involve both arms and legs. Pathologically it is characterized by distal axonopathy (Chapter 17). The reactive metabolite of these two solvents is 2,5-hexanedione (Krasavage et al., 1980).

HEMATOPOIETIC SYSTEM

Benzene is an outstanding example of a solvent affecting this system. It depresses bone marrow in animals and humans, thereby decreases the circulating erythrocytes, leukocytes, and thrombocytes. In humans exposed to benzene, leukemia has been reported (Infante et al., 1977; Goldstein, 1988).

CARCINOGENESIS

As noted above, a number of chlorinated hydrocarbons are known to produce liver tumors. Benzene is carcinogenic in animals and produces leukemia in humans. In addition, dioxane is also a liver carcinogen and has produced nasopharyngeal cancers (Andrews and Snyder, 1996).

Diethylene glycol induced bladder tumors in rats fed large doses of the solvent. In all the tumor-bearing rats, there were bladder stones that were composed of calcium oxalate, a metabolite of this chemical (Fitzhugh and Nelson, 1946). This solvent has thus been considered a secondary carcinogen (Chapter 7).

Other effects

Testicular degeneration and *cardiovascular (CV) abnormalities* have been observed in animals exposed to ethylene glycol monoethyl ether. Methanol may damage the *retina* through its metabolite and affect mainly the part that is responsible for central vision. Methylene chloride causes CNS depression and irritation to the eye and skin. However, it also induces *carboxyhemoglobinemia* because CO is formed in the biotransformation (WHO, 1984). Chloroform may induce *cardiac arrhythmia*, probably as a result of sensitization of the myocardium to epinephrine. This is one of the reasons why chloroform has been discontinued as a general anesthetic.

It should be noted that certain solvents are practically nontoxic. For example, propylene glycol has low toxicities, with LD_{50} values of 32 and 18 ml/kg in rats and rabbits, respectively, and rats fed this solvent at 1.8 ml/kg for two years showed no adverse effects. This chemical has thus been used as a food additive.

Metals

Metals are mined, smelted, refined, and processed for a great variety of uses. Workers are therefore exposed to metals and their compounds in many occupations. The target organs and the nature of toxicity, as described in Chapter 21, depend on the metal and its chemical form. For example, elemental mercury vapor produces excitability, tremor, and gingivitis. On the other hand, the divalent mercuric chloride is corrosive on contact, whereas the monovalent mercurous chloride causes dermal vasodilatation, hyperkeratosis, and hypersecretion of the sweat gland.

Table 24.2 lists the main toxic effects and/or target organs as well as the TLV-TWAs of a number of toxic metals. Additional details are provided in Chapter 21.

Table 24.2 Toxic effects and TLV-TWAs of toxic metals

Metals	Toxic effects	TWA, mg/m³
Arsenic	Cancer (lung, skin)	0.01
Beryllium	Cancer (lung), berylliosis	0.002
Cadmium	Cancer (lung, prostate), kidney lesions Metal fume fever	0.01
Chromium, metal and Cr. III	Skin, irritation	0.5
Cr VI, soluble	Cancer, liver, kidney	0.05
Cr VI, insoluble		0.01
Lead	CNS, GI, blood, kidney, reproduction	0.05
Mercury		
Alkyl	CNS	0.01
Aryl	CNS, neuropathy, eye, kidney	0.1
Inorganic and elemental	CNS, neuropathy, eye	0.025
Nickel, elements	Skin	1.5
Soluble compounds	CNS, skin	0.1
Insoluble compounds	Cancer (lung)	0.2

Source: ACGIH (2000).

Pesticides

Pesticides are widely used in agriculture and in public health programs to control vector-borne diseases. There are several types of pesticides, i.e. insecticides, herbicides, fungicides, rodenticides, and fumigants.

The organochlorine insecticides include aldrin, chlordane, DDT, lindane, and methoxychlor. Their major toxic effects are on the CNS and liver. The organophosphorus insecticides, such as azinphos-methyl, diazinon, malathion, methylparathion, and parathion, inhibit acetyl-cholinesterase (AChE). The inhibition of AChE in the central, peripheral, and autonomic nervous systems produces a variety of adverse effects, as described in Chapter 20. Carbaryl, a carbamate insecticide, also inhibits AChE, but its effects are short-lived.

The herbicides 2,4-D and diquat irritate the skin. Paraquat is stored in the lungs, hence it causes lung edema. The TLV-TWA for this chemical is therefore much lower. The fungicide thiram causes skin irritation and may disturb reproductive function.

Table 24.3 lists the main toxic effects and/or target organs as well as the TLV-TWA of the above-mentioned pesticides. Additional details on their toxicity are provided in Chapter 20. Their acute toxicity in humans is listed in Appendix 24.1.

Table 24.3 Toxic effects and TLV-TWAs of certain pesticides

Pesticides	Toxic effects	TWA, mg/m³
Aldrin	Liver	0.25
Azinphos-methyl	AChE inhibition	0.2
Carbaryl	AChE inhibition	0.5
Chlordane	CNS, liver lesion	0.5
2,4-D	Skin irritation	10
DDT	CNS, liver lesion	1
Diazinon	AChE inhibition	0.1
Diquat	Irritation of eye, skin	0.5
Lindane	CNS, liver lesion	0.5
Malathion	AChE inhibition	10
Methoxychlor	CNS, liver lesion	10
Methylparathion	AChE inhibition	0.2
Paraquat	Lung edema, kidney, liver	0.5
Parathion	AChE inhibition	0.1
Thiram	Skin irritation, reproduction	1

Source: ACGIH (2000).

Miscellaneous toxicants

Particulate matter

As noted above, particulate matter of sizes in the range of 0.01–10 μm are readily inhaled and exert adverse effects. A notable example is asbestos. It was widely used to provide thermal and acoustic insulation as well as fire protection, but causes pulmonary fibrosis (asbestosis), and cancers of the bronchus and mesotheliomas of the pleura and peritoneum (WHO, 1986). Its TLV-TWA is "1 fiber per cc" (ACGIH, 2000).

Other common particulate matter include coal dust, kaolin, silica, and talc. All these substances may induce pulmonary fibrosis. Coke oven emissions cause tracheobronchial cancers. Tobacco smoking enhances the toxic effects of particulate matters, such as asbestos (see Chapter 5) and cement dust (Table 24.4).

Table 24.4 Prevalence of respiratory symptoms in cement workers

Cement dust exposure	Smoking history	Prevalence of respiratory symptoms (%)	Ratio
−	−	1.6	1
−	+	3.3	2
+	−	9.0	5.6
+	+	11.7	7.3

Source: From Lu and Gu (1989), by permission of Academic Press.

Gases

A number of gases, such as CO, CO_2, NO_2, O_3, and SO_2 are encountered in certain occupational settings. But they also occur in the general environment, hence they are described in Chapter 23.

Plastics

There are many types of plastics. They are polymerized monomers, with molecular weights generally in the range of 10,000–1,000,000 daltons, hence inert and nontoxic. However, some monomers are toxic. For example, vinyl chloride has been reported to induce hepatic malignant tumors (angiosarcomas) among exposed workers, (e.g. Creech and Johnson, 1974). It may also cause cancer in the lung, skin and lymphatic and hematopoetic tissues (WHO, 1999). Acrylamide, unlike other monomers, is readily absorbed through the skin and may cause peripheral neurotoxicity. After absorption it releases cyanide and induces CNS toxicity (Drew, 1993).

Among the additives, the catalyst benzoyl peroxide was found to promote the cancer on mouse skin initiated by genotoxic carcinogen (Slaga et al., 1981). Phthalates, used as plasticizers, cause proliferation of peroxisomes, thereby act as nongenotoxic carcinogens (Rao and Reddy, 1987).

Toluene diisocyanate is used in the manufacture of flexible polyurethane foams, surface coatings, fibers, sealants, and adhesives. It is a strong irritant to the eye, skin, and especially the respiratory system, causing allergic asthma. There is an immunologic component in this syndrome with an increased immunoglobulin E (Karol et al., 1994).

Monitoring

To ensure that the specified permissible exposure limits are complied with, both the workplace and some workers are monitored.

Workplace monitoring

In general, using appropriate instruments, the air is monitored for concentrations of air-borne pollutants. These include gases, vapors, dusts (total, inhalable, and respirable), fibers, liquid droplets, and smokes. For details see, for example, Gray (1993).

Biological monitoring

Workers exposed to the same workplace environment may not be equally affected by, or even equally exposed to the toxicants. This is due to differences in age, gender, body build, diet, medication, disease state, etc. In addition, there are differences in work intensity and duration, temperature, humidity, co-exposure to other chemicals, etc. (ACGIH, 2000). ACGIH has therefore published a number of biological exposure indices. The commonly used methods involve monitoring of the exposure to the toxicants or their biological effects.

Effects

Inhibition of acetylcholinesterase in whole blood or plasma is a very sensitive indicator of exposure to organophophorus insecticides, such as parathion and methylparathion, and the carbamates, such as carbaryl.

Zinc protoporphyrin is a sensitive indicator of a minimal effect of lead. Carboxy-hemoglobin is an indicator of the effect of CO.

Exposure

The levels of lead and mercury in blood are good indicators of the extent of exposure to these metals. The level of mercury in urine is also useful. As the volume of urine varies greatly from day to day and between different individuals, the level of mercury in urine is expressed in terms of μg/g of creatinine, since a fairly constant amount of creatinine is excreted daily. The extent of exposure to benzene and carbon disulfide is also determined in urine and expressed in terms of μg/g of creatinine.

Another type of monitoring measures the biochemical reaction products, such as mercapturic acids (N-acetyl-L-cysteine S-conjugates) in wine. This procedure has shown to be useful in monitoring benzene, acrolein, acrylamide, acrylonitrile, trichloroethane, etc. (DeRooij et al., 1998).

References

ACGIH (2000) 2000 Threshold Limit Values for Chemical Substances and Biological Exposure Indices. Cincinnati, OH: Publications Office, American Conference of Governmental Industrial Hygienists.

Andrews, L. S., Lee, E. W., Witmer, C. M., Kocsis, J. J., and Snyder, R. (1977) Effect of toluene on metabolism, disposition, and hematopoietic toxicity of (^{3}H) benzene. Biochem. Pharmacol. 26:293–300.

Andrews, L. S. and Snyder, R. (1996) Toxic effects of solvents and vapors, in Casarett and Doull's Toxicology, C. D. Klaassen (ed.), New York, NY: McGraw-Hill.

Cole, P., Hoover, R., and Friedell, G. H. (1972) Occupation and cancer of the lower urinary tract. Cancer 29:1250.

Creech, J. L. and Johnson, M. N. (1974) Angiosarcoma of the liver in the manufacture of PVC. J. Occup. Med. 16:150–151.

DeRooij, B. M., Commandeur, J. N. M., and Vermeulen, N. P. E. (1998) Mercapturic acids as biomarkers of exposure to electrophilic chemicals: applications to environmental and industrial chemicals. *Biomarkers* 3:239–303.

Drew, R. (1993) Toxicity of plastics, in *Occupational Toxicology*, N. H. Stacey (ed.), London, U.K. and Bristol, PA: Taylor & Francis.

Ecobichon, D. J. (1999) *Occupational Hazards of Pesticide Exposure.* Philadelphia, PA: Taylor & Francis.

Fitzhugh, O. G. and Nelson, A. A. (1946) Comparison of the chronic toxicity of triethylene glycol with that of diethylene glycol. *J. Ind. Hyg. Toxicol.* 28:40–43.

Frankfelder, F. T., Coster, D. J., Drew, R. *et al.* (1990) Ocular injury induced by methylethyl ketone peroxide. *Am. J. Ophthalmol.* 110:635–640.

Furst, A. (1981) Bioassay of metals for carcinogenesis: whole animals. *Environ. Health Perspect.* 40:83–91.

Goldstein, B. D. (ed.) (1988) Benzene metabolism, toxicity and carcinogenesis. *Environ. Health Persp.* 82:3–307.

Gray, C. (1993) Occupational hygiene-interface with toxicology, in *Occupational Toxicology*, N. T. Stacey (ed.), London, U.K. and Bristol, PA: Taylor & Francis, pp. 269–293.

Infante, P. F., Wagoner, J. K., Rinsky, R. A., and Young, R. J. (1977) Leukemia in benzene workers. *Lancet* ii:76–79.

Karol, M. H., Tollerud, D. J., Campbell, T. P. *et al.* (1994) Predictive value of airways hyperresponsiveness and circulating IgE for identifying types of responses to tolerance diiso-cyanate inhalation challenge. *Am. J. Repir. Cont. Care Med.* 143:611–615.

Krasavage, W. J., O'Donoghue, J. L., DiVincenzo, G. D., and Terhaar, C. J. (1980) The relative neurotoxicity of methyl *n*-butyl ketone, *n*-hexane and their metabolites. *Toxicol. Appl. Pharmacol.* 52:433–441.

Levy, J. I., Hammitt, J. K., and Spengler, J. D. (2000) Estimating the mortality impacts of particulate matter: what can be learned from between-study variability. *Envir. Health Perspect.* 108:109–117.

Lu, P. L. and Gu, X. Q. (1989) New challenges for occupational health services facing economic reform in China. *Biomed. Environ. Sci.* 2:17–23.

Meyer, K. H. (1937) Contributions to the theory of narcosis. *Faraday Soc. Trans.* 33:1062–1064.

National Institute for Occupational Safety and Health (NIOSH) (1997) NIOSH Pocket Guide to Chemical Hazards. *DHHS (NIOSH) Publication.* No. 97–140. U.S. Government Printing Office, Washington, DC.

de Raat, W. K., Stevenson, H., Hakhert, B. C., and Van Hemmen, J. J. (1997) Toxicological risk assessment of worker exposure to pesticides. Some general principles. *Regul. Toxicol. Pharmacol.* 25:204–210.

Rao, M. S. and Reddy, J. K. (1987) Peroxisome proliferators and cancer: mechanisms and implications. *Carcinogenesis* 8:631–636.

Reid, W. D. and Krishna, G. (1973) Centrolobular hepatic necrosis related to covalent binding of metabolites of halogenated aromatic hydrocarbons. *Exp. Med. Pathol.* 18:80–99.

Slaga, T. W., Klein-Szanto, A. J. P., Triplett, L. L. *et al.* (1981) Skin promoting activity of benzoyl peroxide, a widely used free radical generating compound. *Science* 213:1023–1025.

Stacey, N. H. (1993) *Occupational Toxicology*. London, U.K. and Bristol, PA: Taylor & Francis.

WHO (1984) Methylene chloride. *Environ. Health Criteria 32*. Geneva: World Health Organization.

WHO (1986) Asbestos and other natural mineral fibers. *Environ. Health Criteria 53*. Geneva: World Health Organization.

WHO (1999) Vinyl chloride. *Environ. Health Criteria 215*. Geneva: World Health Organization.

WHO (2000) Human exposure assessment. *Environ. Health Criteria 214*. Geneva: World Health Organization.

Appendix 24.1 Acute pesticide toxicity, general signs and symptoms in humans

Pesticide	Symptoms and signs
Insecticides	
Organophosphates, Carbamates	*Mild*: Headache, dizziness, perspiration, lacrimation, salivation, blurred vision, tightness in chest, twitching of muscles in eyelids, lips, tongue, face. *Moderate*: Abdominal cramps, nausea, vomiting, diarrhea, bronchial hypersecretions, bradycardia or tachycardia, muscle (skeletal) spasms, tremors, general weakness. *Severe*: Pinpoint pupils, profuse sweating, urinary and/or fecal incontinence, mental confusion, pulmonary edema, respiratory difficulty, cyanosis, progressive cardiac and respiratory failure, unconsciousness leading to coma.
Organochlorines	*Mild*: Systemically, toxic action is confined to the central nervous system with stimulation resulting in dizziness, nausea, vomiting, headache, disorientation. *Moderate to severe*: Hyperexcitability, apprehension, weakness of skeletal muscles, incoordination, tremors, seizures, coma, and respiratory failure (progressive clinical findings related to severity of poisoning).
Pyrethroids	Generally of low toxicity but can cause irritation of oral and nasal mucosa. Some agents cause dermal tingling, stinging, or burning sensation followed by numbness (parethesia). Facial contamination results in lacrimation, pain, photophobia, congestion, and edema of eyelids and conjunctiva. Ingestion of large amounts may cause salivation, epigastric pain, nausea, vomiting, headache, dizziness, fatigue, coarse muscular twitching in limbs, convulsive seizures, loss of consciousness.

(continued)

Appendix 24.1 (continued)

Pesticide	Symptoms and signs
Herbicides Bipyridyls	Irritation of nose and throat, hemorrhage, eye irritation with conjunctivitis and corneal stripping, skin irritation, dermatitis. Ingestion results in initial signs of ulceration of tongue, throat, and esophagus; sternal and abdominal pain; general muscular pain; vomiting; and diarrhea. After 48 to 72 h, signs of renal and hepatic damage (oliguria, jaundice), respiratory difficulty (cough, dyspnea, tachypnea, pulmonary edema), and progressive respiratory failure.
Phenoxyacids Ureas Triazines Chloroaliphatics Arylcarbamates	Generally of low toxicity but, during handling, may cause irritation of eye, nose, throat, and skin. Ingestion may cause gastroenteritis, nausea, vomiting, diarrhea. Respiratory symptoms include burning sensation, cough, chest pain. Muscle weakness and muscle twitching may be encountered, and central nervous system signs include dizziness, weakness, anorexia, and lethargy.
Fungicides Dithiocarbamates Phenolics Chlorobenzenes Benzimidazoles Thiophanates	Generally of low toxicity but local contamination of skin may cause itching, rash, and dermatitis. Ingestion of large amounts may cause nausea, vomiting, diarrhea, and muscle weakness. The dithiocarbomates exert a disulfiram-like effect in the presence of alcohol, causing flushing, sweating, dyspnea, hyperpnea, chest pains, hypotension.
Rodenticides Fluorinated agents Zinc phosphide Strychnine α-Naphthylthiourea Anticoagulants	Accidental rodenticide poisoning is difficult to achieve because agents are packaged as baits attractive only to the pest. When ingested, these agents may cause nausea, vomiting, intestinal cramps, diarrhea, excitation, abnormal cardiac rhythms, muscle spasms, seizures. The anticoagulants require laboratory assessment of coagulation status and treatment with vitamin K_1.

Source: Ecobichon (1999).

Chapter 25

Toxicologic evaluation

Assessment of safety/risk

CONTENTS

Introduction

Importance and reasonableness

Descriptions in prior chapters make it abundantly clear that chemicals differ greatly in the nature and potency of their toxicity. Since human exposure to chemicals is not always avoidable (it may even be desirable in certain cases), toxicological evaluation of many chemicals must be carried out to determine the level of exposure (or intake in the case of food and water) under which no risk is likely to occur. A comprehensive review by Paustenbach (2000) covers risk assessment. Because of the gaps in our knowledge, it is prudent to be conservative in assessing the safety/risk. But when undue caution is incorporated into the process, the public may be denied chemicals of great value and society may be burdened with unnecessary economic costs, such as pollution prevention measures and environmental clean-up. Therefore the most important function of toxicology is to establish the scientific basis for regulating the use (and disposal) of chemicals without undue human health hazards or undue cost.

Historical development

Around the turn of the century, industrialization and urbanization prompted people to move from their farms to cities. Away from the farm, they had to consume stored and processed food. Food adulteration became a serious problem. In the United States, the first U.S. Food and Drug Act was enacted in 1906. Similar action was taken in several other countries. At that time, health hazards were based essentially on *qualitative* assessment; the mere presence of a toxic substance in food was considered adulteration, and "adulterated" food was banned outright.

To permit judicious use of food additives, Lehman and Fitzhugh of the U.S. Food and Drug Administration initiated in 1954 *quantitative* assessment by the use of a "100-fold margin of safety" approach. This assessment of food additives stipulated that "the chemical additive should not occur in the total human diet in a quantity greater than 1/100 of the amount that is the maximum safe dosage in long-term animal experiments" (Lehman and Fitzhugh, 1954).

While this margin of 100 seemed reasonable for food additives, it could not be applied to other chemicals, such as contaminants and pesticide residues, whose levels in food are not readily controllable. Furthermore, it would be impracticable on an international level: there would be marked differences among nations, both in dietary pattern and technological usage. The Joint FAO/WHO Expert Committee on Food Additives therefore coined, in 1961, the term *Acceptable Daily Intake* (ADI). Later that year, this term was adopted by the Joint FAO/WHO Meeting on Pesticide Residues.

In 1977, the U.S. National Research Council (NRC) extended the concept to the assessment of contaminants in water, and EPA extended it to pollutants in air, with slight variation in the terminology.

In carcinogenic chemicals the Delaney Amendment of 1958 to the Federal Food, Drug and Cosmetic Act stipulates that any chemical that has been shown to be carcinogenic in man or animal shall not be used as a food additive. For other chemicals such as veterinary drugs the concept of "negligible residues" were introduced to regulate carcinogenic chemicals. As will be seen in subsequent sections, these measures were no panacea. Mathematical models were then devised to estimate doses that could be considered as "virtually safe" (Mantel and Bryan, 1961).

NRC (1983) divided the management of risk assessment into the following steps:

1 *Hazard identification*, scrutinizing all relevant toxicological and related data to identify the hazard associated with a chemical.
2 *Dose–response assessment*, determining the relationship between the magnitude of the exposure and the probability of health effects.
3 *Exposure assessment*, determining the extent of human exposure.
4 *Risk characterization*, estimating the nature and magnitude of human risk, and the uncertainty of the estimate.

Major approaches

At high enough doses, all chemicals exhibit toxic effects. As the dose is reduced, the severity of the effects as well as the responses diminish. For a majority of the chemicals, there are threshold doses below which they will not elicit adverse effects. There are a variety of reasons for the thresholds. The chemical in question may not reach the site of action because of its limited absorption and distribution or its prompt elimination. Metabolic detoxication often plays an important role. Furthermore, repair and regeneration of affected cells and excess functional capacity may overcome/compensate any minor, temporary effects.

The "safety" of such chemicals can be estimated using the "Acceptable Daily Intake" approach, which involves identification of the most sensitive, yet *appropriate*, indicator of adverse effect and the application of a suitable safety factor to the no-observed-adverse-effect level to compensate for potential differences between animals and humans, and between the relatively small number of test subjects and the large human population which are more heterogeneous.

Genotoxic carcinogens, on the other hand, probably have no threshold doses. The rationale is that a cancer cell can be induced by a single change in the cellular genetic material, and the cancer cell has the capacity of self-replicating. Therefore, theoretically, a single molecule of such a chemical can induce a cancer. In the absence of threshold doses, it would be impossible to identify a no adverse effect level, thus rendering the ADI approach impracticable. Mathematical models have been designed to estimate, from the dose–response relationship and a variety of assumptions, a "virtually safe dose," exposure to which would result in an extremely small risk, say 10^{-6} (one risk in a million).

Acceptable daily intake (ADI/RfD)/safety assessment

Definition and usage

As has already been noted, the term *acceptable daily intake* (ADI) was coined by the Joint FAO/WHO Expert Committee on Food Additives in 1961 (WHO, 1962a). It has been adopted by the Joint FAO/WHO Meeting of Experts on Pesticide Residues (WHO, 1962b). This term has been used at all subsequent meetings of these two international expert bodies in their toxicologic evaluation, and reevaluation, of large numbers of food additives and pesticides that leave residues in food. The term has also been adopted by a number of other bodies in the toxicological evaluation of chemicals in food, water, etc., as a basis for setting standards, e.g. U.S. EPA (Cotruvos, 1988).

ADI is defined as "the daily intake of a chemical which, during an entire lifetime, appears to be without appreciable risk on the basis of all the known facts at the time." It is expressed in milligrams of the chemical per kilogram of body weight (mg/kg). It is worth noting that the ADI is qualified by the expressions "appear to be" and "on the basis of all the known facts at the time." This caution is in keeping with the fact that it is impossible to be absolutely certain about the safety of a chemical and that the ADI may be altered in the light of new toxicologic data.

Toxicologic evaluations of food additives and pesticides, in terms of ADIs by these international expert bodies, have been used by the regulatory agencies in many countries as an important consideration in the formulation of national regulations. ADIs have also been used collectively by national authorities in the framework of the Codex Alimentarius Commission. The Commission is an intergovernmental body with more than

150 countries as members. Its principal function is to elaborate international food standards for the protection of the health of the consumer and to facilitate international food trade. These food standards contain provisions for food additives that are accepted by the Commission only when ADIs have been allocated by the Expert Committee on Food Additives. The latter goal is achieved through the removal of "non-economic" trade barriers based on unjustified claims of health hazards alleged to be associated with certain additives or pesticides. Additional details about the Codex Alimentarius Commission are given in an article by Lu (1988). The close relationship between the Commission, member governments, academia, and industry are shown in Figure 25.3.

There are a number of variations of the terminology. For instance, in dealing with food contaminants, the Joint FAO/WHO Expert Committee on Food Additives in 1972 coined the term "Provisional Tolerable Weekly Intake." The procedure used in arriving at such intakes is identical to that for ADIs. The Committee, however, felt that, unlike food additives which serve certain useful purposes, contaminants do not. Therefore they are not acceptable but merely "tolerable." Furthermore, the intakes were expressed in terms of "weekly" because the contaminants dealt then (mercury, lead, and cadmium) are cumulative, and vary (especially mercury) in the *daily* intake, but less so on a *weekly* basis.

Another variation is used by U.S. EPA which assesses "Reference Doses" (RfD) instead of ADIs, using essentially the same procedure, except that the safety factor is called "uncertainty factor." It might be noted that the term ADI is widely used on an international level as well as by regulatory agencies in many nations, including U.S. FDA.

Procedures for estimating ADIs

The following steps are involved in estimating ADIs:

Collection of adequate relevant data

As noted in previous chapters, chemicals possess different toxicity. Consequently a great variety of toxicity studies must be done (see Chapter 19). Furthermore, pharmacokinetic studies facilitate the assessment of the effects on humans from findings obtained in experimental animals. In addition, the data must be obtained from *relevant* studies. For example, findings of epithelial hyperplasia in the forestomach of rats given an irritant fumigant by gavage have little, if any, bearing on the possible adverse effects on humans consuming food that has been fumigated by the fumigant (see Lu and Coulston, 1996).

The assessment of certain chemicals required less data for establishing their ADIs. Examples are food additives obtained from edible animals, plants, and microbes. The extent of testing and the reasons thereof have been described by WHO (1987).

No-observed-adverse-effect level (NOAEL)

This is the maximum dose level that has not induced any sign of toxicity (adverse effect) in the most susceptible but appropriate species of animals tested, and using the most sensitive indicator of toxicity. As a rule, this level is selected from a long-term study. However, certain signs of toxicity, such as cataract, delayed neurotoxicity, and effects on reproduction, are demonstrable in short-term studies. The NOAEL is not necessarily an absolutely no-effect level; rather it is a "no-observed-adverse-effect-level," because the use of a more sensitive indicator of toxicity or a more suscept-ible animal species may reveal a lower NOAEL. Hence these chemicals are re-assessed whenever significant new toxicologic data become available. In addition, an effect might well be demonstrable if a sufficiently large number of animals were used in the tests. However, using experimental data and mathematical extrapolation, Lu (1985) and Lu and Sielken (1991) showed that increasing the number of animals would only reduce the NOAEL slightly. It should also be noted that part of the safety factor is intended to compensate for the limited number used in most tests.

On the other hand, certain effects are generally considered as physio-logic, adaptive, or otherwise "nontoxic." These effects are therefore excluded in establishing the NOAEL. For example, liver enlargement may result from stimulation in the activity of hepatic mixed-function oxidases and the *de novo* protein synthesis in the smooth endoplasmic reticulum. A decrease of body weight may follow reduced food consumption, which in turn may be a result of unpalatability of the chemical. Feeding large amounts of inert substances such as mannitol and cellulose derivatives may cause diarrhea and malnutrition. However, before disregarding these effects in evaluating the toxicity of a chemical, care must be taken to ensure that these are not manifestations of toxicity. Additional studies may have to be done to elucidate the nature of the effect. These various points have been elaborated in several WHO reports and summarized in a review article (Lu, 1988).

Safety factors

To extrapolate from the NOAEL in animals to an acceptable intake in humans, a safety factor of 100, originally proposed by Lehman and Fitzhugh (1954), is generally used. This factor is intended to allow for dif-ferences in sensitivity of the animal species and humans, to allow for wide variations in susceptibility among the human population, and to allow for the fact that the number of animals tested is small compared to the size of the human population that may be exposed (WHO, 1958, 1974a; Food Safety Council, 1973).

While the factor 100 is often used, the WHO expert committees have used figures that ranged from 10 to 2,000. The size of the safety factor is determined according to the nature of the toxicity. In addition, a larger figure is used to compensate for slight deficiencies in toxicity data, such as relatively small numbers of animals on test. On the other hand, minimal, reversible, and inconsequential effects such as slight inhibition of acetyl-cholinesterase by an organophosphorus pesticide may justify the use of a smaller safety factor. In addition, available human data may warrant the use of a smaller figure, i.e. 10, since they obviate the need for interspecies extrapolation.

Biochemical data relating to the absorption, distribution, and excretion of the toxicant and its biotransformation (detoxication and bioactivation) in various species of animals and in humans are often useful in determining the size of the safety factor. These and other bases for altering the safety factor are elaborated in two WHO documents (WHO, 1987, 1990). The reasons for the use of different safety factors by WHO in the evaluation/reevaluation of the 230 pesticides in the past three decades are noted and explained in a recent review (Lu, 1995).

Some toxicologists prefer the use of individual uncertainty (safety) factors in extrapolating from a NOAEL to the corresponding reference dose (RfD). These usually include a factor of 10 for intraspecies differences, a 10 for interspecies differences, a 10 for NOAEL derived from short-term toxicity studies, etc. (Dourson and Stara, 1983).

Assessment of exposure acceptability

The ADI is used as a yardstick to check the acceptability of the proposed uses. This is done by comparing the ADI with the "potential daily intake" (PDI). PDI is the sum of the products of the amounts of the food (calculated on the basis of the average per capita consumption) and the permitted use levels of the additives in them.

$$PDI = (F_1 \times L_1) + (F_2 \times L_2) + (F_3 \times L_3) \ldots$$

$F_1, F_2, F_3 \ldots$ = per capita consumption of food commodities

$L_1, L_2, L_3 \ldots$ = use levels of food additives or maximum residue levels of pesticide residues or other contaminants

If the potential daily intake exceeds the ADI, the use levels may be lowered or some of the uses may be deleted. The Commission follows the same procedure in accepting the maximum limits for pesticide residues in food. The use of the "potential daily intake" and other estimated intakes by WHO in assessing the acceptability of food additives and pesticides is provided in some detail in a WHO document (1989), and summarized by Lu and Sielken (1991).

Margin of safety

The ADI approach is not designed to provide quantitative information on the risks involved at intakes higher than the ADI. This is because of the wide "gray area" between the NOAEL and the ADI. However, the margin of safety between the estimated intake and the ADI, is sometimes used to indicate the degree of confidence in the safety at a specified intake.

Mathematical models/risk assessment

As discussed in Chapter 7, there are genotoxic and nongenotoxic carcinogens. It is generally agreed that there are probably no thresholds for genotoxic carcinogens. In view of the theoretical absence of threshold doses and in the absence of a reliable procedure to determine a threshold for a carcinogen for an entire population, estimating the levels of risk has been considered to be more appropriate.

Estimation of risks

Definition

Risk has been defined as the expected frequency of undesirable effects arising from exposure to a pollutant. It may be expressed in absolute terms as the risk due to exposure to a specific pollutant. It may also be expressed as a relative risk, which is the ratio of the risk among the exposed population to that among the unexposed (WHO, 1978).

The term was first adopted by the International Commission on Radiological Protection (ICRP, 1966) in evaluating the health hazards related to ionizing radiation. The use of this term stems from the realization that often a clear-cut "safe" or "unsafe" decision cannot be made.

Risks levels and virtual safety

Estimation of risks involves development of suitable dose–response data and extrapolation from the observed dose–response relationship to the expected responses at doses occurring at actual exposure situations. A number of mathematical models have been proposed for this purpose. Such models are also used to estimate the dose that is expected to be associated with a specific level of risk.

Mantel and Bryan (1961) first introduced the concept of virtual safety. The

Table 25.1 Estimated risks for certain activities and natural occurrences

Activity	Risk*
Smoking (10 cigarettes/day)	1/400
All accidents	1/2,000
Driving (16,000 km/year)	1/5,000
All traffic accidents	1/8,000
Work in industry	1/30,000
Natural disasters	1/50,000
Being struck by lightning	1/1,000,000

Source: Adapted from Royal Commission on the Environment, 1976. By permission of the Controller of Her Majesty's Stationery Office, London.

Note
*Risk is expressed as probability of death of an individual for a year of exposure and is given in round figures.

term was defined as a probability of carcinogenicity of less than 1/100 million (10^{-8}) at a statistical assurance level of 99%. The U.S. Food and Drug Administration, however, found that the doses associated with such a low risk level were too small to be enforceable in most actual situations and thus adopted a risk level of 10^{-6} (FDA, 1977). These levels of risk are so low that the doses associated with them are referred to as virtually safe doses (VSD).

Commonplace activities and their risks

In order to place the risk levels in perspective, risks associated with certain commonplace activities and natural occurrences are sometimes cited. Table 25.1 includes a number of estimates of such risks. The risks in Table 25.1, apart from lightning, are considerably greater than 10^{-6}. Estimates of risks associated with other common activities and occupations have been compiled by others, for example, Wilson (1980).

The acceptability of a risk depends on, apart from its magnitude, the nature of the activity. In general, risks associated with voluntary, pleasurable, and/or beneficial activities, such as smoking and driving, are more acceptable to the individual. On the other hand, risks associated with activities that are perceived as having no benefit and those that are not controllable by the individual tend to be rejected, such as food colors suspected of being carcinogenic.

Models for estimating risk/VSD

A number of mathematical models have been developed for the purpose of estimating risk. In general, they involve extrapolating from the observed dose response to either of the following:

1   The risks at a specific exposure level.
2   The "risk specified dose" (RSD) is the dose associated with a specified risk. When the specified risk is low enough, e.g. 10^{-5} or 10^{-6}, the dose associated with it is generally known as the virtually safe dose (VSD).

Probability models

As noted above, Mantel and Bryan (1961) first introduced the concept of virtual safety, and developed a model based on the assumption that the responses (tumor formation) will be the same as most other quantal (all-or-none) toxicologic responses, namely, normally distributed among the subjects.

This S-shaped dose–response curve can be straightened, as described in Chapter 6, by plotting the points on a *probit* basis. Variations of this probit model include *logit and Weibull*. These are also known as "tolerance models," as they are based on the probability of individuals in a population whose tolerances to the carcinogen will be exceeded.

Mechanistic models

Several other models have been designed based on presumed mechanisms of action of carcinogenesis. The *one-hit* model assumes that a critical hit in a cell by a carcinogen may induce a cancer through initiation, promotion, and progression. On the other hand, the *multihit* model assumes that several hits are required for a response to occur. The *multistage* model is built on the assumption that the induction of a carcinogenic response follows random biological events, the time rate of occurrence of each event being in linear proportion to the dose rate.

The conservativeness of these models is achieved through the use of upper confidence limits to responses on the risk estimated, shallow slopes, or the lower confidence limits on the VSD estimated. Figure 25.1 shows the observed responses, the upper confidence limit, and the linear interpolation.

Several U.S. regulatory agencies, including EPA (1986), use the linearized multistage model (Anderson, 1986). With this model, it is presumed that no threshold dose exists, a multistage process is involved in chemical carcinogenesis, and the time rate of occurrence of each event is linearly proportional to the dose.

Based on a set of aflatoxin B_1 carcinogenesis data, low-dose extrapolation was done with various models. The marked difference among them is clearly visible in Figure 25.2. The one-hit and multistage models yielded the most conservative estimates, whereas the probit model yield the least conservative figure. According to the calculations of the Food Safety Council (1980), the VSDs at a risk of 10^{-6} are 3.4×10^{-5} ppb (one-hit),

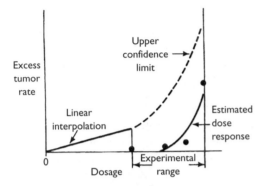

Figure 25.1 Linear extrapolation showing the observed responses, the upper confidence limit of the response at the lowest experimental dose, and the linear interpolation.

Source: Gaylor and Kodell, 1980.

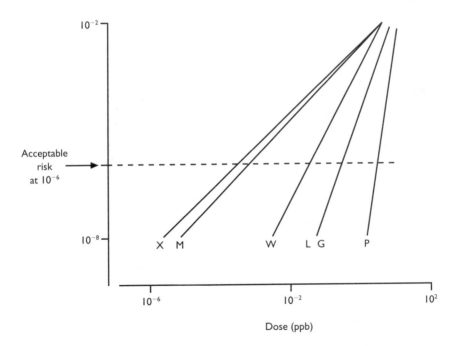

Figure 25.2 The low dose–response relationships based on a set of aflatoxin B_1 data, using different models: X = one-hit, M = multistage, W = Weibull, L = logit, G = multihit, and P = probit model.

Source: Adapted from Krewski and Van Ryzin, 1981.

7.9×10^{-4} (multistage), 4.0×10^{-2} (Weibull), 0.28 (multihit), and 2.5 (probit) respectively.

In addition, *physiologically based pharmacokinetic* (PB-PK) modeling has been developed to utilize toxicokinetic differences between the test animals and humans. For example, the target concentration of dichloromethane was about 150-fold higher in mice than in humans; these data provided a much lower, probably more realistic estimate of the risk of this toxicant (Andersen *et al.*, 1987). For additional examples, see Andersen and Krishnan (1994), and Dallas *et al.* (1995). A modified version, the *biologically based pharmacodynamic* model, also incorporates data on the interaction of the toxicant with tissues and the response of the tissues (Conolly and Andersen, 1991). While such modeling has certain advantages, it involves complex mathematical equations, and the fact that the physiological parameters regarding various species and strains, disease states and the like are often ill-defined.

Other variation

The *time-to-response*, instead of the response itself, has also been proposed for use in the mathematical models (Chand and Hoel, 1974; Sielken, 1981). The importance of this approach has been pointed out by the SOT ED_{01} Task Force (1981). *Background responses*, that is, those occurring also among the unexposed, are often observed. They can also be incorporated into mathematical models (Hoel, 1980).

The response of an organism to a toxicant is related to the dose and the duration of exposure. It is also affected by *competing risks*. Kalbfleisch *et al.* (1983) proposed mathematical models that will take these three factors into account.

Since many carcinogens require bioactivation, the importance of incorporating *metabolic data* in evaluating their risks is obvious. For example, vinyl chloride is carcinogenic after bioactivation. Gehring *et al.* (1978) showed that the tumor incidence in rats exposed to various concentrations of this chemical was proportional to the metabolized amount rather than the exposure concentration (Table 25.2).

Risk assessment

Risk assessment is done by estimating the risk associated with a toxicant at an ascertained level of exposure, using an appropriate mathematical model described above. Where the risk level is low, e.g. 10^{-6} or lower, the exposure might be considered acceptable. However, where the risk is higher, various *risk management* decisions may have to be taken. The options consist of lowering the exposure level, shortening the exposure duration, suspending the manufacture/use of chemical, and others.

Table 25.2 Correlation between exposure concentration of vinyl chloride (VC), metabolism, and induction of hepatic angiosarcoma in rats

Exposure concentration (ppm of VC)	μg of VC/liter of air	μg of VC metabolized	Percentage liver angiosarcoma
50	128	739	2
250	640	2,435	7
500	1,280	3,413	12
2,500	6,400	5,030	22
6,000	15,360	5,003	22
10,000	25,600	5,521	15

Source: Adapted from Gehring et al., 1978.

Other procedures

Noncarcinogenic chemicals

Not all chemicals require the whole gamut of toxicologic testing as described for estimating ADIs. For example, for chemicals to which humans are not likely to be exposed to an appreciable extent, such as indirect food additives and certain pesticides, a *toxicologically insignificant amount* may be estimated on the basis of toxicologic data that include at least 90-day feeding studies in two species of mammals, and by the use of a larger safety factor (generally 1,000) (NAS, 1965). Variations of this principle have been adopted by U.S. FDA and EPA administratively.

Furthermore, a *decision to reject a chemical* may be made on much more limited data, especially in the course of developing new chemicals. Such data include extreme acute toxicity, positive response in short-term mutagenesis tests, or undesirable features in biochemical studies or short-term feeding studies in animals.

As discussed in the next section, most, if not all nongenotoxic carcinogens are assessed by the ADI approach.

Carcinogenic chemicals

Chemicals with questionable data

The Joint FAO/WHO Expert Committee on Food Additives at its second meeting (WHO, 1958) recommended that "no proved carcinogen should be considered suitable for use as a food additive in any amount." This principle has been followed at subsequent meetings of the Committee and at the Joint FAO/WHO Meetings on Pesticide Residues in not allocating ADIs to proved carcinogens. *Temporary or conditional ADIs*, however, have been estimated for chemicals with equivocal carcinogenicity data, such as nitrites and amitrole. On the other hand, *discontinuation* of the use of chemicals without essential functions has been recommended. The basis for the decisions on these and other such chemicals has been reviewed and summarized (Lu, 1979). The principle of considering both the soundness of the carcinogenesis data and the usefulness of the chemical is consistent with the policies of many national regulatory agencies (e.g. Somers, 1986).

Secondary and nongenotoxic carcinogens

The concept of *secondary carcinogens*, which induce tumors only after certain noncarcinogenic effects, has been accepted by many toxicologists. For example, a WHO scientific group (WHO, 1974b) pointed out that the urinary bladder cancers in rats treated with Myrj 45 (polyoxyethylene monostearate) were caused by the bladder calculi rather than the chemical directly and that a NOEL can therefore be established. A variety of other types of nongenotoxic carcinogens have been discussed in Chapter 7. Many investigators (e.g. Reitz *et al.*, 1990), have suggested that the predominant mechanism whereby a chemical elicits a carcinogenic response should be considered in extrapolating laboratory data to humans.

International activities in toxicological evaluation

Chemicals in food

As noted in Chapter 19, the World Health Organization (WHO) and the Food and Agricultural Organization of the United Nations (FAO) have jointly established the Joint FAO/WHO Expert on Food Additives and Contaminants (JECFA) and the Joint FAO/WHO Meeting on Pesticide Residues (JMPR). JECFA deals with food additives, contaminants and residues of veterinary drugs, and JMPR deals with residues of pesticides.

The principles of evaluation followed by these two expert bodies, culminating in the assessment of ADIs, are described in details in two WHO documents (WHO, 1987, 1990). An outline of the principles, along with the historical background of these expert bodies, is provided in an article by Lu (1988). In this article, Lu emphasized two factors contributing to the wide acceptance of the ADIs assessed by JECFA and JMPR. First, there exists a close collaboration between these expert bodies and the research scientists in academia, government, and industry. Second, the ADIs assessed by these expert bodies are used as a basis in the elaboration of international food standards, the Codex Alimentarius. Figure 25.3 depicts the relationship between JMPR and research scientists and that between

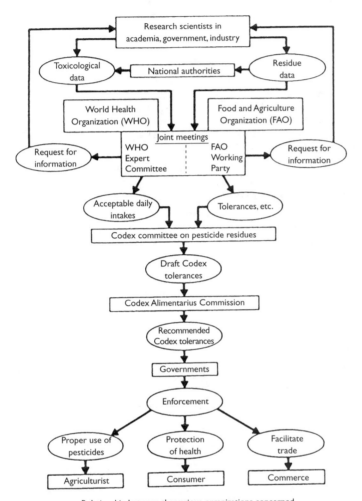

Relationship between the various organizations concerned
with the evaluation and control of pesticide residues

Figure 25.3 The elaborate procedure involved in the allocation of ADIs and tolerances (maximum residue levels) of pesticides (or other food chemicals)
by the expert committee as well as the inputs from worldwide research
scientists are depicted in the upper part of the diagram. The lower part
outlines the role of the governments of member states of the inter-
governmental organization, The Codex Alimentarius Commission, as
well as their impact on the consumer and others. A similar arrangement exists for the handling of food additives and contaminants.

Source: Lu, 1988.

376 Toxic substances and risk assessment

JMPR and the Codex Alimentarius Commission. Similar relationships exist for JECFA. Copies of the Codex Alimentarius and the Procedural Manual of the Codex Alimentarius Commission are available from FAO, Rome, Italy.

Other chemicals

WHO, in conjunction with UNEP (United Nations Environment Program), and ILO (International Labor Organization) have compiled, evaluated, and published more than 200 documents in the "Environmental Health Criteria" series. In general, they deal with subjects such as identity, sources of human exposure, environmental transport, environmental levels, and human exposure, kinetics, and metabolism in animals and humans, effects on laboratory animals and *in vitro* systems, effects on humans, and evaluation of human health risks. These topics are critical reviews and summaries of the literature, plus citations of references. These documents are thus a good source of toxicological and related topics on environmental and occupational toxicants.

As air, water, and soil are not traded internationally, definitive toxicological assessments are, in general, not included in these documents.

References

Andersen, M. E. and Krishnan, K. (1994) Physiologically based pharmacokinetics and cancer risk assessment. *Environ. Health Persp.* 102(Suppl. 1):103–108.

Andersen, M. E., Clewell, H. J., Gargas, M. L., Smith, F. A., and Reitz, R. H. (1987) Physiologically based pharmacokinetics and risk assessment process for methylene chloride. *Toxicol. Appl. Pharmacol.* 87:185–205.

Anderson, P. (1986) *Ninth Symposium on Statistics and the Environment.* Washington, DC: National Academy of Sciences.

Chand, N. and Hoel, W. (1974) A comparison of models for determining safe levels of environmental agents, in *Reliability and Biometry*, F. Proschan and R. J. Serfling (eds), Philadelphia, PA: SIAM, p. 681.

Conolly, R. B. and Andersen, M. E. (1991) Biologically based pharmacodynamic models: tools for toxicological research and risk assessment. *Ann. Rev. Pharmacol. Toxicol.* 31:503–523.

Cotruvos, J. A. (1988) Drinking water standards and risk assessment. *Regul. Toxicol. Pharmacol.* 8:288–299.

Crump, K. S. (1984) A new method for determining allowable daily intakes. *Fundam. Appl. Toxicol.* 4:854–871.

Dallas, C. E., Chen, X. M., Muraledhara, S. *et al.* (1995) Physiologically based pharmacokinetic model useful in prediction of the influence of species, dose, and exposure route on perchloroethylene pharmacokinetics. *J. Toxicol. Environ. Health* 44:301–317.

Dourson, M. L. and Lu, F. C. (1995) Safety/risk assessment of chemicals by different groups. *Biomed. Environ. Sci.* 8:1–13.

Dourson, M. L. and Stara, J. F. (1983) Regulatory history and experimental support of uncertainty (safety) factors. *Regul. Toxicol. Pharmacol.* 3:224–238.

EPA (1986) Guides for carcinogenic risk assessment. *Fed. Reg.* 51:33992–34003.

EPA (1989) *Biological Data for Pharmacokinetic Modeling and Risk Assessment.* EPA/600/3-90/019, Washington, DC.

FDA (1971) Food and Drug Administration Advisory Committee on Protocols for Safety Evaluation: Panel on Carcinogenesis report on cancer testing in the safety evaluation of food additives and pesticides. *Toxicol. Appl. Pharmacol.* 20:419–438.

FDA (1977) Chemical compounds in food-producing animals: criteria and procedures for evaluating assays for carcinogenic residues in edible products of animals. *Fed. Reg.* 42(35):10412–10437.

Food Safety Council (1973) Proposed system for food safety assessment. *Food Cosmetics Toxicol.* 16:1–136.

Food Safety Council (1980) Proposed system for food safety assessment. *Food Cosmet. Toxicol.* 16(Suppl. 2).

Gaylor, D. W. and Kodell, R. L. (1980) Linear interpolation algorithm for low dose risk assessment of toxic substances. *J. Environ. Pathol. Toxicol.* 4:305–312.

Gehring, P. J., Watanabe, P. G., and Park, C. N. (1978) Resolution of dose–response toxicity for chemicals requiring metabolic activation: example vinyl chloride. *Toxicol. Appl. Pharmacol.* 44:581–591.

Hart, R. W. and Fishbein, L. (1985) Interspecies extrapolation of drug and genetic toxicity data, in *Toxicological Risk Assessment*, vol. I, D. B. Clayson, D. Krewski, and I. Munro (eds), Boca Raton, FL: CRC Press.

Hoel, D. G. (1980) Incorporation of background in dose–response models. *Fed. Proc.* 39:73–75.

ICRP (1966) *Recommendations of the International Commission on Radiological Protection.* ICRP Publication No. 9. Oxford: Pergamon Press.

Kalbfleisch, J. D., Krewski, D., and van Ryzin, J. (1983) Dose–response models for time to response toxicity data. *Can. J. Stat.* 11:25–49.

Krewski, D. and Van Ryzin, J. (1981) Dose–response models for quantal response toxicity data, in *Statistical and Related Topics*, J. Csorgo, D. Dawson, J. N. K. Rao, and E. Shilah (eds), New York, NY: Elsevier/North Holland.

Lehman, A. J. and Fitzhugh, O. G. (1954) 100-fold margin of safety. *Q. Bull. Assoc. Food Drug Officials U.S.* 33–35.

Lu, F. C. (1979) The safety of food additives. The dynamics of the issue, in *Toxicology and Occupational Medicine*, W. B. Deichman (ed.), New York, NY: Elsevier/North-Holland.

Lu, F. C. (1985) Safety assessment of chemicals with thresholded effects. *Regul. Toxicol. Pharmacol.* 5:460–464.

Lu, F. C. (1988) Acceptable daily intakes: inception, evolution and application. *Regul. Toxicol. Pharmacol.* 8:45–60.

Lu, F. C. (1995) A review of the acceptable daily intakes of pesticides assessed by WHO. *Regul. Toxicol. Pharmacol.* 21:352–364.

Lu, F. C. and Coulston, F. (1996) A safety assessment based on irrelevant data. *Ecotoxicol. Environ. Safety* 33:100–101.

Lu, F. C. and Seilken, R. L. (1991) Assessment of safety/risk of chemicals:

inception and evolution of the ADI and dose–response modeling procedures. *Toxicol. Lett.* 59:5–40.

Mantel, N. and Bryan, W. R. (1961) "Safety" testing of carcinogenic agents. *J. Natl. Cancer Inst.* 27:455–470.

Munro, I. C. (1988) Risk assessment of carcinogens: present status and future direction. *Biomed. Environ. Sci.* 1:51–58.

National Academy of Sciences (NAS) (1965) *Report on "No Residue" and "Zero Tolerance."* Washington, DC: National Academy of Sciences.

National Academy of Sciences (NAS) (1984) *Toxicity Testing: Strategies to Determine Needs and Priorities.* Washington, DC: National Academy of Sciences.

National Research Council (1977) *Drinking Water and Health*, vol. 1. Washington, DC: National Academy of Sciences.

National Research Council (1983) *Risk Assessment in the Federal Government: Managing the Process.* Washington, DC: National Academy Press.

Paustenbach, D. J. (2000) The practice of exposure assessment: a state-of-the-art review. *J. Toxicol. Environ. Health*, Part B 3:179–291.

Ramsey, J. C. and Gehring, P. J. (1980) Application of pharmacokinetic principles in practice. *Fed. Proc.* 39:60–65.

Reitz, R. H., Mendrala, A. L., Corley, R., Quast, A., Cargas, M. L., Andersen, M. E., Staats, D. A., and Conolly, R. B. (1990) Estimating the risk of liver cancer associated with human exposure to chloroform. *Toxicol. Appl. Pharmacol.* 105:443–459.

Sielken, R. L., Jr. (1981) Re-examination of the ED_{01} study: risk assessment using time. *Fundam. Appl. Toxicol.* 1:88–123.

Somers, E. (1986) The weight of evidence: regulatory toxicology in Canada. *Regul. Toxicol. Pharmacol.* 6:391–398.

SOT ED_{01} Task Force (1981) Re-examination of the ED_{01} Study. *Fundam. Appl. Toxicol.* 1:26–128.

Wilson, R. (1980) Risk–benefit analysis for toxic chemicals. *Ecotoxicol. Environ. Safety* 4:370–383.

WHO (1957) *General Principles Governing the Use of Food Additives.* First Report of the Joint FAO/WHO Expert Committee on Food Additives. WHO Tech. Rep. Ser. No. 129.

WHO (1958) *Procedures for the Testing of Intentional Food Additives to Establish Their Safety in Use.* Second Report. WHO Tech. Rep. Ser. No. 144.

WHO (1962a) *Evaluation of the Toxicity of a Number of Antimicrobials and Antioxidants.* Sixth Report. WHO Tech. Rep. Ser. No. 228.

WHO (1962b) *Principles Governing Consumer Safety in Relation to Pesticide Residues.* Report of a Joint FAO/WHO Meeting on Pesticide Residues. WHO Tech. Rep. Ser. No. 240.

WHO (1974a) *Toxicological Evaluation of Certain Food Additives with a Review of General Principles and of Specifications.* Seventeenth Report. WHO Tech. Rep. Ser. No. 539.

WHO (1974b) *Assessment of the Carcinogenicity and Mutagenicity of Chemicals.* Report of a WHO Scientific Group. WHO Tech. Rep. Ser. No. 546.

WHO (1978) *Principles and Methods for Evaluating the Toxicity of Chemicals.* Environmental Health Criteria 6. Geneva: World Health Organization.

WHO (1987) *Principles for the Safety Assessment of Food Additives and Contaminants in Food.* Environ. Health Criteria No. 70.

WHO (1989) *Guidelines for Predicting Dietary Intakes of Pesticide Residues.* Geneva: World Health Organization.

WHO (1990) *Principles for the Toxicological Assessment of Pesticide Residues in Food.* Environ. Health Criteria, 104.

Chemical index

AAF (*see* 2-Acetylaminofluorene)
Acetaldehyde 35, 65
Acetaminophen: bioactivation 31, 32,
  38; hepatic 184, 186; immunologic
  159; mechanisms 46; renal 200
Acetyl ethyl tetramethyl tetralin 241
2-Acetylaminofluorene (AAF) 38, 58,
  94, 117
Acetylcholine 50
Acridine 212
Acrylamide 240
Actinomycin 159
Adrenocorticotropin 45
Adriamycin 46, 159, 238
AETT (*see* acetyl ethyl tetramethyl
  tetralin)
Aflatoxin 8, 9 epoxide 38, 94
Aflatoxins: action level 281;
  carcinogenicity 38, 62, 95, 100;
  dose–response 80, 371; exposure
  111, 278; hepatotoxicity 184
Alcoholic beverage 100, 134, 187, 242
Aldehyde dehydrogenase 35
Aldrin 355
Alkaline phosphatase 190
Alkylmercury 20, 279
Aluminum 238
Aminoazo dyes 34
Aminobenzoic acid 212
Aminoglycosides 200
6-Aminonicotinamide 135, 243
p-Aminophenol 100
Aminopterin 135
Aminopyrine 59
Amitrole 46, 98, 292
Ammonia 170

Amoxallin 159
Amphetamine 64
Amphotericin-b 200, 201, 202
Anatoxin-s 241
Androgen 134
Angiotensin 50
Aniline 57
ANIT (*see* α-naphthylisocyanate)
Anthracene 212
Arsenic: carcinogenicity 100;
  mechanism 46, 48; occurrence and
  toxicity 172; skin 342; TLV 354;
  vascular damage 262, 316
Arsenic trioxide 159
Asbestos 65, 99, 100, 172, 338
Aspirin 202, 329
Atropine 65
Azathioprine 98, 100, 159
Azide 238
Azinphos-methyl 355

BaP (*see* Benzo[a]pyrene)
BaP-7, 8-epoxide 38, 160
Barbiturates 52, 238
Barium 321
Benomyl 290
Benzene 94, 100, 160, 350, 351, 352
Benzidine 100
Benzo[a]pyrene 38, 66, 94, 214, 217,
  256
Benzoates 161
Benz[c]acridine 214
Benzodiazepine 51
Benzoic acid 15
Benzylpenicillin 277
Beryllium: dermal 316; hepatic 159;

Subject index